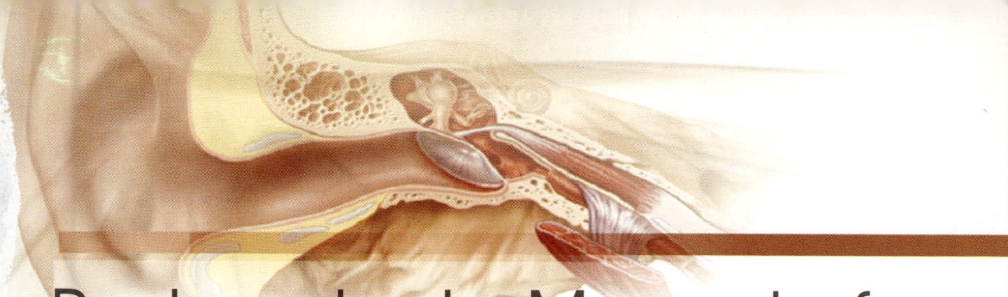

Postgraduate Manual of

Temporal Bone Dissection and Ear Microsurgery

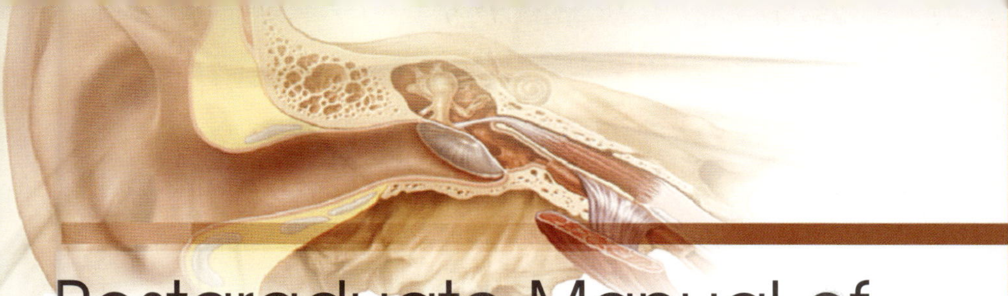

Postgraduate Manual of Temporal Bone Dissection and Ear Microsurgery

Editor-in-Chief

Dipak Ranjan Nayak MS, FICS, Fellow of UICC
Former Professor and Head
Department of ENT–Head and Neck Surgery
Kasturba Medical College, Manipal

Co-Editors

Produl Hazarika DLO, MS, FACS, FRCS
Former Professor and Head
Department of ENT–Head and Neck Surgery
Kasturba Medical College, Manipal

Sampath Chandra Prasad Rao MS, DNB, FACS, FEB-RLHNS, FEAONO
Senior Consultant and Cranial Base Surgeon
Bangalore Head and Neck Sciences

Guest Editors

PSN Murthy
Shankar Medikeri
R Balakrishnan
HN Udaybhanu

CBSPD

CBS Publishers & Distributors Pvt Ltd

New Delhi • Bengaluru • Chennai • Kochi • Kolkata • Lucknow • Mumbai
Hyderabad • Jharkhand • Nagpur • Patna • Pune • Uttarakhand

Disclaimer
Science and technology are constantly changing fields. New research and experience broaden the scope of information and knowledge. The editors have tried their best in giving information available to them while preparing the material for this book. Although, all efforts have been made to ensure optimum accuracy of the material, yet it is quite possible some errors might have been left uncorrected. The publisher, the printer and the editor will not be held responsible for any inadvertent errors, omissions or inaccuracies.

Postgraduate Manual of
Temporal Bone Dissection and Ear Microsurgery

ISBN: 978-93-5466-456-4

First Edition: 2025

Published by **Satish Kumar Jain** and produced by **Varun Jain** for

CBS Publishers & Distributors Pvt Ltd
4819/XI Prahlad Street, 24 Ansari Road, Daryaganj, New Delhi 110 002, India.
Ph: 011-23266838, 23289259
Website: www.cbspd.com
e-mail: delhi@cbspd.com

Corporate Office: 204 FIE, Industrial Area, Patparganj, Delhi 110 092
Ph: 011-4934 4934 Fax: 011-4934 4935 e-mail: publishing@cbspd.com; publicity@cbspd.com

Branches

- **Bengaluru:** Seema House 2975, 17th Cross, KR Road, Banasankari 2nd Stage, Bengaluru 560 070, Karnataka, India
  Ph: +91-80-26771678/79 Fax: +91-80-26771680 e-mail: bangalore@cbspd.com
- **Chennai:** 18/8B, Subbarayan Street, Shenoy Nagar, Chennai 600 030, Tamil Nadu, India
  Ph: +91-044-42032115, 26681266 e-mail: chennai@cbspd.com
- **Kochi:** 42/1325, 1326, Power House Road, Opp KSEB, Power House, Ernakulum Kochi 682 018, Kerala, India
  Ph: +91-484-4059061-65,67 Fax: +91-484-4059065 e-mail: kochi@cbspd.com
- **Kolkata:** 147, Hind Ceramics Compound, 1st Floor, Nilgunj Road, Belghoria, Kolkata-700056, West Bengal, India
  Ph: +033-25633055, 033-25633056 e-mail: kolkata@cbspd.com
- **Lucknow:** Basement, Khushnuma Complex, 7 Meerabai Marg (Behind Jawahar Bhawan), Lucknow-226001, UP, India
  Ph: +0522-4000032 e-mail: tiwari.lucknow@cbspd.com
- **Mumbai:** PWD Shed, Gala no 25/26, Ramchandra Bhatt Marg, Next to JJ Hospital Gate no. 2, Opp. Union Bank of India, Noorbaug, Mumbai-400009, Maharashtra, India
  Ph: 022-66661880/89 e-mail: mumbai@cbspd.com

Representatives

- **Hyderabad** 0-9885175004
- **Jharkhand** 0-9811541605
- **Nagpur** 0-8692091830
- **Patna** 0-9334159340
- **Pune** 0-9664372571
- **Uttarakhand** 0-9716462459

Printed at: Goyal Offset, Works Pvt. Ltd, Kundli, Sonipat, Haryana

Contributors

Ajay Bhandarkar MS (ORL)
Associate Professor
Department of Otorhinolaryngology–Head and Neck Surgery
Kasturba Medical College, Manipal

Ananth Chintapalli MS (ORL)
Consultant ENT-Skull Base Surgery
Star Hospital, Hyderabad

Apoorva N Reddy MS (ORL)
Head and Neck Oncology Fellow
HCG, Bangalore

Asheesh Dora MS (ORL)
Assistant Professor
Department of ENT
Pratima Medical College, Karimnagar

Balakrishnan Ramaswamy MS, DNB (ORL)
Professor and former Head
Department of Otorhinolaryngology–Head and Neck Surgery
Kasturba Medical College, Manipal

Chinmoy Sundar Ray MS (ORL)
Associate Professor, ENT
PRM Medical College
Baripada, Odisha

Dipak Ranjan Nayak MS (ORL), FICS, UICC Fellow
Former Professor and Head
Department of Otorhinolaryngology–Head and Neck Surgery
Kasturba Medical College, Manipal
Senior Consultant ENT
Head and Neck Surgery
Utkal Hospital
Bhubaneswar, Odisha

Kabikanta Samataray MS (ORL)
Professor and Head
Department of Otolaryngoglogy–Head and Neck Surgery
Kalinga Institute of Medical Sciences
Bhubaneswar, Odisha

Kailesh Pujary MS (ORL), DNB
Professor and Head
Department of Otorhinolaryngology–Head and Neck Surgery
Kasturba Medical College, Manipal

K Devaraj
Associate Professor
Department of ENT–Head and Neck Surgery
Kasturba Medical Manipal

Khageswar Rout MS (ORL)
Professor
Department of ENT-HNS
Kalinga Institute of Medical Sciences
Bhubaneswar, Odisha

Madhuri Gore MSc, PhD
Deputy Technical Director
Dr SR Chandrsekhar Institute of Speech and Hearing, Bangalore

Manushrut MS (ORL), Fellowship in Implant Otology
Consultant ENT and Cochlear Implant Surgeon
Yashoda Hospital, Hyderabad

Mario Sanna MD
Professor and Director of Otolaryngology Clinic
University of Cheiti
Founder and Director Gruppo Otologico
Piacenza-Rome, Italy

Nikitha Periaswamy MS (ORL)
Consultant
Vega ENT Hospital
RS Puram, Coimbatore, Tamil Nadu

P Satyanarayan Murthy MS (ORL), DLO
Former Professor
Department of Otorhinolaryngology–Head and Neck Surgery
Kasturba Medical College, Manipal
Former Dean and Professor
Dr P Siddhartha Institute of Medical Sciences and Research Centre
Chinnautapalli, Gannavaram, AP

Produl Hazarika DLO, MS, FRCS
Former Professor and Head
Department of Otorhinolaryngology–Head and Neck Surgery
Kasturba Medical College, Manipal
Consultant ENT Surgeon
Nemcare Hospital, Guwahati, Assam

Rashmi A Deshpande MSc, PhD
Chief Audiologist
Medikeri's Superspeciality ENT Center
Basavanagudi, Bangalore

Rajalaxmi Panigrahi MS (ORL)
Professor and Head
Department of Otorhinolaryngology–Head and and Neck Surgery
Hi-Tech Medical College and Hospital
Bhubaneswar, Odisha

Rohit Singh MS (ORL)
Additional Professor
Department of Otorhinolaryngology–Head and Neck Surgery
Kasturba Medical College, Manipal

Sankar B Medikeri MS (ORL)
Sr Consultant, ENT and Cochlear Implant Surgeon
Medikeri's Superspeciality ENT Center
Basavanagudi, Bangalore

Sanjeev Mohanty MS (ORL)
Former Prof & Head SRMC
Chennai
Sr Consultant, ENT–Head and Neck Surgery
MGM Health Care
Chennai, Tamil Nadu

Santosh Mishra MS (ORL)
Professor of ENT and Dean
MKCG Medical College
Berhampur, Odisha

Sampath Chandra Prasad Rao MS, DNB, FACS, FEB-ORLHNS, FEAONO
Sr Consultant, ENT–Skull Base Surgery
Bangalore Head and Neck Sciences
Consultant, Skull Base Surgery
Manipal Hospital, Bangalore

Santosh Pani MS (ORL)
Professor
Department of ENT
Institute of Medical Science
SUM Hospital, Bhubaneswar, Odisha

Satyajeet Mishra
Professor and Head
Department of ENT–Head and Neck Surgery
Bhima Bhoi Medical College and Hospital
Balangir, Odisha

Sauvagini Acharya MS (ORL)
Professor and Head
Department of ENT
Head and Neck Surgery
VSS Institute of Medical Sciences
Burla, Odisha

Smruti Swain MS (ORL)
Professor and Head
Department of Otorhinolaryngology–Head and and Neck Surgery
SCB Medical College, Cuttack, Odisha

Subrat Behera MS (ORL)
Former Head
ENT-Head and Neck Surgery
SCB Medical College, Cuttack
Professor and Head
ENT–Head and Neck Surgery
Jajati Kesari Medical College, Jajpur, Odisa

Suresh Pillai DNB (ORL)
Professor
Department of Otorhinolaryngology–Head and Neck Surgery
Kasturba Medical College, Manipal

Swetapadma Nayak MS (ORL)
Senior Resident
Department of Otorhinolaryngology–Head and Neck Surgery
SCB Medical College, Cuttack, Odisha

HN Udaybhanu MS (ORL)
Fellowship Otology Lateral Skull Base Surgery
Gruppo Otologico, Italy
Professor of ENT
Akash Institute of Medical Sciences
Bangalore

Foreword

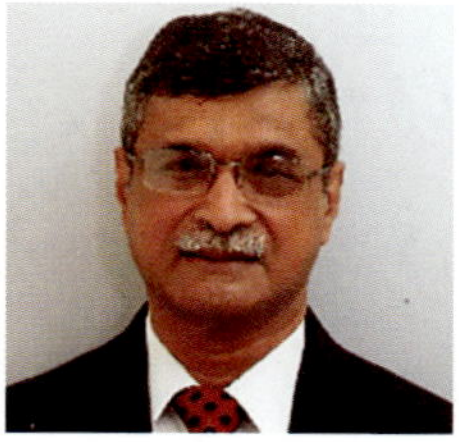

Temporal bone anatomy and surgery are fascinating, a realm where precision, skill, and profound understanding converge to restore hearing, alleviate pain, and enhance quality of life. In this meticulously crafted compendium, we embark on a journey through the intricacies of the temporal bone, exploring its anatomy, pathologies, and the delicate procedures that define modern otologic and neurotologic surgery.

Temporal bone surgery stands as a pinnacle of surgical excellence, demanding mastery of both art and science. Within these pages, a consortium of esteemed Indian and international experts illuminate the complex terrain of the temporal bone, drawing upon their wealth of experience and expertise to offer invaluable insights and techniques.

From the fundamental principles of anatomy to the intricacies of myringoplasty, mastoidectomy, cochlear implants, and beyond, each chapter is a testament to the relentless pursuit of excellence in patient care. Whether you are a novice eager to delve into the world of otology or a seasoned practitioner seeking to refine your skills, this book serves as an indispensable guide, offering a comprehensive overview of temporal bone surgery in all its dimensions.

As we navigate through the nuances of tympanoplasty, stapedectomy, ossiculoplasty, and the translabyrinthine approach, we are reminded of the profound impact these procedures have on the lives of individuals afflicted by auditory and vestibular disorders. Through meticulous dissection and innovative surgical approaches, the contributors to this volume epitomize the spirit of innovation and dedication that defines the field of otolaryngology.

Moreover, this book transcends geographical boundaries, bridging the expertise of Indian and international surgeons in a collaborative endeavor to advance the frontiers of temporal bone surgery. By fostering a global dialogue and sharing best practices, it enriches our collective understanding of the subject.

In an era defined by rapid technological advancements and evolving surgical techniques, it is imperative for practitioners to stay abreast of the latest developments in the field. This book serves as a beacon of knowledge, offering a comprehensive resource that empowers surgeons to navigate the complexities of temporal bone surgery with confidence and precision.

I extend my heartfelt gratitude to Dr Dipak Ranjan Nayak, Dr Produl Hazarika, Dr Sampath Ch Prasad Rao and all those who have contributed to this monumental work. May this book serve as a guiding light for generations of otologic and neurotologic surgeons, inspiring excellence and innovation in the noble pursuit of restoring hearing and improving lives.

Milind V Kirtane
Professor Emeritus
Seth GS Medical College and KEM Hospital
Mumbai

Preface

The anatomy of the temporal bone is complex that houses the organ of hearing and balance with major and vital structures passing through or related to it. Thus it necessitates comprehensive understanding of intricate anatomy and the physiological functions of the structures within, before venturing into microsurgical dissections.

This manual aims to provide a concise yet thorough anatomical understanding of the temporal bone. It also delves into the significance of a temporal lab, detailing methods for extraction and preservation of temporal bones, and offers guidance for the development of microsurgical skills essential for an aspiring otologist. Step by step descriptions of various basic and advance surgical techniques, including lateral skull base surgery that can be performed in a cadaveric temporal bone are presented to facilitate reader comprehension.

Contemporary topics including middle ear surgeries (myringoplasty, tympanoplasty, ossiculoplasty, stapes surgery), inner ear surgeries (translabyrinthine approach, cochlear implant surgery, MIRA-minimally invasive retrosigmoid approach), lateral skull base surgery, temporal bone resection for temporal bone malignancies, management of complications of temporal bone surgeries have been described elaborately by distinguished surgeons with decades of expertise in these specialised areas.

It is imperative for learners to engage in repeated dissections to attain a thorough knowledge of the anatomy and the necessary surgical skills and expertise in various surgical procedures before applying them to live patients. It would be advisable to carry this manual to the lab while doing the temporal bone micro dissection as it serves as a comprehensive reference, providing step-by-step guidance and anatomical insights crucial for successful dissections. Having it readily accessible ensures learners can consult it for clarification and guidance throughout the intricate process, facilitating a more effective learning experience and enhancing surgical proficiency.

We would also like to express our sincere gratitude to Prof Millind V Kirtane, Padmashree awardee and one of pioneer in the field of cochlear implant and endoscopic sinus surgery who has contributed immensely in the field of endoscopic sinus surgery and cochlear implant surgery, for writing the Foreword for this book.

Editior-in-Chief
Dipak Ranjan Nayak
Co-Editors
Produl Hazarika
Sampath Chandra Prasad Rao

Acknowledgements

This book would not have been completed without the blessings of our great teachers and the mentors. We would like to thank all our great teachers and mentors including who have given us the foundation to grow and develop our skills and knowledge.

We are grateful to our founder beloved Dr Ram Das M Pai, Chancellor of MAHE, Prof HS Ballal, Pro Chancellor, Lt. Gen. Prof MD Venkatesh, Vice Chancellor, Prof Sarath Rao, Pro Vice Chancellor of Manipal and Prof Kailesh Pujary, Head, Department of ENT–Head and Neck Surgery, who kindly permitted us to carry on the work on this book in this institution lacking which, we fear, it would not have been possible to bring this work to light. We deeply appreciate Padmashree Prof MV Kirtane, Professor Emeritus, Seth GS Medical College and KEM Hospital, Mumbai, for writing the Foreword to this book. He has tremendous contribution in inspiring many young ENT enthusiasts to take up interest in otology and endoscopic sinus and skull base surgery through his mesmerizing surgical skills.

We are grateful to all our guest editors Prof PSN Murthy, Dr Sankar Medikeri, Prof R Balakrishnan, Dr HN Udaybhanu, for their valuable contributions in editorial assistance.

We are extremely thankful to all our authors, especially Prof Mario Sanna a renowned Otologist and Skull Base Surgeon, Founder and Director, Gruppo Otologico, Italy, for his contribution.

We immensely thank all our contributing authors. All the contributors deserve applaud for whatever contribution they have made, whether it is big or small, without which it would not have been possible to finish this stupendous task in time. We thank all our faculties of MAHE for their contribution and constructive criticism.

A lot of people have helped in various ways while preparing the manuscript. They are our past and present postgraduate students. We thank Dr Nishanth, Dr Nikhil, Dr Abhinay, Dr Prashant, Dr Pooja, Dr Reshmi, Dr Nithu, Dr Jalwa, Dr Aditi, Dr Ishan Sardesai, Dr Faria, Dr Tejashwi, Dr Vidhi, Dr Shyam, Dr Mihika, Dr Aiswarya, Dr Majitha, Dr Akshaya K, Dr Akshay P, Dr Jigisha, for their timely help.

Special thanks to Dr Swetapadma Nayak for doing a tireless proofreading and also contributing to key illustrations.

We would be failing in our duty if we do not appreciate the contribution of our parents. Special thanks to our spouse and children for their help and guidance. We sincerely thank Mr Bhaskar, Mr Sudhakar, for their assistance in operating room, Mrs Latha for secretarial assistance, Mr Sitharam, Mrs Mangala, Mr Shreekant, our OPD technicians, Mrs Baby, OPD sister, Mrs Usha, OT sister and all other non-teaching staff of the Department of ENT, KMC, Manipal, for their kind help.

Editior-in-Chief

Dipak Ranjan Nayak

Co-Editors

Produl Hazarika

Sampath Chandra Prasad Rao

Contents

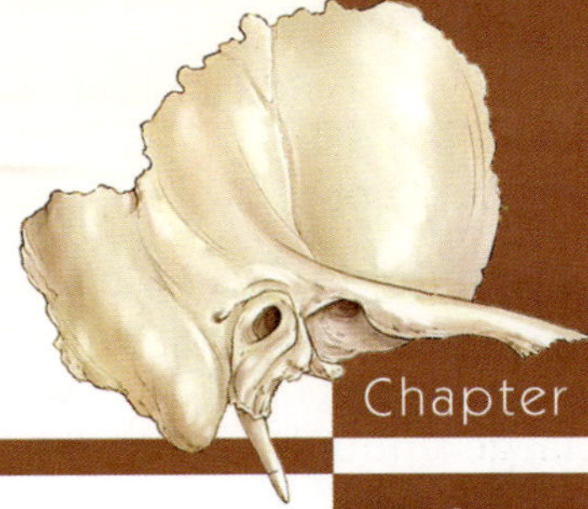

Chapter

1

Temporal Bone Dissection Laboratory Setting

Dipak Ranjan Nayak • Produl Hazarika • P Satyanarayan Murthy

Surgery of the temporal bone and skull base is a challenging task in executing invasive procedure (Gulya and Schuknecht, 2007). It requires a thorough knowledge because of the complicated three-dimensional anatomy (Irugu et al 2016). Cadaveric temporal bone is one of the most important source of learning for residents and surgeons in the field of otology and lateral skull base surgery (Fig. 1.1). A well-equipped temporal bone laboratory is perhaps one of the greatest assets in achieving the microsurgical skill and understanding the temporal bone anatomy. Repeated microsurgical dissection under operating microscope allows the surgeon to acquire the requisite microsurgical skill and the knowledge of the complicated neurovascular anatomy that surrounds or passing through the temporal bone. Virtual learning method can also be adopted to improve learning the three-dimensional anatomy (Wang, 2006). The setting of a good temporal bone laboratory necessitates a lot of equipment and instruments that are used in a standard otologic operating room. This gives the surgeon, the ease and comfort while doing long hours of micro-dissection and to replicate easily the skill acquired to be used in the operating room.

Historical Perspective Microsurgery of Ear

The term 'microscope' came from the Greek word, where a system uses lenses for magnification. Although microscope was introduced in 17th century, the first microsurgery in the history of otology was done by Swedish otologist Carl-Olof Nylén (1921) by using a mono-ocular microscope. In the year 1922, Holmgren used binocular operating microscope for ear surgery. Until 1951, although various models were developed, the most suitable and perfected one for microsurgery for ear was developed by Littmann and Zeiss company (Murdy, 2000). Schwartz (1873) used gouge, chisel and mallet for mastoid surgery. Macewen introduced the electrical dental burr for mastoid surgery, but it remained largely unrecognised. At the beginning of the 1950s, the systematic use of the microscope in ear surgery allowed generalised use of the drill and improvement of the suction-irrigation system (Murdy, 2000).

Equipment

Bench/Table (Figs 1.1 and 1.2): A bench or a suitable table is extremely important for a temporal bone laboratory. It should be large enough (about 30 to 33 inches) in height to allow the surgeon's knees to fit comfortably while using otologic drill for micro-dissection of temporal bone. The length can vary depending on whether single or multiple units/stations are being used simultaneously, where additional microscope and instruments are required to be accommodated. Each station requires separate, water tap necessary for proper functioning of microscope, drill system, irrigation and suction facility, etc.

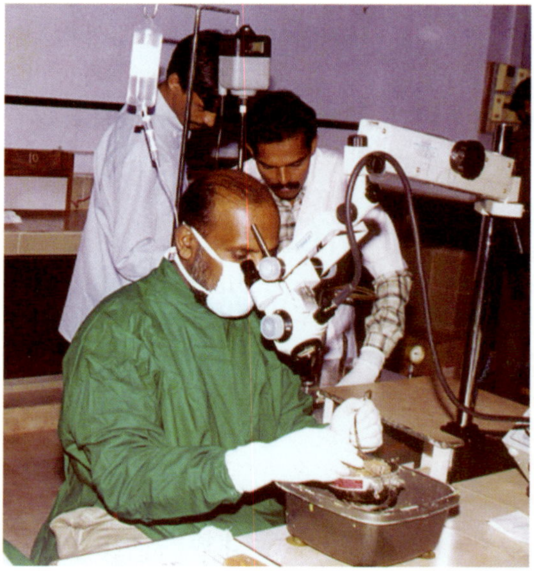

Fig. 1.1: Temporal bone dissection in progress

Chair: A specially designed height adjustable chair with back rest is important for doing long hours of microsurgery (Fig. 1.1). A well padded operation stool with a foot pedal is recommended. Chair with wheels for mobility are very comfortable and allows the surgeon to move closer or farther away.

Drill: This should resemble the equipment in the operation theatre and should have varying sizes and types of burr points like cutting burrs, polishing burrs and diamond burrs. For a right handed dissector, the drill is held in the right hand and the suction in the left hand. The system should allow enough room for movement of drill (Fig. 1.2A).

The drill unit consists of a motor, handpiece and burrs of various types and sizes.

a. **Motor:** The micromotor type is commonly being used with a range of 30000–40000 rpm. The other types are being hanging motor type, stand type and table top type with a range of 12000 to 20000 rpm. Recently multipurpose high speed drill cum debridor developed by Storz and Xomed are available with very high speed drill. Use of low speed drill used to give a different tactile response and a change in sound while touching of burr over critical structure like dura and blood vessels. However, with modern high speed drill the need

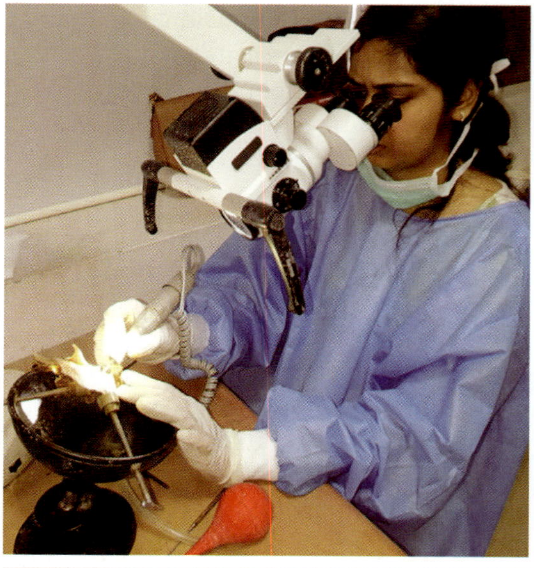

Fig. 1.2A: Temporal bone is fixed to the temporal bone holder while temporal bone dissection is in progress with a straight handpiece micromotor drill

for digging and chatter has been reduced although at the expense of tactile and sound feedback.The high speed drill requires practice.

b. **Handpieces:** Two types are available:
   i. ***The straight type:*** It is preferred most of the time and especially at the beginning of surgery. It gives better hand control (Fig. 1.2B).
   ii. ***Contrangular type*** *(Fig. 1.3)*

c. **Burrs:** Three types are used.
   i. Cutting (Fig. 1.4)
   ii. Polishing diamond burrs
   iii. Cutting (coarse) diamond burrs (Fig. 1.5).

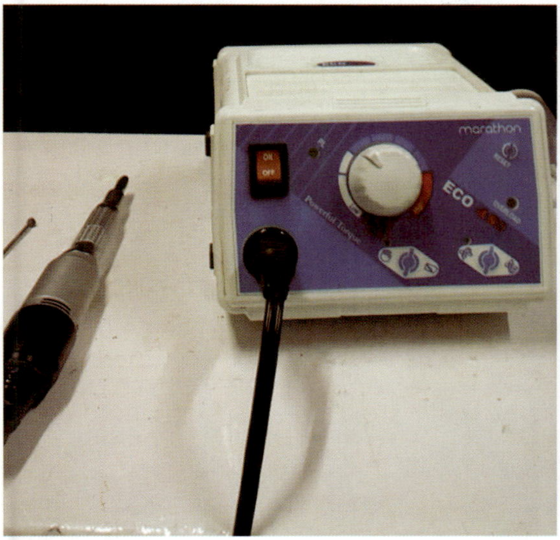

Fig. 1.2B: Straight handpiece attached to the micromotor

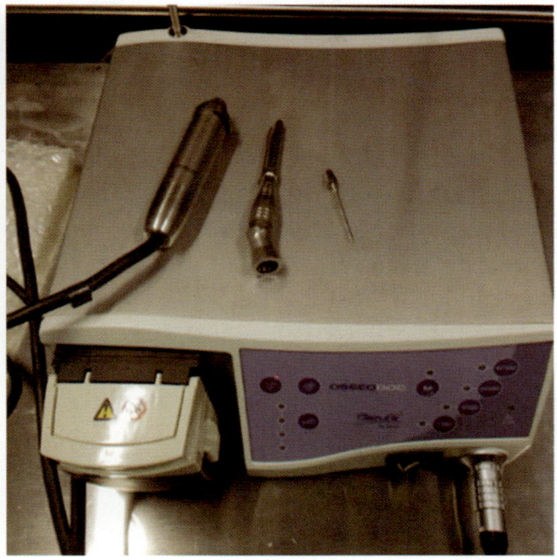

Fig. 1.3: Contrangular type handpiece

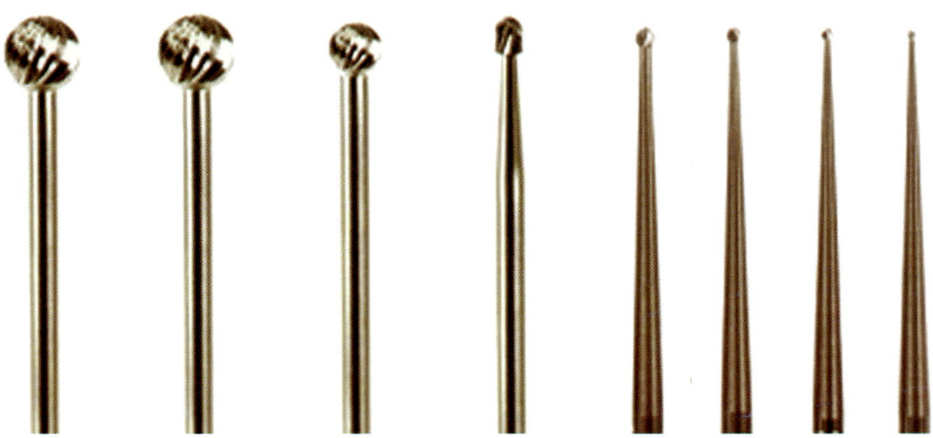

Fig. 1.4: Cutting burrs of various sizes for ear microsurgery

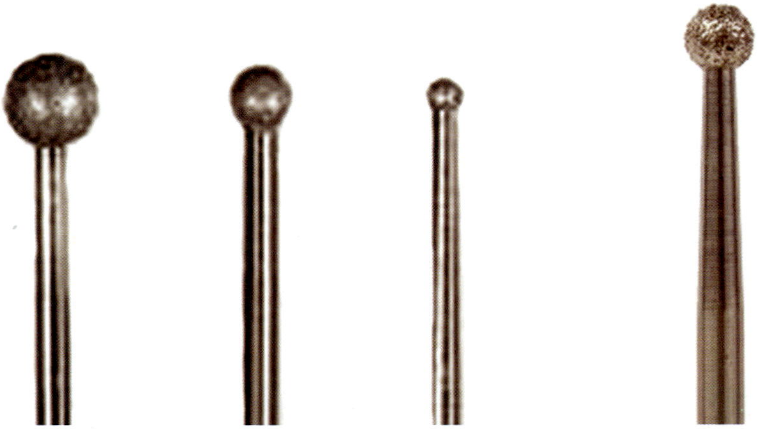

Fig. 1.5: Polishing and coarse cutting diamond burrs

Each of them is available within a size range of 1 to 10 mm. Tungsten carbide is used as the cutting edges in all of them. These again may be of the ordinary type or of the gear fitting type.

For smooth drilling and prevention of accumulation of bone dust, irrigating fluid will be required during drilling. In live operations, ringer lactate or any other isotonic solution may be used for this purpose. The drill handpiece should be held closer to the rotating shaft of the burr for better control without compromising the field of vision. To prevent jumping of drill and to drill with a smooth motion, the burr should be brushed along the bone surface in a direction, opposite to the burr rotation (Fig. 1.6).

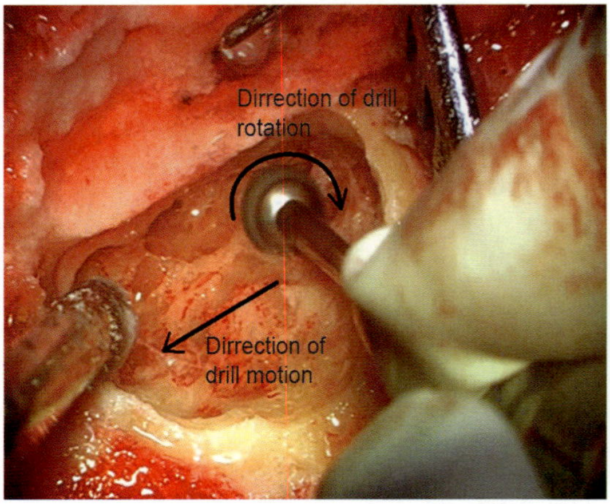

Fig. 1.6: Correct method to hold the handpiece and drilling while doing temporal bone dissection. Note the direction of rotation of burr and the motion of drilling

Piezoelectric electric device: Recently piezoelectric bone surgery is gaining popularity in mastoid surgery. The device has two piezoelectric handpieces and two inserts that are attached to the main unit. The device supplies power and has holders for the handpiece and peristaltic pumps with irrigation fluids for cooling during surgery with a jet of physiological solution that discharges from the inserts (Salami et al, 2007). Piezo electric bone surgery is very selective in cutting that recognizes tissue hardness and works only on mineralized structures, without soft-tissue damage, so facial nerve, chorda tympani can be spared without thermal damage while doing bone removal.

Operating Microscope (Fig. 1.7)

Basic Principles

Although many different types of microscopes are available in the market, the same general principles are applied in most cases. Most of the microscopes are designed to the par

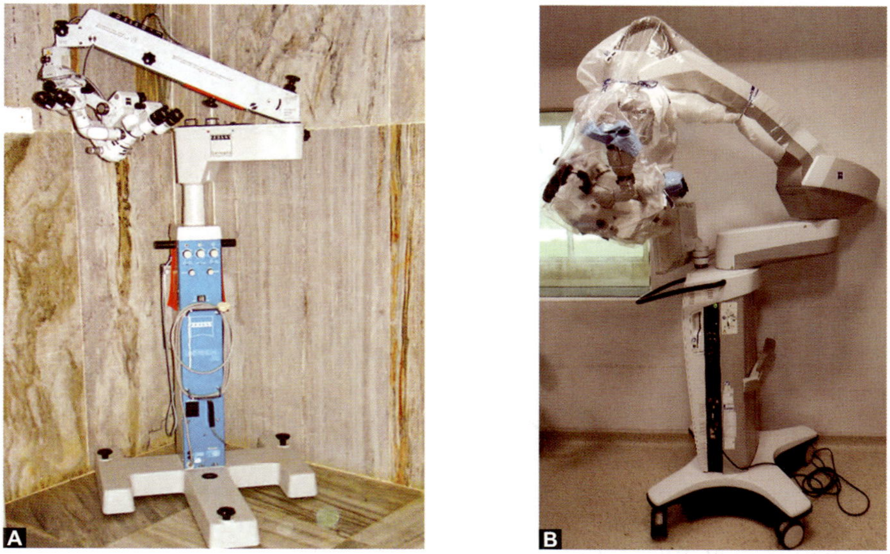

Fig. 1.7: **(A)** Zeiss operating microscope and the headpiece, **(B)** advanced Zeiss operating microscope with autofocus is draped before surgery

focal, but this ideal is not always achieved and one may find it necessary to make minor adjustments in focus while moving from one magnification to another.

Parts of a Basic Microscope

a. Optical system or optics
b. Lighting or illumination
c. Stand

The optical system consists of the following:

i. Binocular assembly
ii. Magnification changer
iii. Objective lens

Binocular assembly: This consists of 2 eyepieces. Various eyepieces with different magnifications are available. They include 10x, 12.5x, 16x, 20x and others. Generally 12.5× is used. These eyepieces have a diopteric scale of +5 to –5 and this can be adjusted according to the refractive error of the dissector.

Magnification changer: Magnification changer or the turret is a rotating device between the object and binocular assembly. With this the magnification can be changed from 6 to 40. For routine ear work a magnification of 10 is used. For finer work a magnification of 16 is used. As the magnification becomes higher, the field of vision becomes narrower. Nowadays zoom and magnification can be controlled through foot control or hand grips pannel attached to the microscope.

Objective lens: This is fitted at the bottom of the head. It can be easily screwed and unscrewed. The focal length of the microscope is the distance between this lens and the object. For the ear surgery it is usually 200 mm/250 mm, for the nose it is 300 mm and for the larynx it is 400 mm.

Illumination: Adequate illumination is necessary for good microscopic work. The lighting should not be too bright. Usually incandescent lamps of 6 V 50 W bulbs are used if brighter light is needed. Other sources are:
(i) Halogen lamp, and (ii) Fiberoptic source

Stand: The microscope should run easily on the stand and can be fixed on the stand tightly with knobs provided. The arms and their control are arranged on the stand that the head of the microscope can be tilted in any direction at any level convenient to the operator.

Microscope Suspension System

Proper Usage

i. Interpupillary distance is adjusted to get a single image with the binoculars.
ii. Dioptric adjustment should be made accordingly if needed. Those with astigmatism should wear suitable glasses.
iii. Focusing can be done by moving the microscope and with the fine focus control.
iv. One should note that under higher magnification the margin of error is less than one millimeter while drilling doing exploration or dissection in the important areas like facial canal, endolymphatic sac decompression, translabyrinthine approach, jugular bulb and carotid artery for infratemporal fossa approaches.

Photography Through the Microscope

A surgical microscope by its inherent design, naturally lends itself to photo differentiation. The operative field is defined by the view obtainable through the microscope and is well illuminated. There is no need for separate focusing and composition of operative photograph. No extra personnel are needed and asepsis is never compromised.

High quality, reasonably priced equipment is available to facilitate photo documentation by 35 mm photography, video recording and 18 × 16 mm cinematography. The images so produced may be used for many purposes including documentation of findings and teaching at a number of different levels and later analytical review. With the dynamic studies (video and movies), surgical techniques can be analyzed and improved upon.

Use of video also offers a major improvement in the operating room environment, because this technology allows the entire surgical staff to participate in the surgical procedure. Combination of a small field and physical barrier of the operating microscope itself often isolated the surgical assistants and the scrub nurses from a view of the operating field. So isolated, attention of these surgical personnel may wander, especially during the long procedures. The use of continuous closed circuit televised viewing of the operation reverses this. Attention is fostered when assistants can see the surgery on video monitors in the operation theatre, and they are thus able to again anticipate the needs of the surgeon and assist him accordingly. An additional advantage is that, the ability to achieve an 'instant replay' via a video tape is seen. This on occasions has defined a problem, such as the site of intraoperative facial nerve damage and aided the surgeon in dealing with it properly.

Use of dual photo-adapter with the help of additional internal beam splitter allows both 35 mm and videography to be done simultaneously with various focal length combinations.

The use of high speed film and improved sensitivity of the video cameras has helped for good photography with additional illumination facility. The flask information system may be used in the laboratory without moving the flask closer to the field. This system consists of an eyepiece mounted, light emitting diode (LED), which enables the surgeon to be aware of the flash status signal normally appearing in the camera's view finder. The flash when charged sends a signal which makes the LED bulb glow steadily. If the flash is totally discharged by the exposure the LED is extinguished, the surgeon may be informed when the next picture may be taken by the glowing LED. With the addition of the winder, the film is advanced automatically and multiple sequences are possible.

Color video cameras have improved remarkably in the last few years and a number of small light weight cameras, which are suitable for microsurgical applications are readily available. Apfelbaum RI recommends Hitachi 9017 camera for excellent resolution with reasonable price.

Three-Dimensional Microsurgical Videos

The use of 3-dimensional technologies can be divided into 4 areas. The first area is in developing better teaching methods. Second in the development of better imaging technology, the third area is that of adapting procedures now done in 2D or 3D. The last area for the future of 3D technology is merging technology. With the use of stack computer arrays, 3D images can be created and manipulated.

Bone Holders

There are many bone holders available. These include:

1. The Houston urban stainless steel bone holder
2. Dr Mahadeviah's bone holder
3. Vijaya's bone holder
4. Prabhu's bone holder
5. Hazarika's temporal bone holder designed by Prof Produl Hazarika, Co-author and former Head, Department of ENT–Head and Neck Surgery, Kasturba Medical College, Manipal.

This holder has the following features:

- It is made of brass
- Has 3 points for firm holding
- Has a lead base for stability
- The bowl is placed on a sports ring ball made up of rubber for easy maneuverability

Suction Irrigation

Ideally both suction and irrigation should be provided on the same handpiece. The hand-piece is held in the left hand and is advantageous in the sense that there is no need for an assistant to pour the saline or irrigation fluid. However, simpler set ups incorporating separate suction apparatus and irrigator can also be used but requires an assistant to do the suction while the dissector is performing the drilling work. This can be used to continuously irrigate the field with a separate irrigation channel during dissection.

Surgical Instruments

1. Suction cannula of various sizes
2. Sickle knife
3. Bone curette
4. Alligator forceps

5. Scalpel
6. Straight pick
7. Right angle pick
8. Aditus seeker
9. Periosteal elevator

Bone

Both dry and wet bones can be used for dissection. It is better to start dissection with dry bones first. Dry bones are soaked in decalcifying agents to soften the bones. Details of various decalcifying agents are given later. Stapedectomy, facial nerve decompression, etc. are better done with fresh bones or wet bones.

Fresh bones can be usually obtained during postmortem examinations, without mutilating the external appearance of the cadaver using proper technique of removal. Temporal bones cut from specimens should include mastoid air cells, a small portion of squamosal part of the bone, the tympanic ring and petrous tip. The collected temporal bones should be fixed in a 10% neutral buffered formalin solution for a period of 2 weeks at 4°C temperature or in a high concentration of alcohol (Fennessy et al., 2009).

Procedure for Removal of Temporal Bones

Legal issues still a problem in harvesting and transporting temporal bone in India besides preservation and infection transmission being the major issues. Because of this problem, newer modalities like simulation and virtual reality are being used as teaching tool which may replace the existing system. It can be collected in supervision of forensic department based on anatomy act as published under the government gazette. The cadaveric temporal bone gives the opportunity to study anatomical variations (Naik et al, 2014). Temporal bones may be removed by either the use of block method or the core method while performing postmortem (Fennessy, 2009). The great demand of dissection of temporal bone by the otologists made it essential to establish a temporal bone laboratory in institutes and hospitals.

Block Method

It requires four bone cuts to remove temporal bone to help remove single temoral bone. Walvekar et al. 2010 described a modified block method, where two temporal bones can be removed from the cadaver with just four cuts.

Block method is preferred over the Core method (Shambaugh) (Fig. 1.8) because:

i. More structural features are retained in a larger sample
ii. Eustachian tube can be removed
iii. Related cranial nerves can be viewed
iv. It is easier to teach on a larger sample

Steps

1. Skull cap is removed in such a way as to leave two pyramidal eminences anteriorly and posteriorly to avoid slipping of the cap over the skull bone later on.
2. Brain is removed

Four saw cuts are made to remove the temporal bone. 1st and 2nd cuts are at right angles to superior angle of the petrous bone.

1st cut is made near the apex of the bone as the size and shape of the posterior cranial fossa permits (well anteromedial to the cochlea). The further forward it is made, larger the portion of the Eustachian tube removed. 2nd cut is made roughly

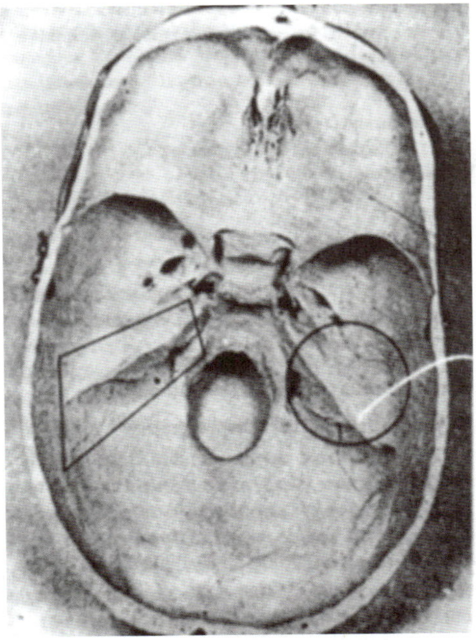

Fig. 1.8: Outline marked for Block and Core method of temporal bone removal

parallel to cut 1 and through the middle mastoid region as near to its lateral wall as the saw can be held.

Cut 3 is made vertically in the floor of the middle cranial fossa about one inch in front of the petrous ridge and laterally as close to the cranial wall as possible. This should join the forward ends of cuts 1 and 2. If done correctly this lies 3/8 inches laterally and in front of the tympanic membrane. The block tissue removed includes the deeper part of the osseous external auditory canal.

Cut 4 is an undercut of block tissues outlined by the above 3 cuts. It is made along an anatomical horizontal plane as near to the floor of the posterior cranial fossa as the saw can be placed. Posterolateral end of this cut is made first and then advanced slowly to apex of the petrous bone.

The removal of the block outlined above is the most difficult job and is accomplished with the help of a lion-jaw forceps. The block is grasped by placing the prongs of the jaw of the forceps in cut 4 and closing down the other jaw in such a manner that its prongs grasp the superior angle of the petrous bony pyramid, because this region of the surface is usually more free of underlying pneumatised or narrow spaces than the more lateral positions of the superior surface.

With gentle back and forth movement of the handle, the unsevered connections are broken without damage to inner structures. After the bone becomes completely loose, it is elevated with the forceps to allow insertion of a knife along cuts 3 and 4 to severe the dense connections remaining. A wide sharp chisel is useful especially in the region of the styloid process.

After the removal of the bone the following two important steps are carried out:

i. The internal carotid artery is grasped and ligated
ii. The external auditory canal is sutured with silk with a piece of muscle plugged in between the sutures

iii. Any defect in the bone of the skull is filled with plaster of Paris to prevent leakage of embalming fluids. This method of removal of the temporal bone leaves no external deformity of the skull.

Core Bone Plug Cutter Method

Cylindrical block of bone is removed by centering a 'Bone plug Cutter' on the acoustic eminences as shown in Fig. 1.9A and B. The block is removed in the same way as described above for block method.

Use of Decalcifying Agents for Dry Temporal Bone

It is often difficult to get wet cadaveric temporal bone. A dry temporal bone can be used to understand basic surgical anatomy of temporal bone. But it is very difficult to drill in such bone to open up the mastoid antrum and perform common surgical procedure.Use of gouge/chisel and mallet can cause crack and break the specimen before being used (Tremble, 1930). Decalcifying agent can make the job easy in such situation. These agents can be classified broadly into three main types:

1. **Based on strong mineral acid:** Can be used as 5–10% for a period of 12–14 hr for temporal bone to prevent total demineralization. Can be used as 10% nitric acid in 5% in distilled water. Hydrochloric acid also can be used but should be washed of formalin preserved bone before used.
2. **Based on weaker organic acids:** Formic acid aqueous solution or in combination of formalin can be used. Alternatively acetic acid can also be used. Bone can also be put in simple vinegar for 48 hr. before taking it for temporal bone dissection when standard acid is not available.
3. **Composed of chelating agents:** EDTA is commonly used for this purpose, in the form of its disodium salt. However, it can bind only ionized calcium and hence can act only on the outer layer.

Factors affecting the rate of decalcification:

1. **Concentration of the active reagent:** In general, more the concentration, more rapid is the decalcifying process. Steady concentration of the active reagent can be maintained

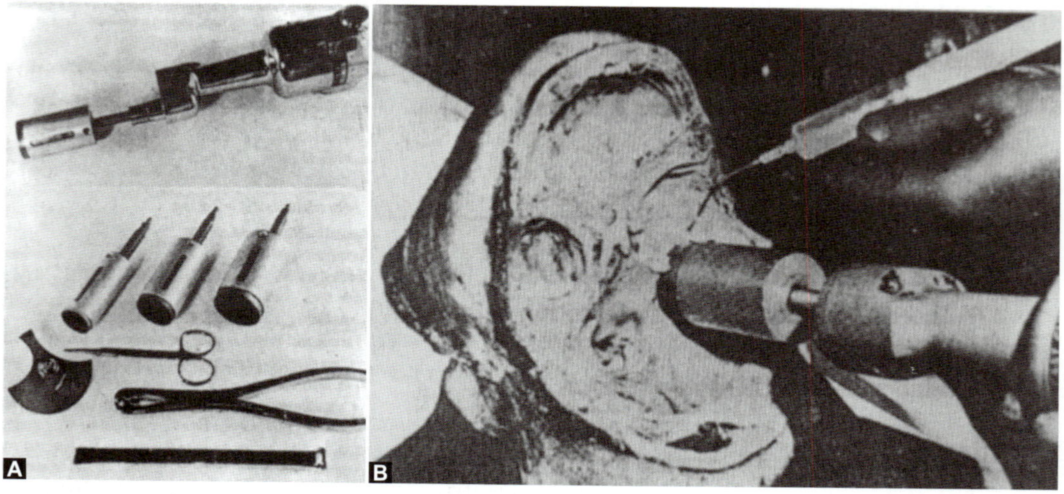

Fig. 1.9: (A) Instruments to cut and remove temporal bone, (B) Core method of temporal bone removal

by using large bulk of this agent compared to the specimen (volume ratio of 20 : 1 approximately) or by renewing the fluid several times during the decalcifying process. It is recommended that strong acids are changed 2–3 times during 24 hours, weak acids daily and EDTA once a week.

2. **Temperature:** Increased temperature hasten decalcification. However, increase beyond an optimum temperature can damage other normal structures. Moreover a partial decalcification helps better temporal bone drilling of dry temporal bone. Wet temporal bone does not require decalcification.

   Optimum temperature for acid decalcification has not been determined properly. Twenty five degree centigrade (summer heat) is a useful standard temperature but in practice the temperature of a working lab is suitable (Smith, 1962). Thus EDTA can be used at a temperature of 60°C with good effect (Brain, 1966).
3. **Agitation:** Hastening effect of agitation on decalcification, though appears logical, is quite controversial. Shaking manually once or twice a day can be done, keeping the above point in mind.

Completion of Decalcification

Constant surveillance will be needed to obtain optimum decalcification. A complete decalcification makes the bone unsuitable for drilling. A partial decalcification with weak acid like formic acid or acetic acid for short period is more suitable for temporal bone dissection.

REFERENCES

1. Bradbury S. The evolution of the microscope. Oxford: *Pergamon*, 1967.
2. Holmgren G. Operations on the temporal bone, carried out with the help of the lens and the microscope. *Acta Otolaryngol (Stockh)* 1922; 4:386–93.
3. Mudry A. The history of microscope for use in ear surgery. *The American Journal of Otology*, 2000; 21(6):877–86.
4. Schwartze H, Eysell C. Uber die kunstliche eroffnung des warzenfortsatzes. *Arch Ohrenheilkd*. 1873;7:157–62.
5. Irugu DVK, et al. Establishing a Temporal Bone Laboratory in Teaching Institutes to Train Future Otorhinolaryngologists and Fundamentals of Temporal Bone Laboratory: Considerations and Requirements; *Indian J Otolaryngol Head Neck Surg* (Oct–Dec 2016) 68(4):451–455; DOI 10.1007/s12070–015-0962–0.
6. Fennessy BG, O'Sullivan P (2009). Establishing a temporal bone laboratory: considerations for ENT specialist training. *Ir Journal of Medical Science* 178:393–5.
7. Wang H, Northrop C, Burgess B, Liberman MC, Merchant SN (2006). Three-dimensional virtual model of the human temporal bone: a stand-alone, downloadable teaching tool. *Otol Neurotol* 27:452–7.
8. Surgery of the Ear. Glasscock and Shambaugh. 4th edition.
9. Theory and Practice of Histopathological Techniques. Bancroft and Stevens. 3rd edition pages 314–20.
10. Temporal Bone Dissection Manual: Nelson (House Ear Institute).
11. Naik SM, Naik MS, Bains NK (2014) Cadaveric temporal bone dissection: Is it obsolete today? *Int Arch Otorhinolaryngol* 18:63–7.
12. Angelo Salami, Tommaso Vercellotti, Renzo Mora, *et al*. Clinical techniques and technology Piezoelectric bone surgery in otologic surgery; *Otolaryngology–Head and Neck Surgery* (2007) 136, 484–5.

13. Walvekar RR, Harless LD, Loehn BC, Swartz W (2010). Block method of human temporal bone removal: A technical modification to permit rapid removal. *Laryngoscope* 120:1998–2001.
14. Learning Ear Surgery by Temporal Bone Dissection: KK Ramalingam.
15. Atlas of Ear Surgery: Miglets Paparella and Sandes. 4th edition.
16. Three-dimensional imaging in Microsurgery Bulletin: Bailey GJ. *American Colleges of Surgeons.* 78:4:1993.
17. Apfelbaum R I. An Optical Switch for Improved Photography through Operating Microscope: *Surg neurol* 6:335–336:1976.
18. Walvekar RR[1], Harless LD, Loehn BC, *et al.* Block method of human temporal bone removal: a technical modification to permit rapid removal. *Laryngoscope,* 2010; 120(10):1998–2001. doi: 10.1002/lary.21052.
19. Tremble GE. Decalcification of temporal bone for dissection; *Arch Otolaryngol.* 1930;11(5):580–582. doi:10.1001/archotol.1930.03560050054003.
20. Stearchi DL. Bone in Bancroft's Theory and Practice of Histological Techniques; edited by Kim S Suvarna, Christopher Layton, John D. Bancroft, 7th edition (2018) Churchi Livingstone.
21. Clayden EC. A discussion on preparation of bone section by paraffin wax method with special reference to control decalcification; *Journal of Medical Lab Technology* (1952)10, 103.

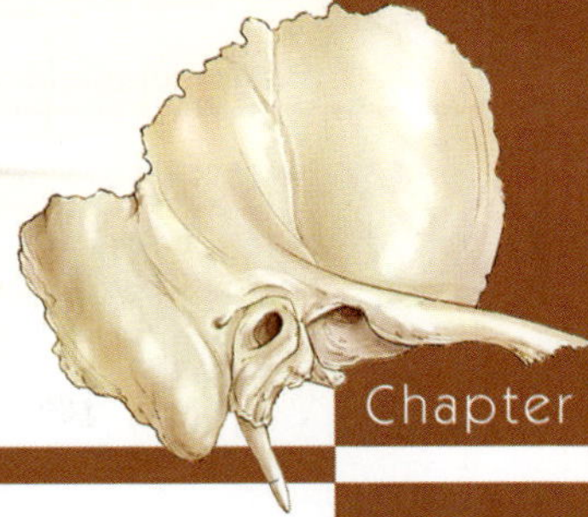

Chapter

2

Temporal Bone Anatomy including Radiology

Dipak Ranjan Nayak • Swetapadma Nayak • Satyajeet Mishra

To achieve skills and competency and understanding of otologic surgery requires dedication, complete depth of anatomical knowledge, repeated practice of surgical dissection over a cadaveric temporal bone under the microscope to understand the micro-anatomy. The introduction of HRCT (high-resolution computed tomography) scanning has revolutionized the understanding the temporal bone anatomy and pathology.

Traditional X-rays with various views have limited role in understanding the structural anatomy of the ear which has been overcome by the HRCT. The inner ear and the neurovascular structures including facial nerve, auditory vestibular nerve including their central connections can be better studied by the MRI (Fig. 2.2B).

Surgical Anatomy of Temporal Bone

Before starting the micro-dissection of the temporal bone the dissector must become well oriented to the surgical anatomy of the temporal bone by reading standard anatomy text

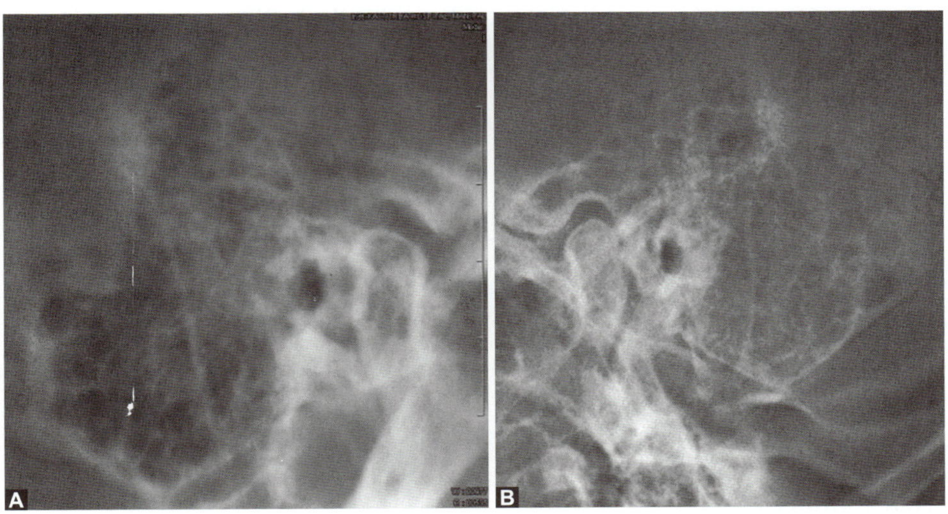

Fig. 2.1A and B: Hazy mastoid air cells on the left side compared to right

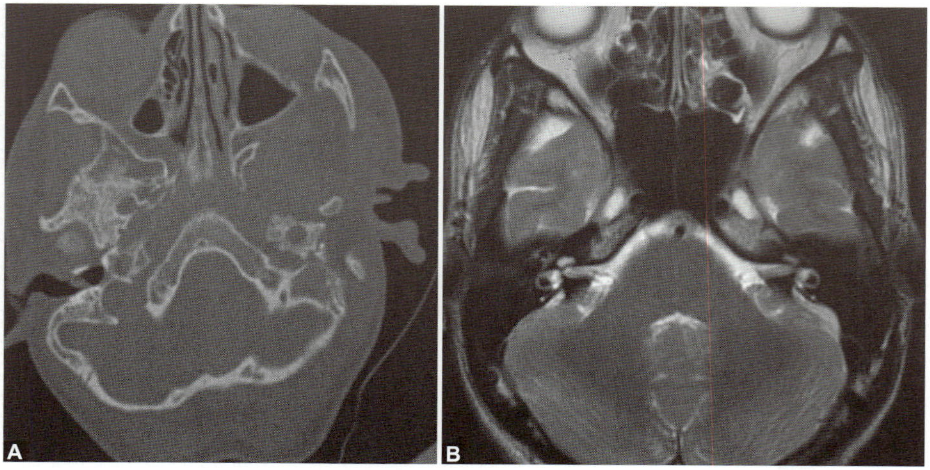

Fig. 2.2: (A) Showing CT scan of temporal bone with left coalescent mastoiditis with subperiosteal mastoid abscess, **(B)** MRI of the temporal bone and brain showing normal membranous cochlea and vestibule with intact central connections

book and basic science related to otology and temporal bone radiology. The temporal bones comprise the lateral skull base, forming portions of the middle and posterior fossae. Each temporal bone is composed of five osseous parts: The squamous, mastoid, petrous, tympanic, and styloid portions. The following basic points of the surgical anatomy of the temporal bone should be known to the dissector. Sir William Macewan (1893) established the concept of the **suprameatal triangle**, also called the **Macewan triangle**.

A. Lateral Surface *(Figs 2.3 and 2.4)*

Lateral surface of the temporal bone shows mastoid, styloid and zygomatic portions. Note the important land marks:

1. Mastoid tip
2. Macewen's triangle
3. Styloid process
4. Anterior and posterior roots of zygoma
5. Articular tubercle
6. Glenoid fossa
7. Petrotympanic fissure
8. Postglenoid tubercle
9. Temporalis line
10. Tympanomastoid suture
11. Foramen of the mastoid emissary vein
12. Tympanosquamous suture

B. Medial Surface

1. Groove for middle meningeal vessels
2. Internal auditory canal
3. Sigmoid sulcus

C. Posterior Surface *(Fig. 2.5A)*

Posterior surface of the temporal bone forms anterior aspect of posterior cranial fossa. Note down the following landmarks:

1. Sigmoid sinus sulcus
2. Subarcuate fossa
3. Internal auditory canal
4. Vestibular aqueduct
5. Sulcus for superior petrosal sinus

Carefully examine the internal auditory canal and its four walls.

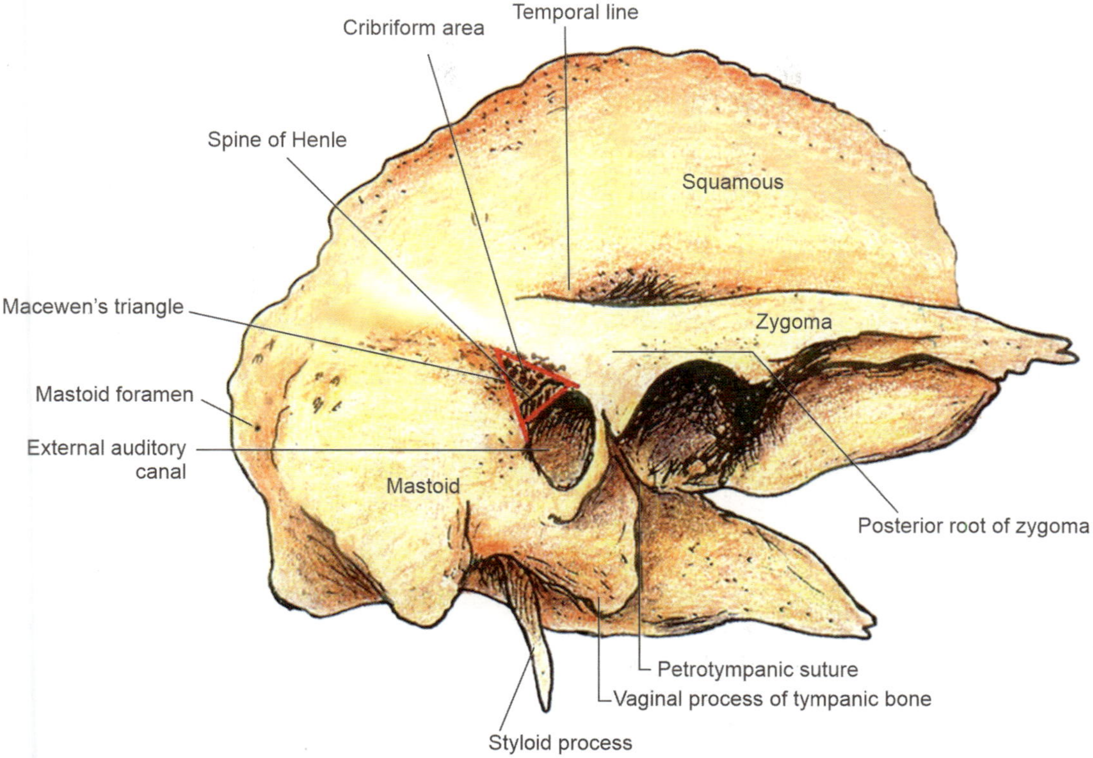

Fig. 2.3: Illustration showing structures on the lateral wall of temporal bone

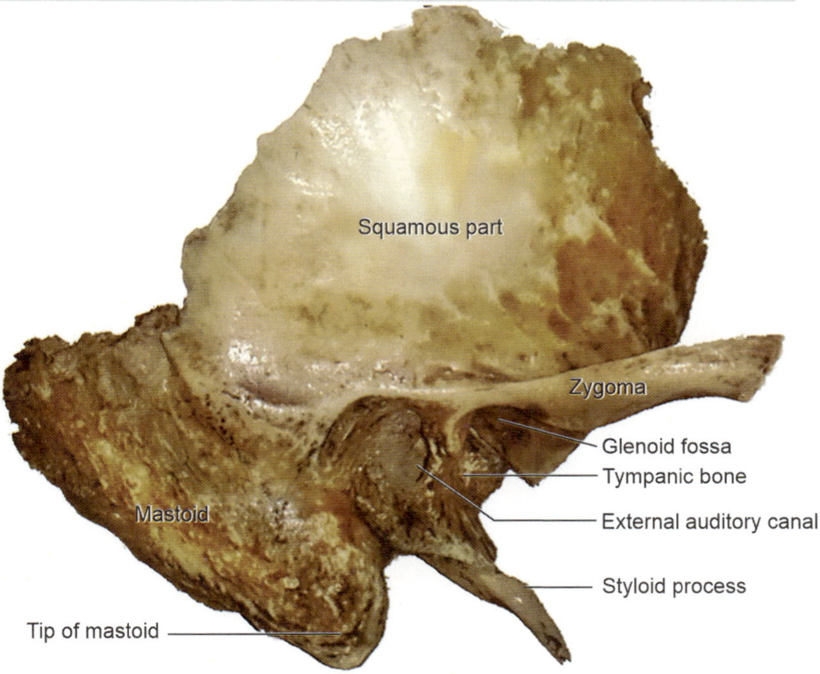

Fig. 2.4: Right temporal bone lateral wall and its parts

D. Superior Surface *(Fig. 2.5B)*

Observe the superior surface of the temporal bone and note the following landmarks.

1. Tegmen plate
2. Arcuate eminence
3. Petrous apex
4. Impression of trigeminal ganglion
5. Hiatus for greater superficial petrosal nerve
6. Carotid canal opening

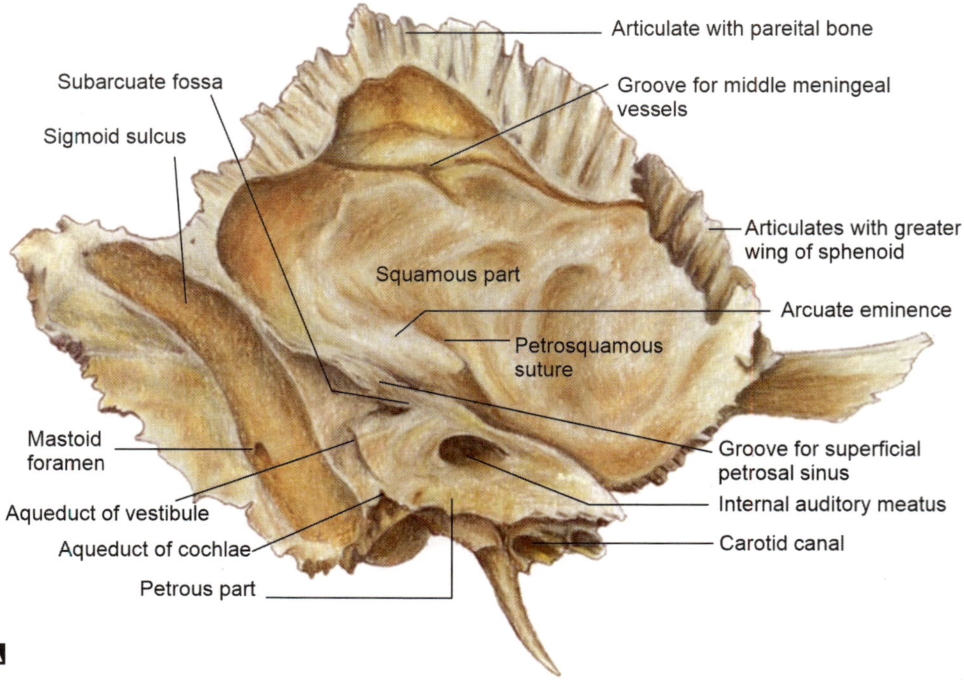

A

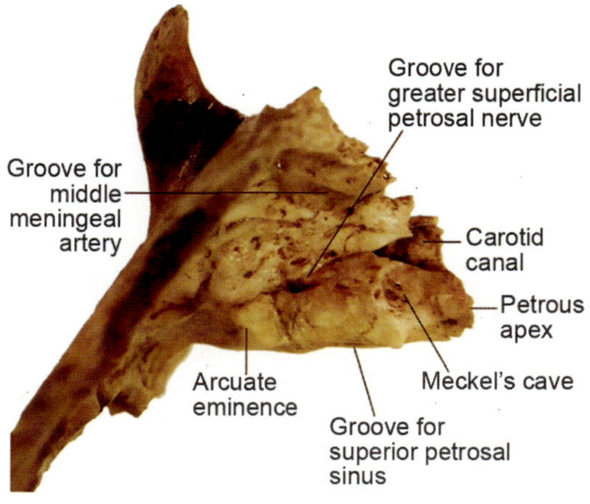

B

Fig. 2.5: (A) Medial and anterior aspect of posterior cranial fossa, **(B)** Superior surface of petrous temporal bone

E. Inferior Surface (Fig. 2.6)

The following landmarks are to be noted:

1. Jugular fossa
2. Carotid canal
3. Stylomastoid foramen
4. Styloid process
5. Digastrics groove
6. Canaliculus for cochlear aqueduct
7. Tympanic nerve canaliculus

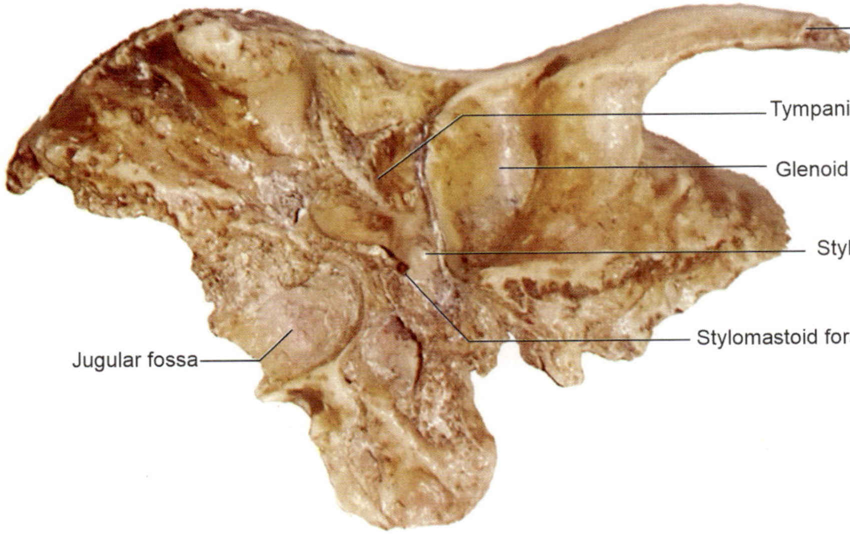

Fig. 2.6: Inferior surface of temporal bone

Petrous Temporal Bone and Petrous Apex

It is a pyramidal structure situated at the medial aspect of temporal bone with apex pointing anteromedially and the base posteromedially that houses the structures of the inner ear.

The anterior surface is related to the middle cranial fossa. It is attached to the squamous part of the temporal bone by petrosquamous suture. Around the mid portion lies the bony prominence of the superior semicircular canal is called **arcuate eminence**. Lateral to this eminence is a depressed area, where the bone is thin and called tegmen tympani that forms the roof of the middle ear cavity. A shallow groove is present posterolaterally to open into the hiatus of the facial canal, just lateral to is another smaller hiatus that lodges the **greater superficial petrosal nerve**. At the apex, the termination of the carotid canal is present.

Posterior surface is related to the posterior cranial fossa. A large opening that leads in to the internal auditory meatus is present medially is about 1 cm in length and transmits the facial, vestibulocochlear nerve and internal auditory branch of basilar artery. Posterior to the opening of internal auditory meatus is a slit like opening that leads to the vestibular aqueduct (Figs 2.5 and 2.13). The **petromastoid canal (subarcuate canal)** joins the mastoid antrum to the posterior cranial fossa, that can be confused on imaging as a fracture line. This canal if persists as a wide canal can transmit infection from the mastoid to the posterior fossa (Fig. 2.7C).

The **inferior surface** forms part of the external part of the base of the skull. Various of foramina can be seen which include opening of the carotid canal anteriorly and the jugular foramen posteriorly and in between a small inferior tympanic canaliculus, through which the tympanic branch of the glossopharyngeal nerve passes. The stylomastoid foramen is situated on the inferior surface just posterolateral to the styloid process.

The petrous bone has three angles. The **superior angle** has a groove, over which lies the superior petrosal sinus. The tentorium cerebelli is attached to this angle of petrous bone and on its medial part lies the trigeminal nerve. The **posterior angle** has a sulcus over which lies the inferior petrosal sinus medially, jugular foramen formed along with the jugular notch of the occipital bone laterally. The anterior angle fuses with the squamous part laterally with petrosquamous suture and articulates medially with the spinous process of the sphenoid bone (Fig. 2.7A and B).

The apex of the petrous bone is pyramidal shaped anteromedial part of the petrous bone that articulate with greater wing of sphenoid and the occipital bone. It should be examined carefully on radiology to look for, petrosphenoid fissure laterally, internal carotid artery anteriorly and the posterior cranial fossa behind, petro-occipetal suture medially in the axial CT (Figs 2.5B, 2.7A and B). On the superior surface laterally is a depression Meckel's cave of trigeminal ganglion.

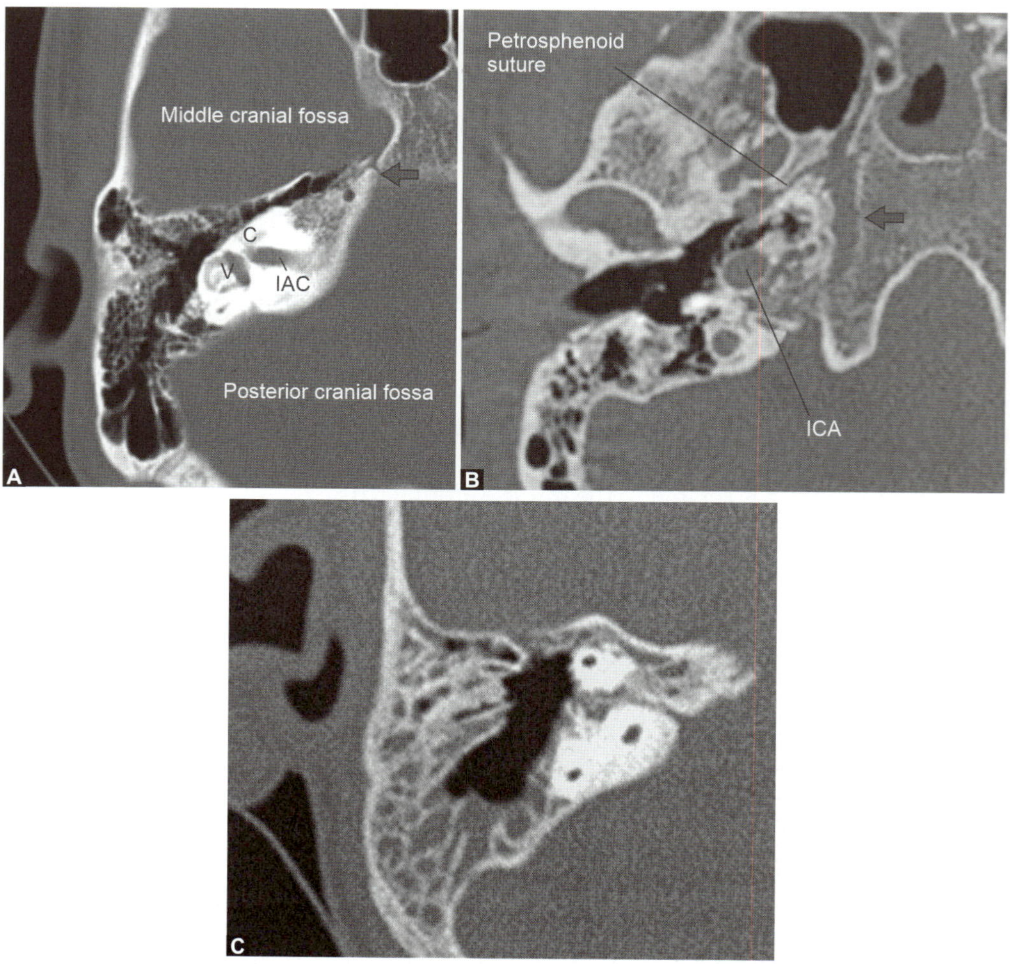

Fig. 2.7: (A) Vestibular labyrinth (V), cochlea (C), internal auditory canal (IAC), Petroclival fissure (black arrow), **(B)** Petrosphenoid suture, internal carotid artery (ICA), petroclival fissure (black arrow), **(C)** Petromastoid canal

External Auditory Canal (Fig. 2.8)

The lateral 1/3rd of the canal is fibrocartilaginous and needs to be removed and prepared before mounting the temporal bone for the drilling. Now the medial 2/3rds can be well visualized which is made up of tympanic part of the temporal bone. If the canal skin is elevated posteriorly, two suture lines can be seen superiorly (tympanosquamous) and inferiorly (tympanomastoid). They are very important land mark, while elevating the tympanomeatal flap and securing of vascular strip before myringoplasty and mastoid surgery. The anterior wall forms the posterior part of the glenoid fossa and is related to the temporomandibular joint while the posterior wall forms the mastoid bone.

Tympanic Cavity (Fig. 2.9)

It is a six wall air filled space within the temporal bone, lying between the tympanic membrane laterally and the cochlea medially. Its upper part extending above the

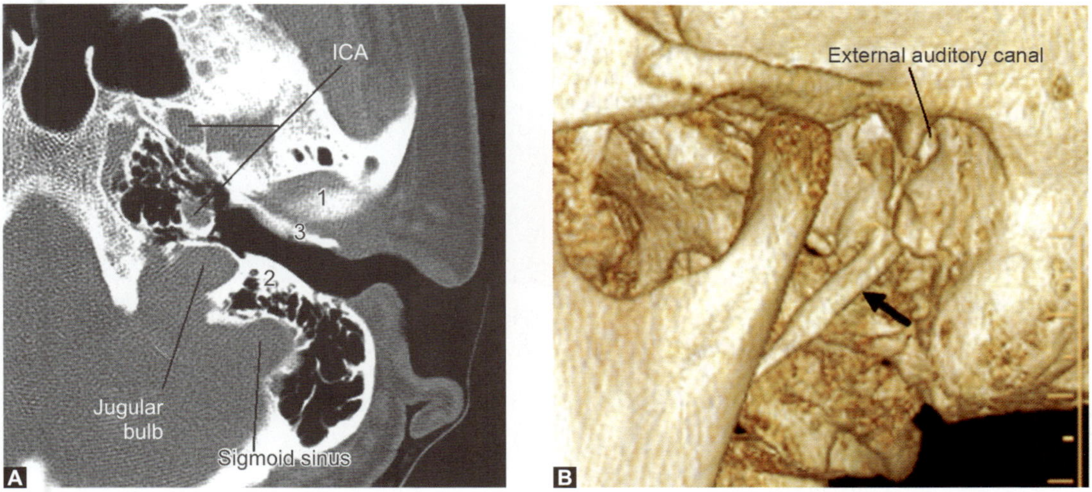

Fig. 2.8: (A) CT temporal bone (left) external auditory canal, middle ear, and temporomandibular joint and related structure. 1: Mandibular condyle; 2: Posterior canal wall; 3: Anterior canal wall; ICA: Internal carotid artery; jugular bulb and sigmoid sinus. **(B)** 3D CT imaging, showing external auditory canal relationship to TM joint. Note the attachment of styloid process (black arrow)

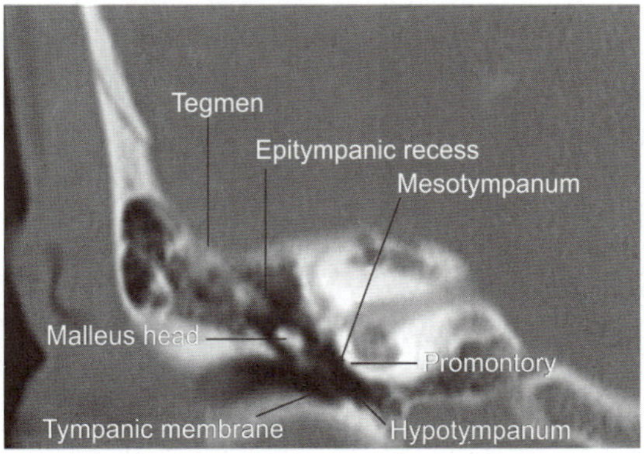

Fig. 2.9: HRCT right temporal bone coronal view showing tympanic cavity and its division

tympanic membrane is known as the epitympanic recess or attic, and the lower part extending below the level of the floor of the external auditory meatus is referred to as the hypotympanum. Area next to the tympanic membrane is known as mesotympanum. The cavity has a vertical length greater than the breadth, narrow in depth, particularly in its central portion where the basal turn of the cochlea forms a bulge on medial wall known as promontory.

Roof of the Tympanic Cavity

It is formed by tegmen tympani which separates it from the dura of the middle cranial fossa. It is formed in part by the petrous and in part by the squamous bone. The levels and slope of the tegmen are approximately represented on the skull surface by fascia which is attached to the supramastoid crest and posterior root of zygomatic process.

Floor of the Tympanic Cavity

The floor separates the cavity from the bulb of the internal jugular vein. The tympanic branch of the glossopharyngeal nerve enters the cavity through the floor. The glomus jugulare (jugular body) is situated in this portion of the jugular bulb.

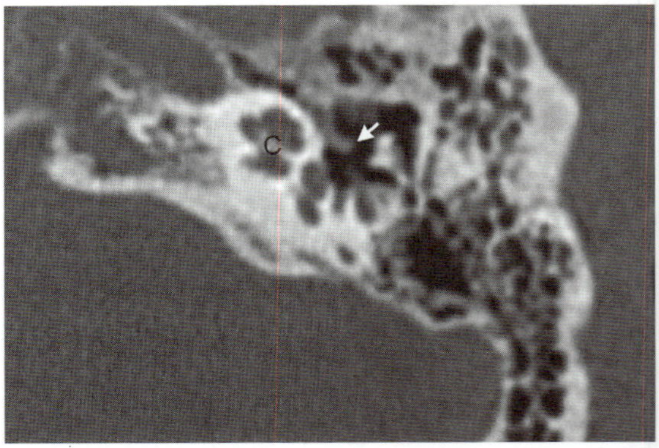

Fig. 2.10: Tensor tympani muscle and tendon (white arrow), cochlea (C)

Anterior Wall

The anterior wall is rather narrow as the medial and lateral walls converge. They are four openings from above downwards

1. Canal of Hugier, through which the chorda tympani escapes from the middle ear
2. Canal for tensor tympani muscle (Fig. 2.10)
3. Tympanic orifice of eustachian tube
4. Petrotympanic suture, containing the tympanic artery and the anterior ligament of the malleus.

Posterior Wall

In its upper part is the aditus that connects the attic to the mastoid antrum. Below the aditus, the pyramid gives exit to the stapedius tendon. Just above the pyramid lies the fossa incudis occupied by the short process of the incus. Below the pyramid, is a depression of the sinus tympani (Fig. 2.11) . The facial nerve, as it bends downwards at the level of the floor of the aditus, is in danger of infection arising from the air cells, and of danger during surgical attempts at air cell extirpation. The anatomy of sinus tympani has been discussed in detail in Chpter 3.

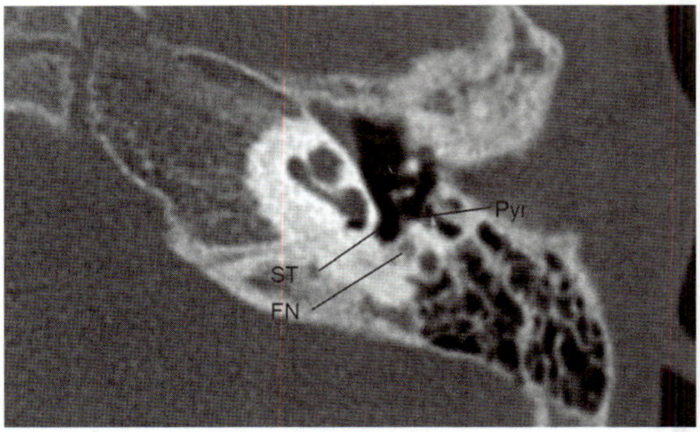

Fig. 2.11: HRCT left temporal bone (axial) showing sinus tympani (ST), FN (FN), pyramid (Pyr)

Posterolateral to the fallopian canal in the aditus lies the rounded prominence of the bony wall of the lateral semicircular canal. Between the tympanic annulus laterally and the facial nerve canal medially, is the facial recess. Running through the wall between the two with a varying degree of obliquity, is the chorda tympani nerve.

Lateral Wall

The lateral wall is formed mainly by the tympanic membrane and the outer bony wall of the attic.

The lateral wall of the epitympanum also includes the part of the tympanic membrane lying above the anterior and posterior malleolar folds—the pars flacida. The lateral bony epitympanic wall on the scutum is thin and its lateral surface forms the superior portion of the deep part of the external auditory canal.

Medial Wall

The medial wall separates the tympanic cavity from the inner ear. It has several obvious features which are:

1. The promontory is a rounded bony elevation covering the basal turn of cochlea.
2. Behind and above the promontory is the fenestra vestibule, closed by the footplate of the stapes and its surroundings annular ligament.
3. The fenestra cochlea or round window, closed by the secondary tympanic membrane, lies below and behind the fenestra vestibule, from which it is separated by a posterior extension of the promontory called subiculum.

Trautmann's Triangle

It is an area of vascular cancellous bone, triangular in shape. It is bounded above by the superior petrosal sinus with the tegmen tympani and antrum covering the middle fossa dura, behind by the caries of this bone leads to formation of perisinus abscess, sinus thrombosis and extradural abscess and can extend into the posterior fossa of the skull.

Mastoid Process

The mastoid process lies behind the tympanic portion of the temporal bone. Its development begins at the end of first year of life and achieves its definite size at puberty. The stylomastoid foramen lies immediately behind the tympanic ring.

80% of the mastoids become honey combed with air spaces. In some people, the marrow persists within the bony structure of the mastoid (diploeic type) while in others, the air cells and marrow spaces are wholly absent (acellular or sclerotic type).

Mastoid Antrum (Fig. 2.13)

It is an air filled sinus within the petrous part of the temporal bone. It communicates with the middle ear by way of the aditus and has mastoid air cells arising from its wall. The antrum is well developed at birth.

The medial wall of the antrum is related to the posterior and horizontal semicircular canals and more deeply and inferiorly is the endolymphatic sac and dura of the posterior cranial fossa. The roof of the tegmen antrum forms part of the floor of the middle cranial fossa separating the antrum from the temporal lobe of the brain. The posterior wall is formed by the bone covering the sigmoid sinus. The lateral wall is part of the squamous portion of the temporal bone, increasing in thickness during life, from 2 mm at birth to 12–15 mm in the adult. The lateral wall in the adult corresponds to the **suprameatal (Macewen's) triangle** (Fig. 2.3) on the lateral surface of the skull. This region can be felt through the cymba conchae of the auricle and is defined by the supramastoid crest (posterior prolongation of the upper border of the root of the zygoma), a vertical tangent through the posterior margin of the external auditory canal, the posterior–superior margin of the external meatus itself.

The floor of the mastoid antrum is related to digastrics muscle laterally and the sigmoid sinus posteriorly. Through the posterior wall and the floor of the antrum it communicates, by several openings with the air cells. The anterior wall of the antrum has the aditus in its upper part, while lower down, the facial nerve passes in its descent to the styloid foramen.

Aditus ad Antrum (Fig. 2.13)

The aditus ad antrum leads backwards from the upper attic space of the epitympanum into the mastoid antrum. The bony prominence of the horizontal semicircular canal lies between its medial wall and floor. The facial nerve lies on a plane below and deep to the opening of the aditus. The short process of the incus is closely related to the facial nerve and lateral semicircular canal.

Facial Nerve (Fig. 2.13)

The facial nerve canal runs above the promontory and fenestra vestibule in an antero-posterior direction. Immediately anterior to the point where the facial nerve turns medially to penetrate the inner ear, is the processus cochleariformis. The facial canal turns vertically downwards at the posterior extremity of the scala vestibule. The nerve then has a slight backwards and lateral inclination that carries it into the posterior wall behind the pyramid and below the fossa incudis.

The ampullary end of the semicircular canal lies just above the second genu of the facial nerve.

Contents of the Tympanic Cavity (Figs 2.12 and 2.13)

1. Ossicles: Malleus, incus and stapes
2. Muscles: Tensor tympani and stapedius
3. Nerves: Chorda tympani and nerve to stapedius
4. Air
5. Tympanic plexus of nerves lies on the promontory, deep to the mucous membrane.

Inner Ear (Figs 2.11 and 2.12)

The inner ear is situated within the petrous part of the temporal bone including cochlea, vestibule and semicircular canal. The osseouus cochlea with its 2 ½ turn including basal, middle and apical turn can be identified on CT (Juliano et al, 2013). The microanatomical structure of the osseous spiral lamina and modiolus can be identified in an HRCT with thin slice (Fig. 2.13A). The lateral part of the basal turn of cochlea, that projected into the middle ear cavity forms the cochlear promontory. The structures of the membranous labyrinth (cochlear duct, utricle, saccule, semicircular

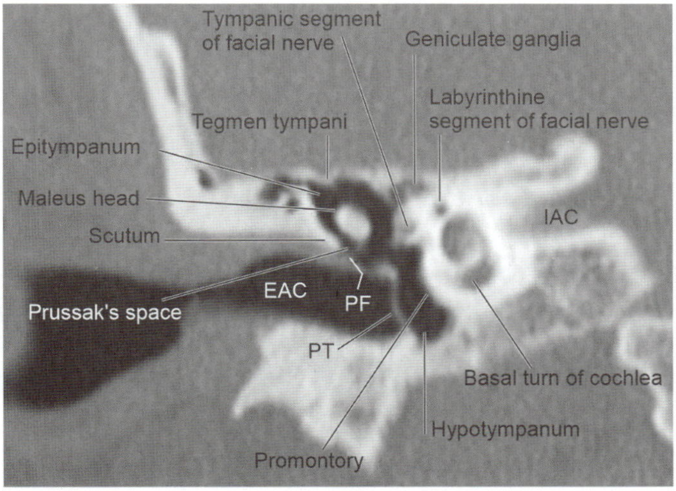

Fig. 2.12: HRCT temporal bone, coronal section at the level of Malleus head, also are PF (pars flacida), PT (pars tensa), IAC (internal auditory canal), Geniculate ganglion tympanic & labyrinthine segment of facial nerve, Basal turn of cochlea

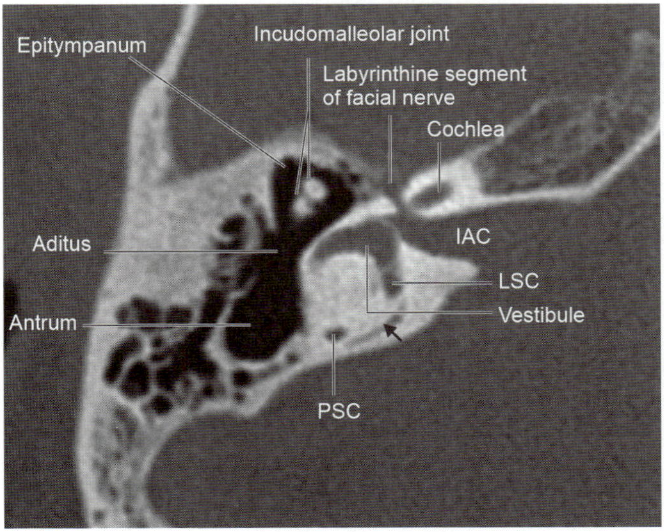

Fig. 2.13: Axial CT at the level of lateral semicircular canal epitympanum, incudomalleolar joint aditus, antrum, labyrinthine segment of facial nerve, internal auditory canal (IAC), posterior and lateral semicircular canal (PSC & LSC), vestibular aqueduct (black arrow)

ducts, and endolymphatic duct and sac) cannot be distinguished in a CT scan, however can be best studied in MRI.

The petrous temporal bone consisting of the inner ear structures that lies medial to the middle ear. The cerebellopontine angle, the facial nerve and vestibulocochlear nerve that passes through the internal auditory meatus (IAC) can be appreciated better in T2 weighted MRI including pathology involved (Fig. 2.14B).

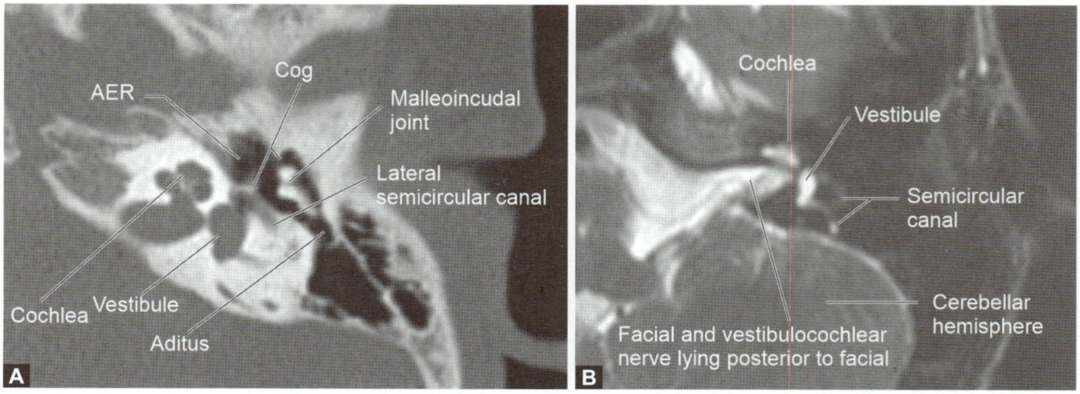

Fig. 2.14: (A) HRCT temporal bone at the level of attic showing cog, malleoincudal joint, inner ear structures including cochlea, vesibule, lateral semicircular canal and internal auditory canal, **(B)** MRI T2 weighted, axial at the level of CP angle, showing facial nerve and the vestibulocochlear nerve lying posterior to it, the cochlea, the vestibule and the semicircular canals

REFERENCES AND FURTHER READING

1. Macewen W. Pyogenic and infective diseases of the brain and spinal cord. Glasgow: MacLehose & Sons; 1893
2. Gulya AJ & Schuknecht H. Anatomy of the Temporal Bone with Surgical Implications, 3rd edition (2007), CRC Press, ISBN 9780849375972-CAT# DK7597
3. Fujii N, Inui Y, Katada K. Temporal bone anatomy: correlation of multiplanar reconstruction sections and three-dimensional computed tomography images. *Jpn J Radiol*. 2010 Nov. 28(9):637–48. [Medline].
4. Juliano AF, *et al*. Imaging review of the temporal bone: Part-1. Anatomy & inflammatory disease and neoplastic process; *Radiology* 2013,v-269(1) p 17–33.
5. Surgery of the Ear–4th edition; Michael E. Glasscock, George E. Shambaugh—Surgical anatomy of the temporal bone, pages 35–53.
6. Scott Brown Diseases of ENT Vol. 1: Basic Science, 5th edition, pages 14–46.
7. Gray's Anatomy, 36th edition
8. Temporal bone dissection guide (International edition)-2nd edition; Howard W Francis & John K Niparko, 2017, Thiem Medical & scientific publication, Private limited
9. Juliano AF et al. Imaging Review of the Temporal Bone: Part I. Anatomy and Inflammatory and Neoplastic Processes. *Radiology*, 2013; 269 (1), 17–33.

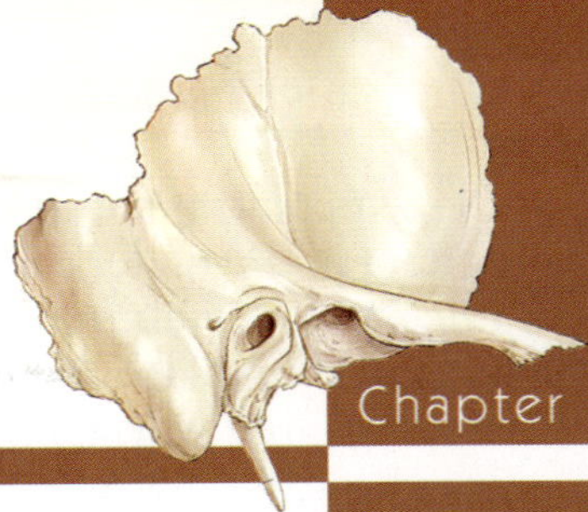

Chapter 3

Endoscopic Surgical Anatomy of the Middle Ear

Sanjeev Mohanty • Nikitha Periaswamy • Dipak Ranjan Nayak

Introduction

Otoendoscopy has revolutionised the armamentarium of otologists worldwide. It has made to understand the complex middle ear anatomy as well as the middle ear spaces due to a better magnification and to facilitated to look "behind the corner" (Marchioni et al., 2010). In addition to having a panoramic view of middle ear anatomy, endoscopy also allows better understanding of middle ear physiology and ventilation pathways and pathology.

Historical Perspective

Since the development of rod endoscope by Hopkins 1966, new interest have been developed its use in diagnostic and therapeutic application in ear surgery. Jaco (1966) and Zini (1967) used micromirror to visualize sinus tympani which was helpful to visualize the disease and was not helpful for removal (Bremon et al., 1990). Mer et al. in 1967 used flexible fiberoptic endoscope for examining the middle ear. Marquet used one 1.7 mm endoscope to visualize the tympanic cavity through the perforation of tympanic membrane (Thomassin, 2016). A needle otoscope with side viewing was subsequently developed by Namura (1982) consisting of a SELFOC® rod lens for observation and a glass fibre bundle for illumination, which can be attached to camera for taking photograph of the middle ear. In 1990, Thomassin described otoendoscopic surgery and its role in managing middle ear cholesteatoma especially sinus tympani. The endoscope was initially used to visualize hidden areas during conventional surgery while dealing with cholesteatoma.

Role of Otoendoscopy in Understanding the Anatomy and Pathology of Middle Ear

Baki et al. (2002), described the endoscopic anatomy of sinus tympani. Exploration of certain important anatomical areas and hidden recesses like the sinus tympani, the anterior epitympanic space, and the protympanic space is possible with magnification and angular vision, which is almost impossible with the traditional microscopic views. Otoendoscopy is not only a less invasive surgical approach, but also allows us to perform a more 'physiologic' surgery of middle ear (Marchioni et al., 2011).

The tympanic membrane forms the lateral wall of the middle ear. Endoscope plays an important role in understanding the tympanic membrane pathology with special reference to attic pathology like retraction pockets and perforation of pars flacida, erosion of outer bony wall of the attic (scutum). Perforation of pars tensa can facilitate visualisation of mesotympanum and status of the incudostapedial joint.

Based on the mesotympanum, the middle ear space can be divided subspaces as mentioned below, to understand the endoscopic anatomy of the middle ear (Fig. 3.2).

Retrotympanum (Figs 3.2 and 3.3)

It is the part of the middle ear space lying posterior to the mesotympanum. The retro-tympanum contains four spaces. Two spaces lie anterior and superior to the *vertical segment of facial nerve,* which is further divided by the ponticular ridge into the sinus tympani inferiorly and the posterior tympanic sinus superiorly. Two spaces lie posterior and inferior to the vertical segment of facial nerve, separated by the chordal eminence into the facial recess superiorly and the lateral tympanic sinus inferiorly.

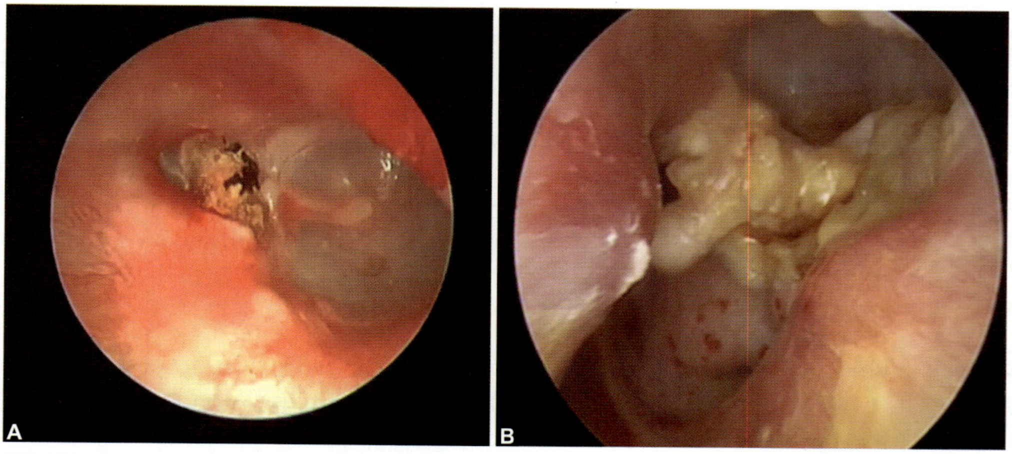

Fig. 3.1: Otoendoscopic pictures showing **(A)** attic cholesteatoma with scutum erosion, **(B)** attic cholesteatoma with otomastoid cavity

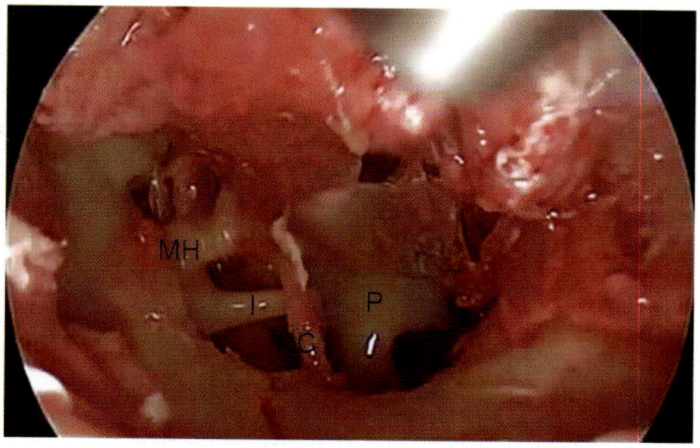

Fig. 3.2: Cadaveric endoscopic view of mesotympanum showing, MH: Malleus head–neck and handle, I: Long process of incus, C: Chorda tympani nerve obscuring the view of incudostapedial joint and stapes suprastructure, P: Promontory

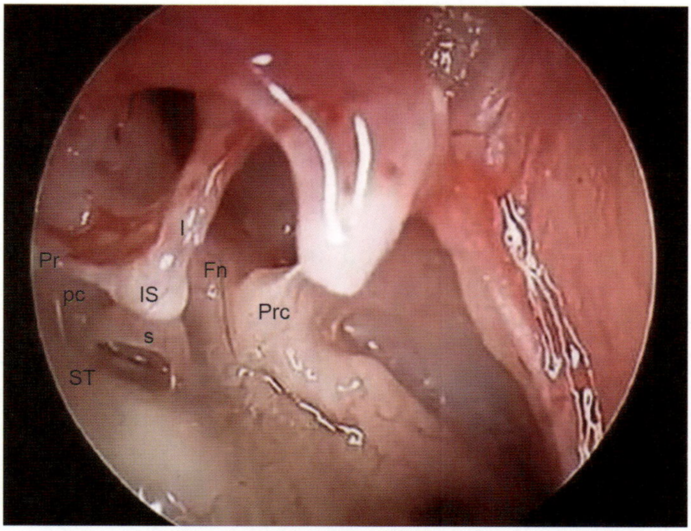

Fig. 3.3: Middle ear structures: ST: Sinus tympani, Pr: Pyramidal eminence with stapedius tendon, pc: Ponticulus, IS: Incudostapedial joint, S: Stapes superstructure, Fn: Facial nerve, Prc: Processus cochleariformis. Note the long process of the incus (I) is partialy eroded

Sinus Tympani

It is bounded by the pyramidal eminence, stapedius muscle and the facial nerve laterally, medially by the posterior semicircular canal, superiorly by the ponticulus and inferiorly by the ridge extending from the styloid eminence to the posterior rim of cochlear window niche.

The sinus tympani is classified into three types based on their depth in relation to the facial nerve on radiological evaluation.

- **Type A:** A small sinus tympani without any medial or posterior extension beyond the facial nerve.
- **Type B:** Medial extension of the medial boundary of the sinus tympani, medial to the facial nerve, but no posterior extension.
- **Type C:** Medial and posterior extension of the medial boundary of the sinus tympani beyond the facial nerve.

Ponticulus is the bony ridge extending from the pyramidal recess to the promontory region, separating the sinus tympani from the posterior tympanic sinus. The *subiculum* is the bony ridge extending from the posterior lip of the round window niche to the styloid eminence, separating the sinus tympani from the subtympanic sinus.

Facial recess: This is an area bounded medially by the facial canal and pyramidal eminence, laterally by the chorda tympani, superiorly the incudal buttress, lodging the short process of incus.

Epitympanic Space

The space superior to the mesotympanum is the epitympanum. The epitympanic diaphragm forms the floor of the epitympanic space and consists of three malleaolar ligamental folds, namely the anterior, lateral and posterior, the posterior incudal ligamental fold and two membranous folds—the tensor tympani fold and the lateral incudomalleaolar fold.

Epitympanic Space is Divided by the Cog

The cog is the bony projection that detaches from the tegmen tympani cranially and extending vertically towards the cochleariform process, into the anterior and posterior epitympanic space (Fig. 3.4). The posterior epitympanic space contains the body and short process of incus along with the head of malleus. The lateral part of the posterior epitympanic space is further divided into a superior and inferior spaces by the lateral incudomalleaolar fold. The inferior lateral attic is also called the Prussak's space. This space is ventilated by a posterior pocket from the mesotympanum and can be associated with retraction pocket and cholesteatoma formation due to blockage (Fig. 3.5).

The rest of the attic is ventilated from the mesotympanum through the tympanic isthmus. The tensor tympani fold separates the anterior attic (epitympanic space) from the mesotympanum thus making the tympanic isthmus the only route of ventilation of

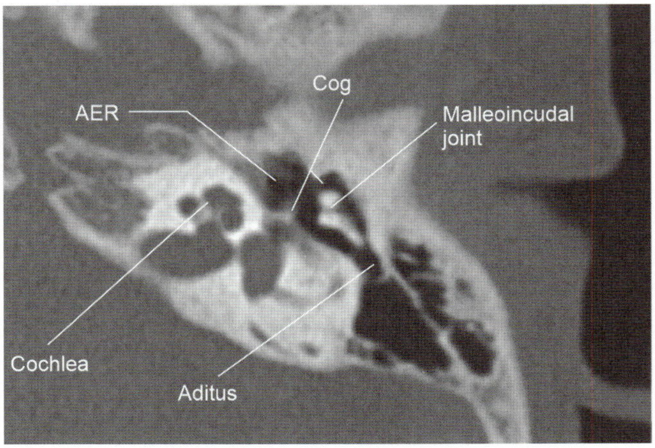

Fig. 3.4: Axial CT showing anterior epitympanic recess (AER), Cog, Malleoincudal joint, aditus and cochlea

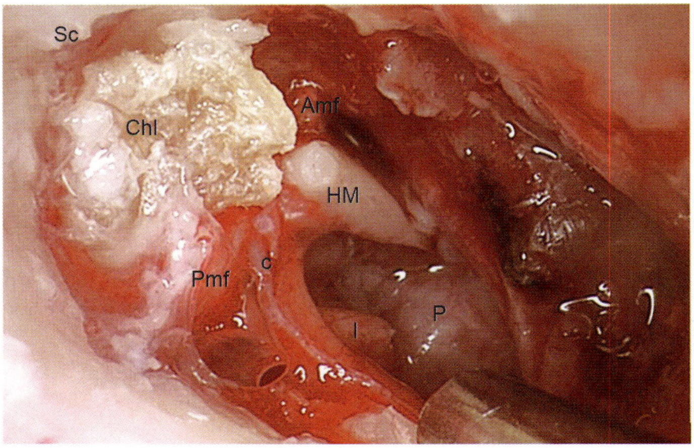

Fig. 3.5: Prussak's space cholesteatoma being exposed by removal of scutum (Sc). Also seen are anterior malleolar fold (Amf), posterior malleolar fold (Pmf), chorda tympani (C), long process of incus (I), promontory (P), handle of malleus (HM)

the anterior attic. However, the tensor tympani fold is deficient in 25% of cases where the anterior attic is directly ventilated by the supratubal recess in the mesotympanum.

Protympanum

Portion of the middle ear space anterior to the mesotympanum, inferior to the anterior attic space and superior to the hypotympanum. It contains the supratubal recess superiorly and the eustachian tube orifice inferiorly. Above and medial to the eustachian tube orifice is the internal carotid artery.

Hypotympanum

The portion of the middle ear space inferior to the mesotympanum. It separates the middle ear space from the jugular bulb. The jugular bulb protrudes into the middle ear space to varying extents. It contains various anatomical details like spines, lamellae, trabeculae and pneumatised cells.

Facial Nerve

To understand the course of the facial nerve through the middle ear in endoscopic approach, it can be divided into two segments, the *pre-cochleariform segment* which lies superior and anterior to the cochleariform process and the *post-cochleariform segment* which lies posterior to the cochleariform process (Fig. 3.3).

The *cochleariform process* is an important landmark to identify the geniculate ganglion which lies in the floor of the anterior attic space, superior and anterior to the cochleariform process. The removal of malleus provides good access to this portion of the facial nerve.

The malleoincudal joint should be disarticulated (Fig. 3.6) before removal of the incus and the head of the malleus, that can provide a clear view of the post-cochleariform segment of the facial nerve.

The only portion of the facial nerve which can be visualized without disrupting the ossicular chain is the posterior most part of the facial nerve related to the second genu and the pyramidal eminence. One has to remember that facial nerve can be dehiscent in this segment (Fig. 3.7).

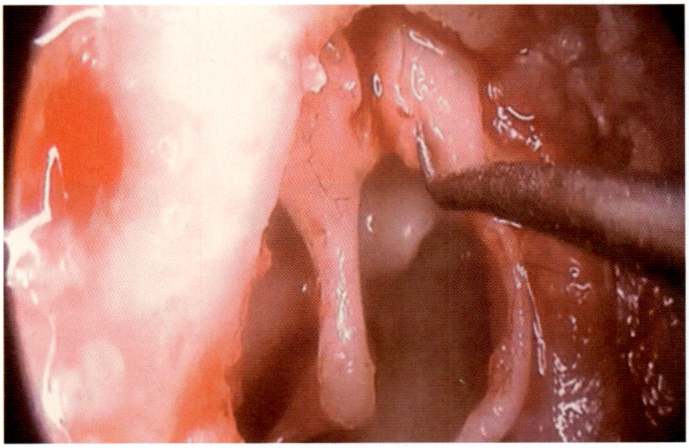

Fig. 3.6: Dislocated malleoincudal joint

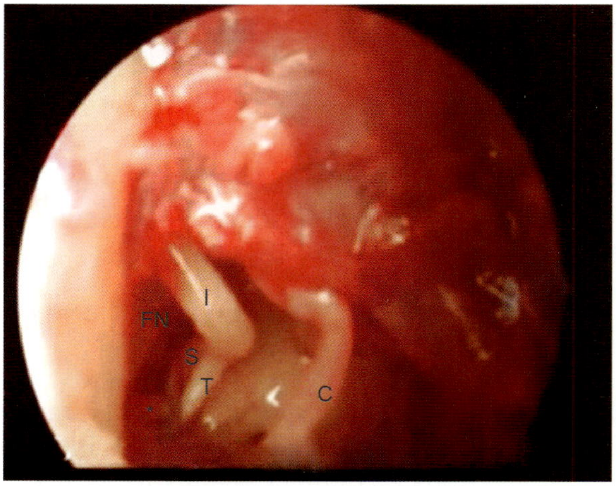

Fig. 3.7: Dehiscent overhanging facial nerve (FN) obscuring the view of the footplate. Posterior crura (*) is visible partially. Also seen are stapes head (S), long proces of incus (I), stapedius tendon (T), chorda tympani (C)

The post-cochleariform segment of the facial nerve is an important landmark for the identification of the aditus and antrum.

Although, it is imperative to master the temporal bone anatomy by the conventional temporal bone dissection, otoendoscopes have added a new dimension to the understanding of intricate anatomy and applied middle ear physiology. Knowledge of middle ear anatomy is the basis for any otologist. Endoscopy of middle ear is the best way to explore the tympanic cavity and to understand the importance of ventilation routes, which is central to the genesis of chronic middle ear disease. Endoscopy allows us to understand isthmus blockage, complete or incomplete tensor fold and mastoid pneumatisation. Endoscopic surgery of the ear is usually done with one hand, with dominant hand used for handling surgical instruments while the other hand is used to hold the endoscope. This issue and the narrow space inside the EAC require training to improve the surgeon's skills to safely apply the technique in patients. In general, the gold standard for surgical training is considered to be cadaveric dissection. In cases of unavailability of cadaveric specimens or local ethical issues, an animal model for the training of endoscopic ear surgery has recently been described. The future trends would probably centre around a good supplementation of both endoscopic and microscopic amalgamation to achieve good patient outcomes.

REFERENCES AND FURTHER READING

1. Marchioni D, Molteni G , Presutti L. Endoscopic anatomy of the middle ear. Indian J Otolaryngol Head Neck Surg. 2011; 63(2): 101–13.
2. *Bremond G*, Magnan J, Chays A, De Gasquet R (*1990*) *Endoscopie* de la trompe d'Eustache. Ann Otol Laryngol (paris); 107, 15–9.
3. Mer SB, Derbyshire AJ, Brushenko A, et al. Fibre optic endoscope for examining middle ear. *Arch Otolaryngol.* 1967 Apr;85(4):387–93.
4. Thomassin JM. The History and Development of Endoscopic Ear Surgery (EES). *Journal of Aryngol Otol* 2016; R 674.3, Vol 130 S3, DOI: https://doi.org/10.1017/S002221511600253X.

5. Nomura, Y. A needle otoscope: An instrument of endoscopy of the middle ear. *Acta Otolaryngol* 1982; 93: 73–9.
6. Thomassin JM, et al. Endoscopic ear surgery, initial evaluation. *Ann Otolaryngol Chir Cervicofac*. 1990;107(8):564–70.
7. Baki FA, El Dine MB, El Said L, et al. Sinus tympani endoscopic anatomy. *Otolaryngol Head Neck Surg*. 2002;127:158–162. doi: 10.1067/mhn.2002.127588.
8. Tarabichi, M. Endoscopic management of limited attic cholesteatoma. *Laryngoscope*. 114(7), 1157–62 (2004).
9. Wang MC, et al. The costs and quality of operative training for residents in tympanoplasty type I. *Acta Otolaryngol*. 2009;129:512–4.

Chapter

4

Cortical Mastoidectomy

Rohit Singh • Dipak Ranjan Nayak • Chinmoy Sundar Ray

Historical Perspective

The first documented incision to drain an infected ear goes to Ambrose Pere in the 16th century and the first documented recommendation of mastoidectomy was found in the writings of Johannes Riolanus in 1671, however, the credit for performing the first mastoidectomy by drilling to remove pus goes to Jean Lois Petit (1774). He use to remove carries bone by using a chisel and hammer.[1] The postauricular incision for ear surgery by William Wilde in 1853 revolutionized the mastoid surgery following postauricular incision and ultimately gave rise to simple mastoidectomy. Von Troeltsch is credited for creating interest in mastoidectomy among German surgeons and motivated his student, Hermann Schwartze to standardize cortical mastoidectomy, who also established clear indications for such procedure.

Preparations

It is important to prepare the bone before dissection. The soft tissue around the external auditory canal and over the mastoid should be removed especially over the root of zygoma carefully to identify the spine of Henle with the help of an elevator. This helps in identifying the landmarks like Macewen's triangle (suprameatal triangle) (Fig. 4.1). All the landmarks have to be identified prior to and during dissection and should be preserved till the landmarks at the deeper levels are located.

Surgical Principle and Instrumentation

A wider approach to the mastoid is most important while doing cortical mastoidectomy. The largest possible burr is used to remove the mastoid cortex. The burr should be preferably angled so that the flukes on the side are hitting directly against the surface. The largest burr should be used especially in areas where smaller burr could plunge into the dural plate. The largest suction irrigator is used during the initial exposure. As there are no important structures in the cortex, the bone can be removed rapidly and safely. Drilling should be done only under good visualization.

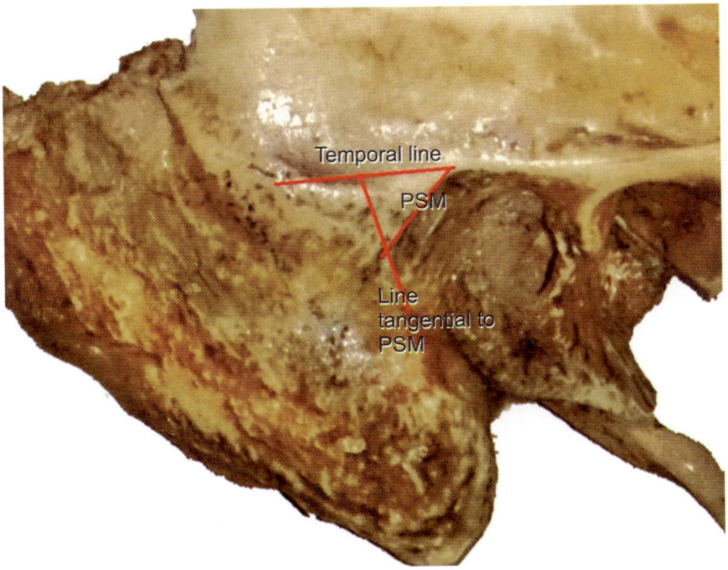

Fig. 4.1: Macewen's triangle formed by (1) temporal line, (2) posterior superior meatal wall (PSM), (3) tangential line to PSM

Surgical Technique

The bone is carefully fixed to the temporal bone holder in the same anatomical position as one does during surgery. The landmarks seen on the mastoid cortex after positioning the bone to the temporal bone holder before dissection are:

a. The external auditory meatus anteriorly
b. The suprameatal spine of Henle at the superoposterior part of the external auditory canal
c. The suprameatal triangle of Macewen behind the spine of Henle
d. The temporal line which is a ridge continuous from the superior border of the zygomatic arch posteriorly onto the mastoid cortex which is the inferior limit of the Temporalis muscle.

The drill is positioned on the mastoid cortex just at an area posterior to the spine of Henle. A straight cut made along the temporal line posteriorly into the sinodural angle marks the limit of dissection. A second cut is made perpendicular to the first and directed toward the mastoid tip just immediately posterior to the posterior canal wall.

Different techniques are used to remove the mastoid cortex and to identify antrum.

One way of opening the cortex is by opening up the air cells and the dissection progressing medially. The line of dissection in this case can be from posterior to inferior as shown in Figs 4.2 and 4.3. This allows the surgeon to pass under the bulge of the middle fossa and toward the antrum.

Another technique is to remove the lateral surface of the cortex from the temporal line above to the mastoid tip below and from the posterior osseous meatal wall in front to the probable extent of pneumatization as seen in the X-ray. Orderly removal of cell tracts will help complete penetration of all accessible cells. This can be done by working from the antrum outward (Shambaugh).

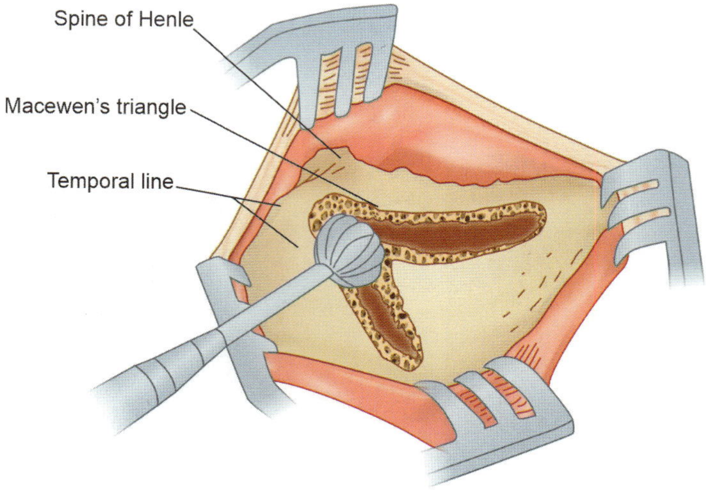

Fig. 4.2: Landmarks and initial step of cortical mastoidectomy

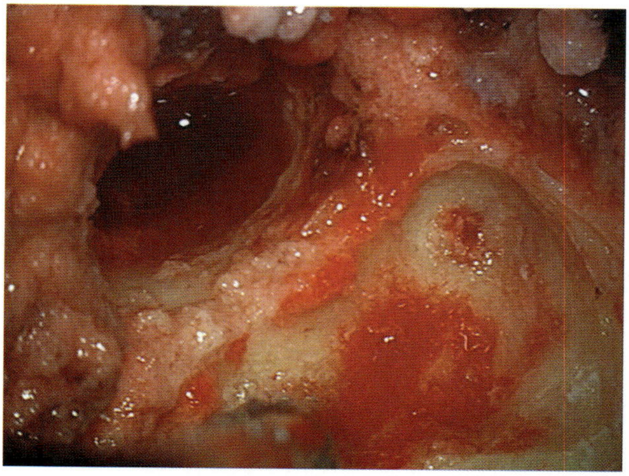

Fig. 4.3: Systematic saucerization of mastoid cortex using largest burr

The mastoid cortex is thus removed in a systematic way of saucerization with deepest portion of penetration at the junction between the two perpendicular lines as mentioned earlier. A wide cortical removal should be done before deeper penetration into the antrum. The opening should be beveled and conical rather than a blind narrow deep hole. The posterior canal wall is thinned so that the shadow of any instrument can be seen through the bone.

It is important to expose the middle fossa dural plate (tegmen tympani) for best possible access into the antrum and the epitympanic areas. The cortex is removed by burring into the area of the linea Temporalis until the bone color changes to show that the middle fossa dura is reached. This plate exposure can be followed into the antrum without lacerating the dura. Smaller burrs are used here to prevent fracture of the thin plate and to prevent dural dehiscence. Thinning can be done by a diamond burr.

The sigmoid sinus is then drilled out along the posterior part of the mastoid cavity. In a well pneumatized bone, drilling may continue until the occiput is exposed. The sigmoid

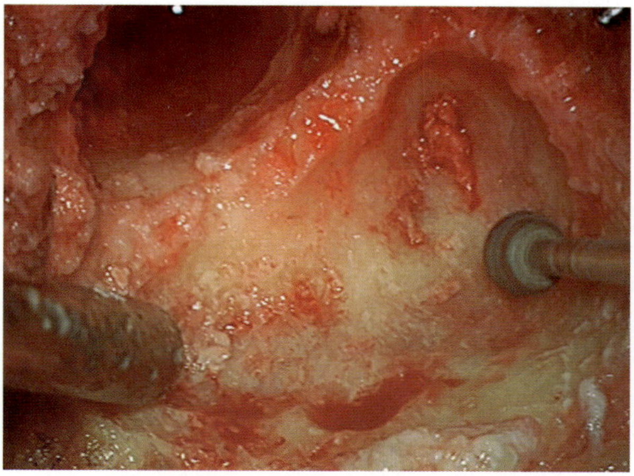

Fig. 4.4: Change of color bone while drilling on the posterior aspect of mastoid confirming sinus plate. One may encounter bleed in from this area from emissary vein that can be controlled easily with diamond burr

sinus appears in the posterior part of the dissection as a blue colored smooth bony plate. Once this is seen, the area between the sigmoid and the middle fossa plate, the sinodural angle can be cleared of cells. Deep penetration of this area leads to exposure of superior petrosal sinus. The sigmoid sinus is usually the posterior limit of a mastoid dissection. Diamond burrs are used here to control bleeding from the bone by pushing the vessel down to its channel (Fig. 4.4).

The mastoid tip cells should be then cleared to gain better exposure to the jugular bulb area. The new landmarks after dissection are shown in Figs 4.5 to 4.7.

a. The middle fossa plate
b. The sinodural angle plate
c. The sigmoid sinus plate
d. Mastoid tip air cells
e. Thinned posterior canal wall

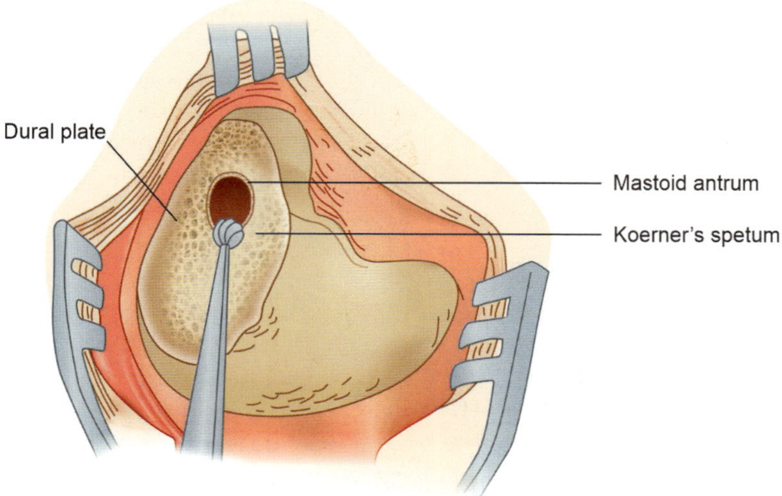

Fig. 4.5: Right cortical mastoidectomy in progress

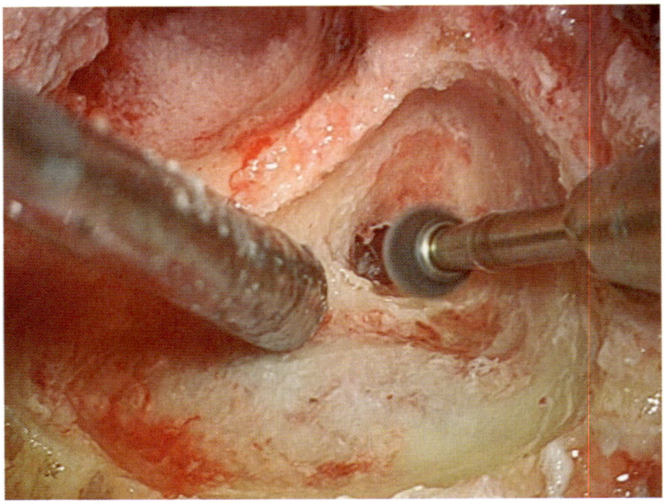

Fig. 4.6: Koerner's septum is being drilled to open the mastoid antrum on the left side. Note the bluish color, change of the sigmoid sinus posterior to suction tip

The mastoid antrum lies just below the deepest point of penetration into the temporal bone, posterior to the spine of Henle. Sometimes the Koerner's septum lies deep to the mastoid cortex and often is mistaken for the hard bone of labyrinth and horizontal semicircular canal. This septum should be drilled through in the anterosuperior part of the dissection and the antrum will be seen as a large cavity (Figs 4.5 and 4.6). At the bottom of the antral cavity lies the smooth, hard labyrinthine bone of the horizontal semicircular canal (Fig. 4.7).

Once this is identified, the fossa incudis, the epitympanum anterosuperiorly and the external genu of the facial nerve inferomedially can be exposed. Cells between the

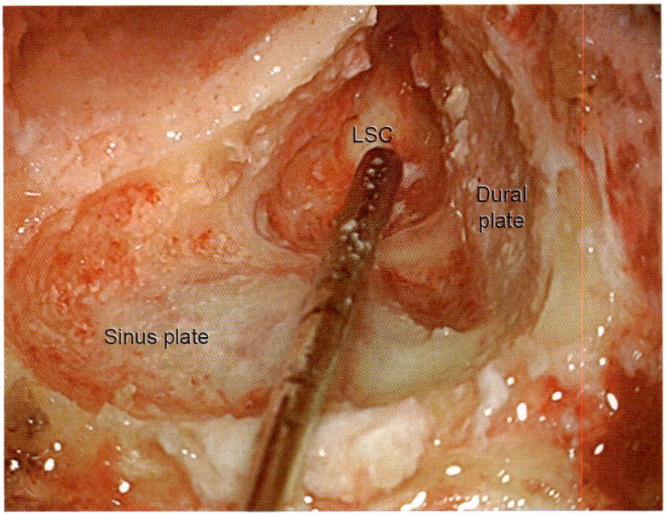

Fig. 4.7: The lateral semicircular canal (LSC) after mastoid antrum is opened. The dural plate and sinus plates are well saucerized

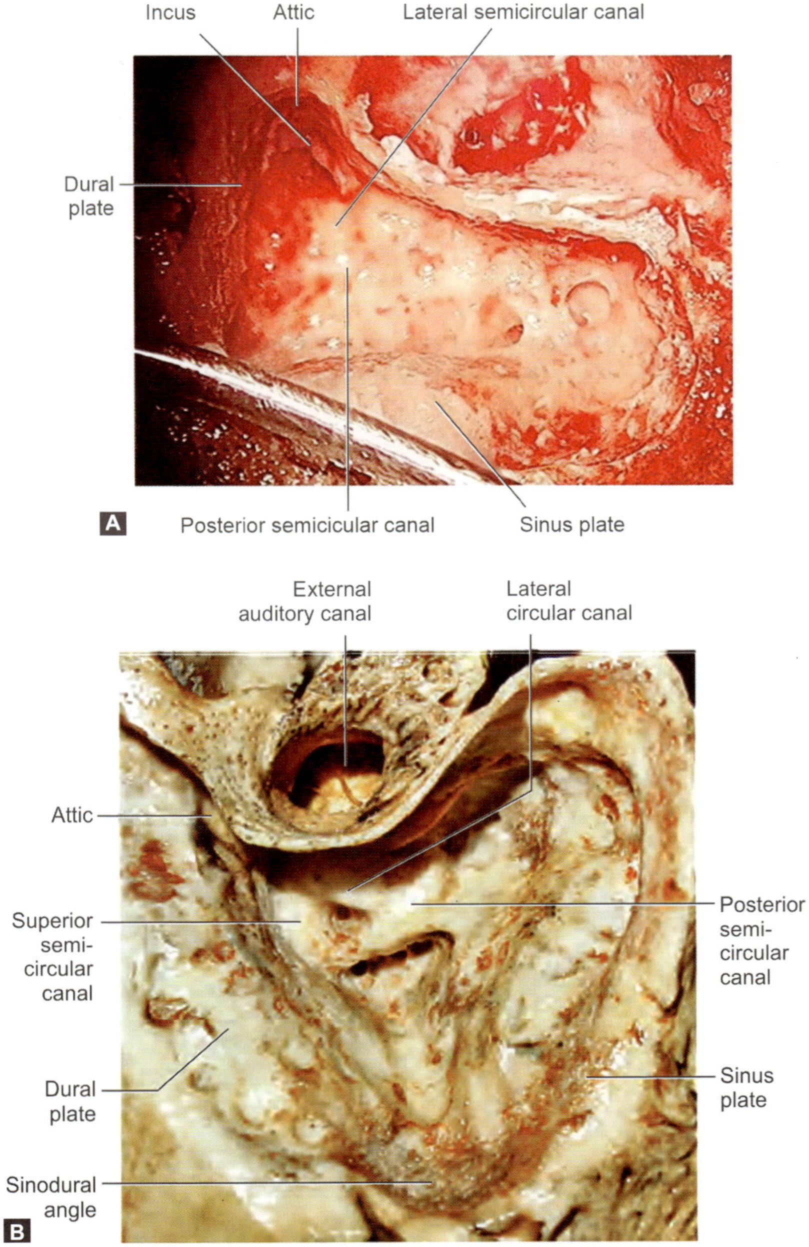

Fig. 4.8: (A) Completed cortical mastoidectomy in live patient and **(B)** in dry cadaveric temporal bone

horizontal canal and the sinodural angle are removed exposing the hard angle/solid angle which are a part of the otic capsule.

At the inferior part of the dissection, the tip of the mastoid can be thinned to expose the periosteum of the digastrics muscle. The periosteum is seen usually as a semilunar shape, turning upwards to blend with the facial nerve sheath at the stylomastoid foramen and thus the facial nerve can be located. Some cells are present in the retrofacial region. The fossa incudis can be easily exposed by removing the bone from the zygomatic root over the antrum. The incus can be exposed. The facial nerve can be located by thinning the posterior canal wall bone and clearing the facial recess which is delineated by the fossa incudis, chorda tympani and the facial nerve in facial recess approach (posterior tympanotomy). A higher grade of magnification of the operating microscope is required here to visualize the region. A cutting burr and good irrigation helps this part of dissection. The facial nerve sheath and blood vessels will show as a white area in the cadaver but pink in the living. Thus the sheath can be followed inferiorly towards the mastoid tip and superiorly and anteriorly into the facial recess. In this way, most of the cells are cleared of the disease and the cortical mastoidectomy is completed.

REFERENCES AND FURTHER READING

1. Bento RF and de Oliveiria Fonseca AC. A brief history of mastoidectomy; *Int Arch Otorhinolaryngol.* 2013 Apr; 17(2): 168–178.
2. Sunder S, Jackler RK, Blevins NH. Virtuosity of the mallet and gouge; The brilliant triumph of the modern mastoid operation; *Otolaryngol Clin North Am.* 2006 Dec;39(6):1191–210.
3. Ralph A Nelson. Temporal bone surgical dissection manual , 2nd revised edition, House Ear Institute,1 983.
4. Glasscock ME, Gulya AJ and Shambaugh GE *Jr. Glascock-Shambaugh Surgery of the ear*, 5th Edition

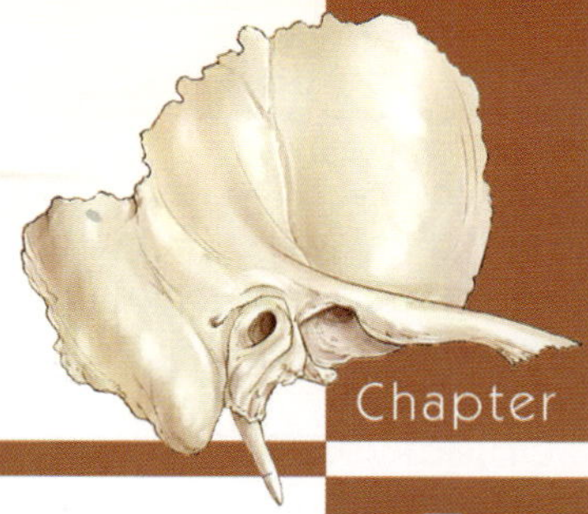

Chapter

5

Modified Radical Mastoidectomy

Dipak Ranjan Nayak • Balakrishnan Ramaswamy • Subrat Behera • Santosh Mishra

Introduction

Modified radical mastoidectomy is one of the most commonly performed procedure for active squamous epithelia type of disease (cholesteatoma). In this procedure the middle ear, attic, aditus and mastoid cavity is converted into a single smooth walled cavity draining through the external auditory canal, while preserving the tympanic membrane, the middle ear mucosa, and the remnant of the stapes. The other ossicles are preserved whenever possible for the purpose of reconstruction of the sound conducting mechanism at a subsequent stage.

Shambaugh and Glasscock advocate repair of the tympanic membrane perforation along with the MRM in the 1st stage and inspection of the cavity for removal of any residual or recurrent disease along with reconstruction of the sound conducting mechanism in the 2nd stage, usually after an interval of 6 months.

Historical Perspective

Worsening of hearing following the radical mastoidectomy lead to the development of modified radical mastoidectomy. Gustave Bondy was credited with improving the procedure that was the precursor of the modified radical mastoidectomy in 1910[1]. Bondy removed the bony external auditory canal up to the attic to facilitate the clearance of the purulent discharge from the attic and antrum. He tried to preserve the pars tensa and the ossicles wherever possible. A meatal skin flap was used to seal the defect between the attic and mesotympanum. When the ossicles were preserved he used this flaps to cover the exposed ossicles. He also developed the criteria for the modified radical mastoidectomy.

Indications

1. Cholesteatoma with chronic or recurrent ear discharge when the cochlear reserve is sufficient for contemplation of future tympanoplasty.
2. In atticoantral disease when the posterior tympanotomy approach is difficult as in small sclerotic mastoids.
3. Cholesteatoma of the attic, antrum or mastoid but not involving the mesotympanum.
4. Surgeons not familiar with the posterior tympanotomy approach.

5. Disease in an only hearing ear.
6. Patients who will not come for regular follow up as and when necessary.
7. Nonreconstructable posterior canal wall.
8. Severe otologic or central nervous system complications.

Objectives

1. To remove safely all bone invading disease;
2. To create an accessible, self cleansing and exteriorized cavity.
3. To promote epithelialization of the cavity with healthy skin.

Procedure

It can be done in two ways.

1. **Outside in approach:** In this approach a standard cortical mastoidectomy is done after which the posterior and superior meatal wall is lowered by drilling to communicate external auditory canal, middle ear cavity, attic, aditus and mastoid into a single cavity. It is a good approach for a well pneumatized mastoid. In case of a primary sclerotic mastoid, this approach is dangerous and can cause injury to sigmid sinus, tegmen plate including dura and lateral semicircular canal. It is still the basic canal wall down mastoid surgery for the postgraduate training.
2. **Inside out approach:** It is suitable for all kind of mastoid and is the preferred approach for endoscopic approach besides microscopic surgery. Needs expertise and can be associated with facial nerve injury in case of distorted landmark following extensive disease. In this approach the drilling is started at the area of pars flacida perforation.

Outside in Approach

After completion of a good cortical mastoidectomy as described earlier an epitympanotomy (atticotomy) is done as follows (Fig. 5.1):

1. Preserving the Canal Skin

This is done by elevating the posterior and superior canal skin along with the posterior annulus and reflecting it anteriorly, to prevent any injury from the burrs.

A pedicle skin flap may be fashioned just as in myringoplasty by incising along the tympanomastoid and tympanosquamous suture lines from near the annulus outwards to the bony cartilaginous junction. A circular incision near and parallel to the annulus connects the above incisions. The flap is reflected out and anteriorly in the canal wall retractor. This pedicle flap is later used to cover the facial ridge and the floor of the operated mastoid cavity.

2. Atticotomy (Epitympanotomy)

After a completion of cortical mastoidectomy, a cutting burr 2–3 mm in diameter is used with a within outwards motion, so as to not injure any underlying structures. Bone is removed in a triangular area above and behind the meatus as shown in Fig. 5.1, whose boundaries are superiorly, a line along the suprameatal crest, inferiorly, a line along the Posterosuperior canal wall and the apex points towards the zygoma.

The depth at which the attic is reached is just lateral to the notch of Rivinus. The bone removal is carried forwards above the meatus into the aditus and attic, thus exposing

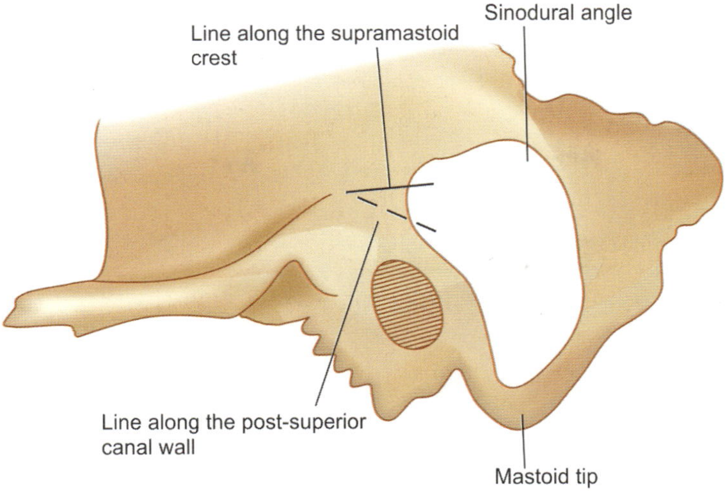

Fig. 5.1: Extent of epitympanotomy after a complete cortical mastoidectomy

the body and short process of incus in the fossa incudis. Further anteriorly, the incudo-malleolar joint and the head of the malleus are seen.

The anterior limit of dissection is the junction of the anterior bony meatal wall and the tegmen. The surgeon should be careful not to injure the middle cranial fossa dura.

If the cholesteatoma extends medial to the ossicles or envelops them, then the incus and the head of malleus should be removed. Usually it is necessary to remove the incus even though it is intact to reach the remaining cholesteatoma. Even if the head of the malleus can be preserved, there is little point in doing so unless there is a wide clearance from the walls of the epitympanum, for it frequently becomes ankylosed to the walls later and prevents free movement of the tympanic membrane—a deterrent to successful reconstruction of a functioning ossicular chain (Figs 5.2 and 5.3).

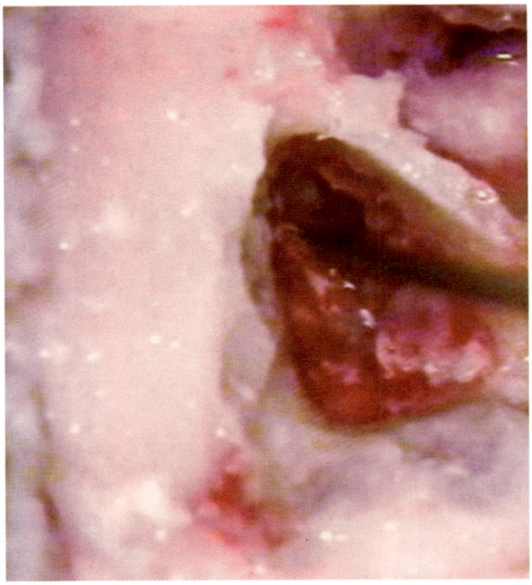

Fig. 5.2: Cortical mastoidectomy with epitympanotomy in progress

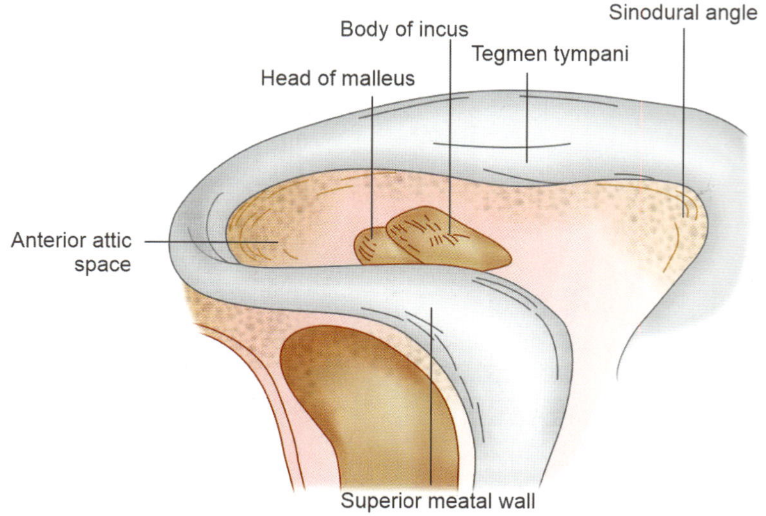

Fig. 5.3: Exposure of malleoincudal joint after epitympanotomy

3. *Removal of the Bridge* *(Figs 5.4 and 5.5)*

The bridge is that portion of the posterosuperior canal wall which overlies the ossicles and bridges across the notch of Rivinus. This is removed with a cutting burr initially (Fig. 5.5) and a diamond burr later. A curette may also be used for the last part, always working outwards and away from the fallopian canal.

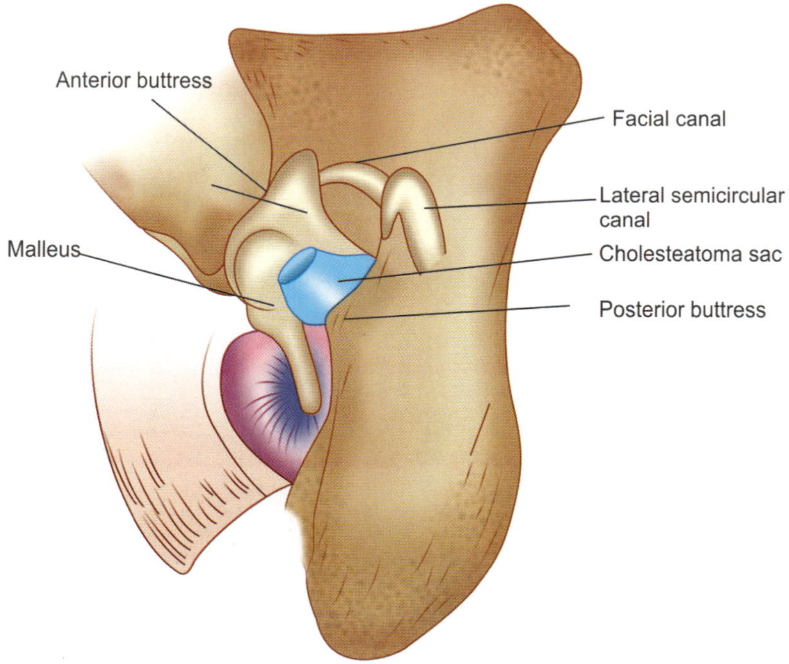

Fig. 5.4: Middle ear structures seen after removal of the bridge

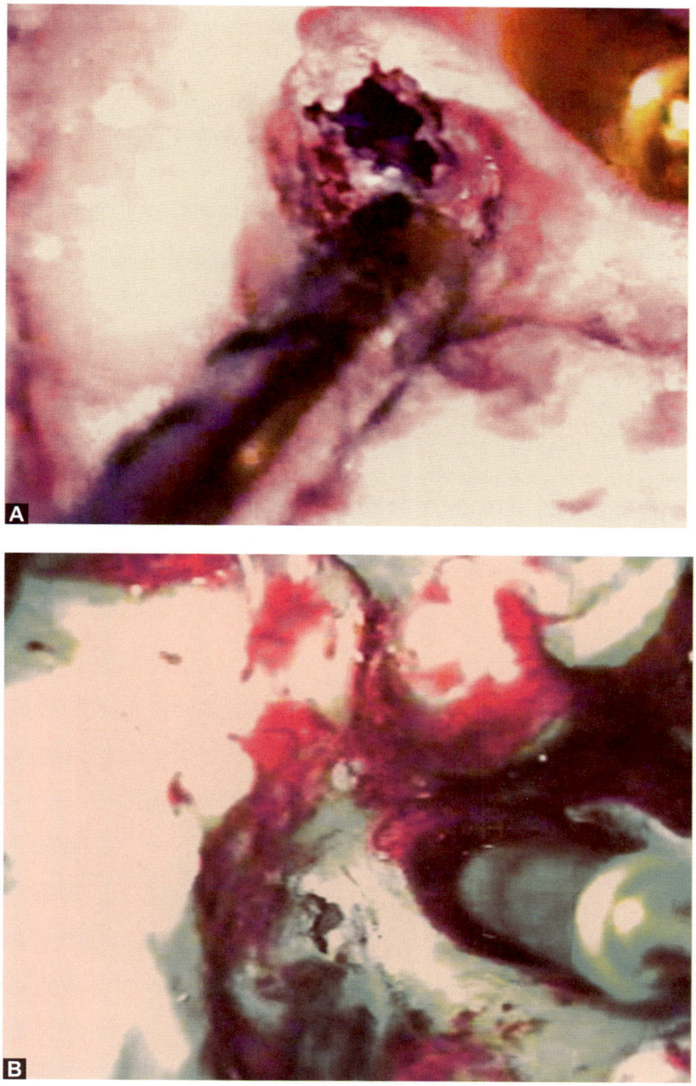

Fig. 5.5: Lowering of facial ridge (A) and removal of facial bridge (B) in the right temporal bone

4. Removal of Anterior Buttress *(Figs 5.6 and 5.7)*

The anterior buttress is that bone where the posterior bony canal wall meets the tegmen.

A diamond burr or curette is used in a within-outwards motion always working away from the facial canal. Once the anterior buttress is removed totally, there will be a smooth curve from the middle fossa tegmen to the middle ear epitympanic tegmen to the anterior wall of the external auditory canal (Fig. 5.8).

5. Removal of Posterior Buttress *(Figs 5.8 and 5.9)*

The posterior buttress is where the posterior canal wall meets the floor of the external auditory canal lateral to the facial nerve. This is best removed by lowering the facial ridge

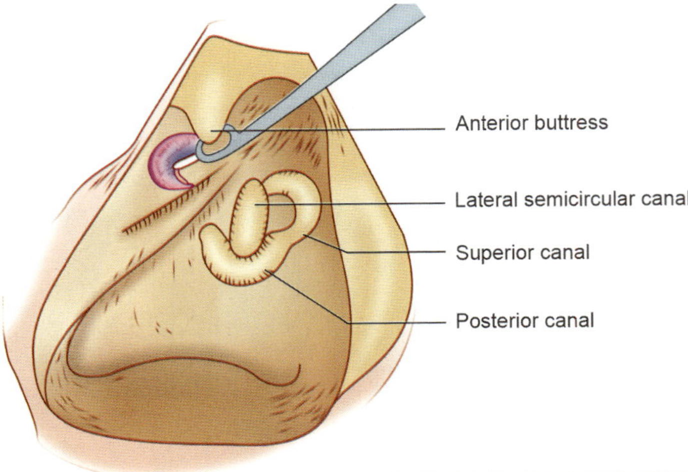

Fig. 5.6: Removal of anterior buttress after removal of facial bridge

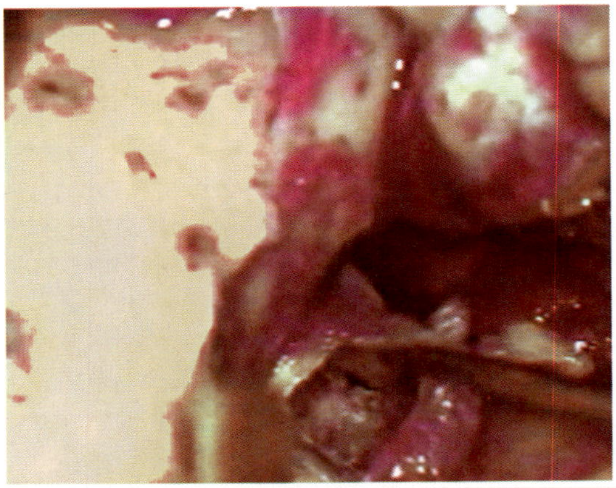

Fig. 5.7: Anterior buttress before removal

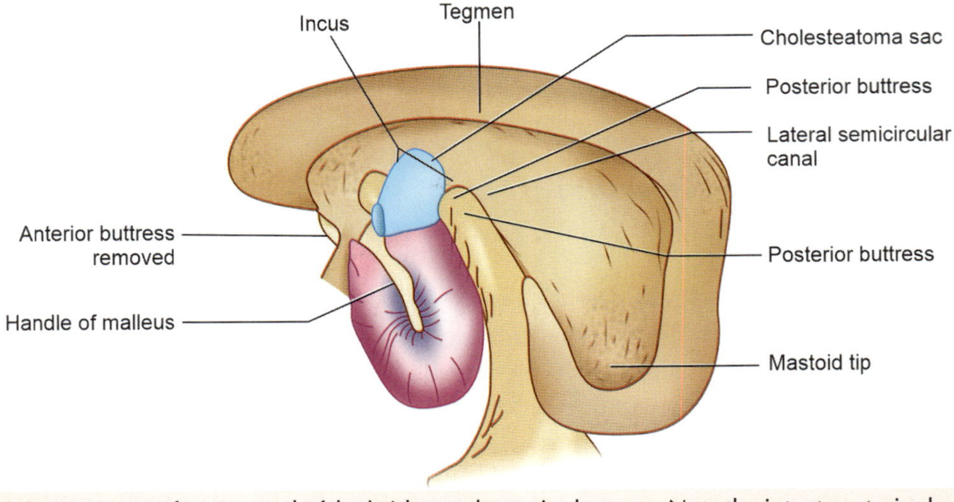

Fig. 5.8: Structures after removal of the bridge and anterior buttress. Note the intact posterior buttress that needs to be removed with a curette

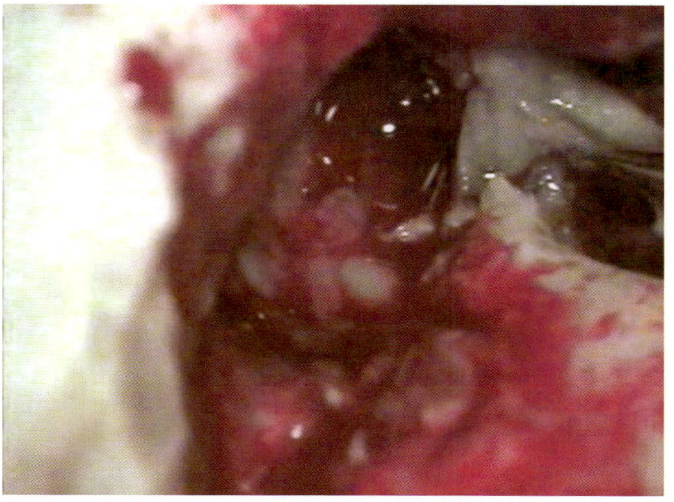

Fig. 5.9: Posterior buttress before removal

by skeletonizing the facial nerve laterally. A diamond burr or fine curette is used in a within-outwards motion. Then, the EAC will slope off gently into the mastoid tip.

If the posterior buttress is left behind, it will result in a deep 'Blind Pocket' at the mastoid tip. The facial nerve will be seen as a whiter strip of bone running above oval window. This serves as a valuable landmark for the next step (Fig. 5.9).

6. Removal of Incus and Head of Malleus

After the removal of the incus by carefully disarticulating the incudostapedial joint, the head of the malleus is removed by using a malleus nipper at the neck of the malleus. In extensive disease, the cholesteatoma might have eroded the stapes suprastructure and handle of malleus. In such cases the disease should be cleared completely from the foot plate in addition to removal of malleus and incus and excenteration of all the diseased cells by a diamond burr. A TORP or cartilage graft from the septal spur can be used for reconstruction. After which, the temporalis fascia can be used for tympanic membrane repair as described under the chapter tympanoplasty (Fig. 5.10).

7. Lowering the Facial Ridge

It is that part of the posterior bony meatal wall, which houses the posterior bend and vertical facial nerve, is called the facial ridge. All bones lateral to the facial nerve between the tegmen and the floor of the EAC is removed, thus eliminating the posterior bony canal wall. Lowering of ridge is done up to the level of the floor of the EAC in the horizontal plane and up to the level of the fallopian canal or annulus in the vertical plane.

This step is done slowly with a drill with a larger burr, stroke by stroke with feather touch and always working parallel to the facial nerve along its course from lateral semicircular canal to the diagastric ridge. Irrigation is very important to prevent thermal damage to the facial nerve and should be done profusely while drilling near the facial nerve.

A pinkish line and bleeding are encountered when the facial nerve is exposed. The facial nerve should not be unnecessarily exposed, as it can lead to a Bell's type of paresis. The lowering of the facial ridge widely exposes the upper part of the facial recess, fully

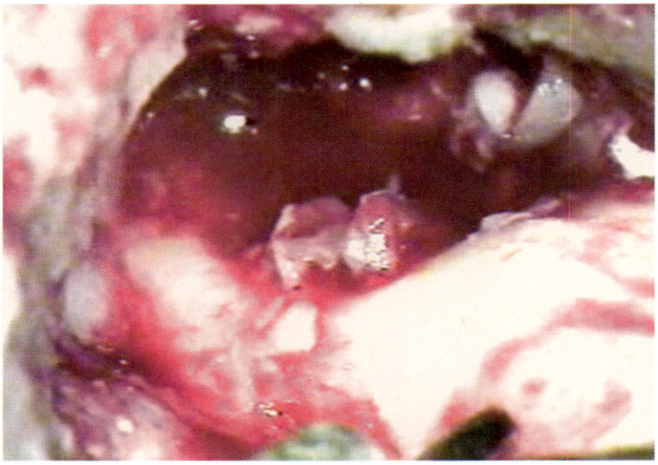

Fig. 5.10: Mastoid cavity with stapedial remnant after removal of cholesteatoma before final clearance. Note the facial ridge has been lowered as described in inside out approach

exposes the pyramid, stapes and chorda tympani. The landmarks which indicate the approximate position of the facial nerve are the bony horizontal semicircular canal, the tympanomastoid suture in the posterior meatal wall, the short process of incus and the digastrics ridge in the mastoid tip.

8. Saucerization of the Mastoid Bowl (Fig. 5.11)

The mastoid cavity should be well saucerized, which allows the soft tissues to obliterate better and shrink the remaining open cavity. Smooth surfaces also allow faster epithelialization of the postoperative mastoid cavity.

In a sclerotic mastoid, the floor of the external auditory canal will be at the same level as the floor of the mastoid cavity, thus allowing dependant drainage from the meatus.

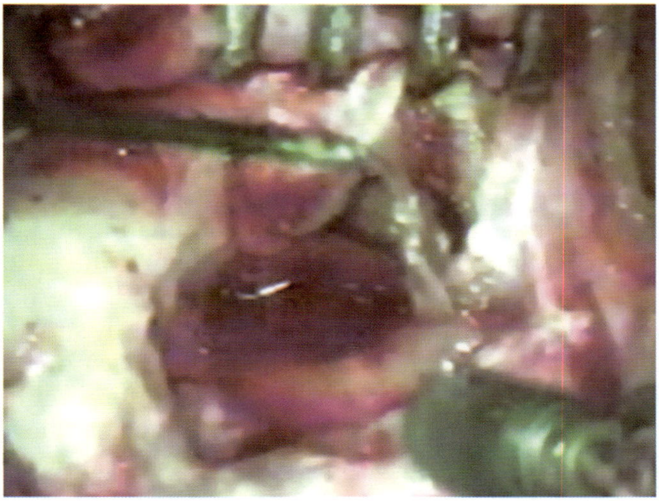

Fig. 5.11: Mastoid is being saucerized using a large conical burr

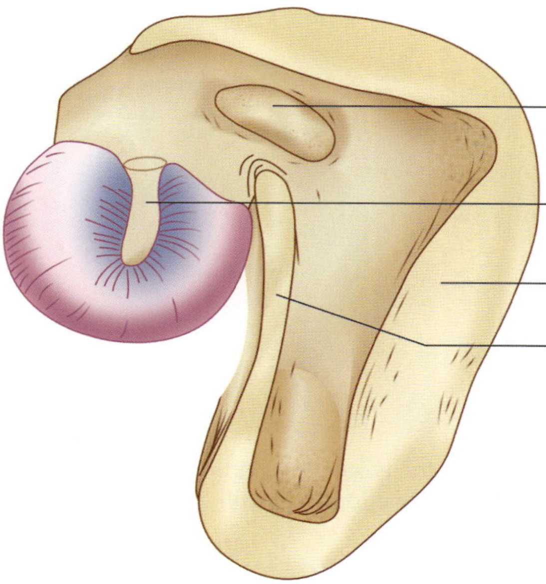

Fig. 5.12: Complete modified radical mastoidectomy (outside in approach)

In a pneumatized mastoid with a well developed tip, it is necessary to remove the mastoid tip lateral to the digastric ridge and the floor of the external auditory canal lateral to the facial nerve. This allows the sternocleidomastoid muscle and soft tissues from the neck to collapse into cavity, thus reducing its size.

Now the completed mastoid cavity (Fig. 5.12) is irrigated with warm saline for hemostasis and for removing any bone particles or other debris. Under the operating microscope, the cavity is inspected minutely for any remaining osteitis or cholesteatoma.

9. Placement of the Meatal Flap

The flap of meatal skin is turned back to cover the facial ridge and floor of mastoid cavity.

10. Adequate Soft Tissues Meatoplasty

This is done by excising conchal cartilage after raising a posterior canal skin flap, to allow better aeration of the mastoid cavity and easy visualization of the entire cavity to facilitate postoperative care and self cleaning. Many techniques are described:

1. Korner's
2. Fisch's
3. Yanagisawa's
4. Sieberman's
5. Portmann's

Inside Out Approach

Epitympanotomy (Fig. 5.13)

The bony external auditory meatus is gradually widened starting from the region of outer attic wall towards outer external auditory canal and isthmus and spine of Henle. This allows a wider exposure for easy drilling directly under vision while straightening the

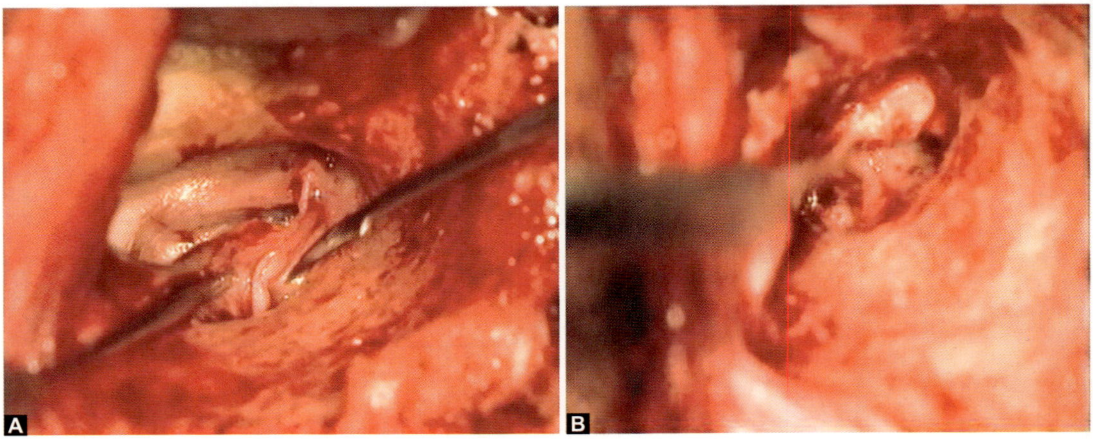

Fig. 5.13: (A) Exposed cholesteatoma sac in the posterior superior quadrant, also note the chorda tympani nerve and **(B)** exposure of attic and posterior canal wall and middle ear before inside out mastoidectomy

external auditory meatus. Then the outer attic wall is removed with a 2–3 mm burr to thin out the outer attic wall which is then removed with a small curette from inside outward to expose the cholesteatoma sac close to the tegmen tympani superiorly. Bone is drilled anteriorly till the extent of cholesteatoma. While drilling one should avoid touching the ossicular chain to prevent sensorineural hearing loss.

Epitympanomastoidectomy *(Fig. 5.14)*

A 4–5 mm burr is used in a circular motion posteriorly to uncap the bone overlying the incus, while exposing the posterior limit of the cholesteatoma. The incus is an important landmark that stays lateral to the facial nerve and helps to stay away from the facial nerve while exteriorizing the cholesteatoma. If the incus is eroded, the facial canal is identified and stapes remnant is visualized by lifting the epitympanic part of the cholesteatoma and the bone is removed within outward, away from the facial. The posterior canal wall is lowered further after knowing its position. If the cholesteatoma is extended posteriorly, the bone is further drilled along the remaining lateral attic wall and curette is used to remove the overlying bone away from the facial nerve. This allows the exposure of aditus and the lateral semicircular canal.

Removal of Disease *(Fig. 5.15)*

The cholesteatoma sac is exteriorized completely. A small cotton ball is used to dissect out the cholesteatoma from the underlying structure and removed in its entirety. In case of cholesteatoma is extensive and involves the middle ear and sinus tympani, further clearance is done as described under outside in approach.

Reconstruction *(Figs 5.16 and 5.17)*

After the disease is removed completely along with incus, which is frequently involved, suitable reconstruction is done by using cartilage, TORP/PORP as described under tympanoplasty. The senior author (DRN), uses grommet as PORP in the reconstruction of ossicular chain.

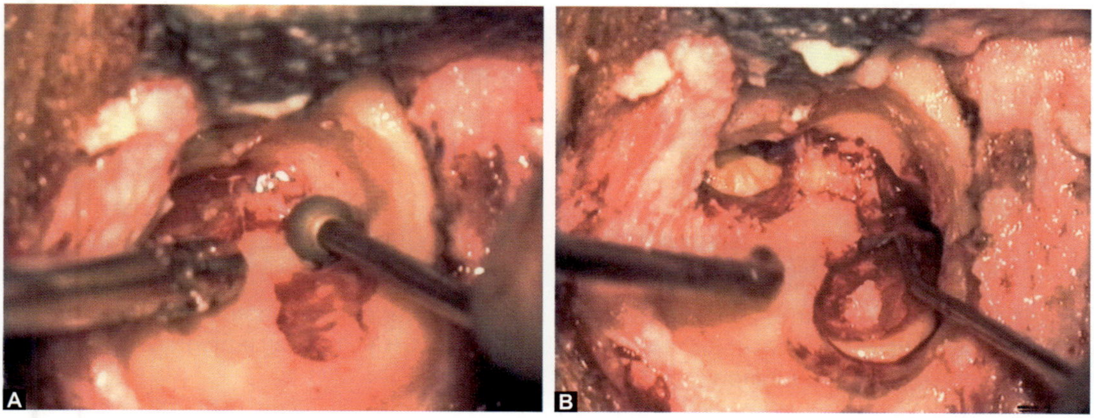

Fig. 5.14: (A) Inside out mastoidectomy with removal of facial bridge in progress and **(B)** after facial bridge is removed with exposure of anterior and posterior buttress

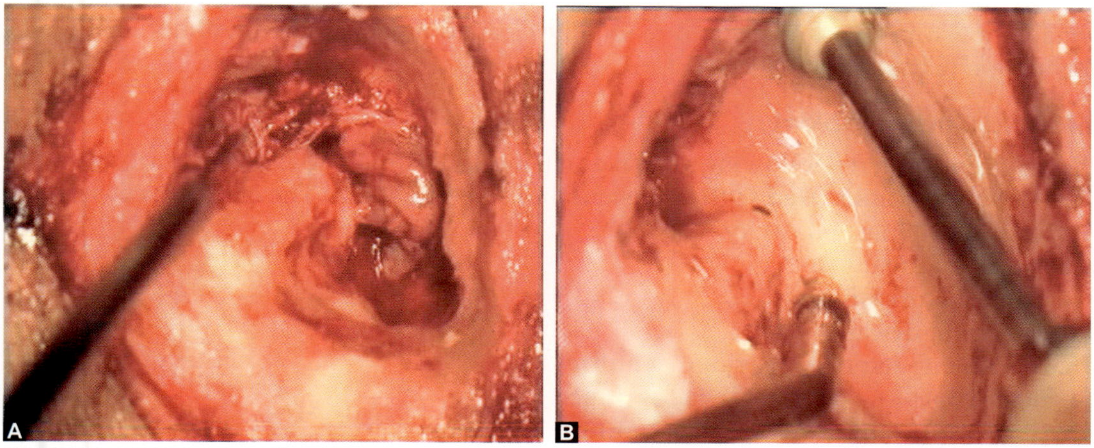

Fig. 5.15: (A) exposure of cholesteatoma sac in the region of aditus after removal of anterior buttress and **(B)** complete removal of anterior and posterior buttress and clearance of cholesteatoma

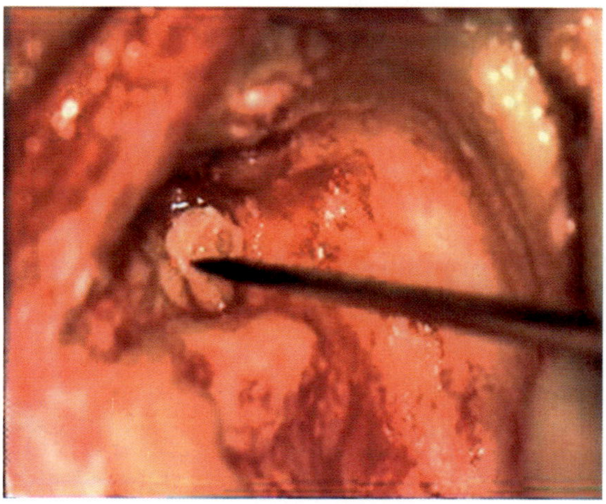

Fig. 5.16: Cartilage is used as a TORP

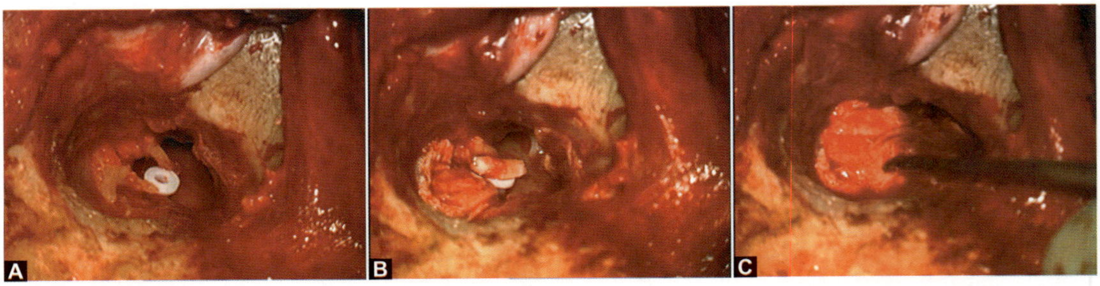

Fig. 5.17: Reconstruction of attic and ossicular chain, **(A)** after epitympanotomy with grommet, **(B)** conchal cartilage used cover the grommet and attic defect, **(C)** Underlay temporalis fascia graft is placed to cover the perforation

Meatoplasty

Meatoplasty is performed as the end stage of a canal wall down mastoidectomy to provide adequate enlargement of the external auditory meatus that leaves the patient with a smaller mastoid recess that could readily be cleaned and examined without anatomical restriction (Choi et al, 2009).

Mastoid Cavity Problem

Problem encountered following a canal down mastoid surgery that does not achieve a dry ear and may be associated with persistent foul smelling drain. The common causes are:

1. Too large a mastoid cavity
2. Improper meatoplasty
3. Residual disease
4. Recurrent disease
5. Inadequate removal of bridge or buttress
6. Inadequate lowering of the facial ridge
7. Lining by respiratory mucus-secreting epithelium

Complications of Modified Radical Mastoidectomy

1. Intraoperative

1. Bleeding from dural vessels, sigmoid sinus, middle ear or facial nerve
2. Facial nerve injury: Identifying the nerve is the safest way of avoiding injury into it
3. Labyrinthine injury: Should be sealed with fascia and bone dust immediately to preserve residual function.

2. Postoperative

1. Mucous or chocolate cyst
2. Cholesteatoma (recurrent and residual)
3. Persistent otorrhea

3. Late

1. Stenosis of mastoid cavity (neo-osteogenesis)
2. Meatal stenosis and closure
3. Postauricular depression
4. Mastoid-cutaneous fistula

REFERENCES AND FURTHER READING

1. Heath C. The restoration of hearing after removal of the drum and ossicles by a modification of the radical mastoid operation for suppurative ear disease. *Lancet*. 1904;164:1767–9.
2. Pappas D G. Bondy's modified radical mastoidectomy revisited. *Ear Nose Throat J*. 1994;73(1):15–8.
3. House WF. The Struggles of a Medical Innovator: Cochlear Implants and Other Ear Surgeries [place unknown] CreateSpace; 2011. 208 p.
4. Surgery of the Ear, 4th edition, Glasscock and Shambaugh. Chapter 10: The Open Cavity mastoid Operations.
5. Choi IJ, Song JJ, Jang JH, Chang SO. A novel meatoplasty method in canal wall down tympanomastoidectomy: a perichondrial posterior fixation technique. *Clin Exp Otorhinolaryngol*. 2009;2(4):164–8.
6. Sculerati N, Bluestone CD, Pathogenesis of cholesteatoma. *Otolaryngological Clinics of North America*. Volume 22, No. 5, October 1989.
7. Lee K J, Editor, *Surgical Atlas of Otology and Neuro-otology*. 1983 edition. pgs 229–260
8. Manual of Temporal Bone Dissection. Nelson, House Ear Institute. Pg.86-89.
9. Learning ear surgery by temporal bone dissection. Prof. K. K. Ramalingam
10. Atlas of Ear Surgery. 4th edition 1986, Miglets, Paparella, Saunders. Pg.194-201
11. Diseases of the Nose, Throat, Ear, Head and Neck. John Jacob Ballenger. 14th edition 1991. Chapter 55: Surgery in Chronic Ear Disease.
12. Kinney SE. The problem mastoid cavity-Medical and Surgical Management. Laryngoscope, 1977; 87(11):1853–60.

Chapter

6

Radical Mastoidectomy

Kailesh Pujary • P Satyanarayan Murthy • Dipak Ranjan Nayak

Introduction

Radical mastoidectomy is not very popular in modern days because of the non-feasibility of future reconstruction of the middle ear and is reserved for skull base osteomyelitis, neoplasm unresectable cholesteatoma, etc.

Radical mastoidectomy is an operation performed to eradicate middle ear and mastoid disease in which, mastoid antrum, tympanum and external auditory canal are converted into a common cavity exteriorized through the external auditory meatus (this operation involves removal of all the structures excepting the foot plate of the stapes and does not involve any reconstructing or grafting procedure)—Sheehy, 1988.

Historical perspective: The radical surgery of the mastoid was evolved 1880s to tackle intracranial complications. Ernst Küster (1988) and von Bergmann (1889) were, both general surgeon, credited with developing the radical surgery, by converting the spaces of the attic, antrum, and middle ear into a single large cavity (Bento et al, 2013). Zaufal (1890) improved this technique by dissecting from antrum to attic and suggested removal of posterior meatal wall following simple mastoidectomy. These exposures were followed by complete clearance of the middle ear structures, including the drum, and the fashioning of meatal flaps to improve access to the residual cavity which was to be lined with skin growing from the raw edges of these flaps. Zaufal advocated closure of postauricular wound. Thiersch grafts to the walls of the cavity followed in the 1890s.

Indications for Radical Mastoidectomy

1. Unresectable cholesteatoma extending to eustachian tube.
2. Promontory cochlear fistula due to cholesteatoma
3. Chronic perilabyrinthine osteitis or cholesteatoma that cannot be removed and must be cleaned and inspected periodically
4. Carcinoma of external auditory meatus and middle ear
5. Childhood necrotizing acute otitis media leading onto secondary acquired cholesteatoma.

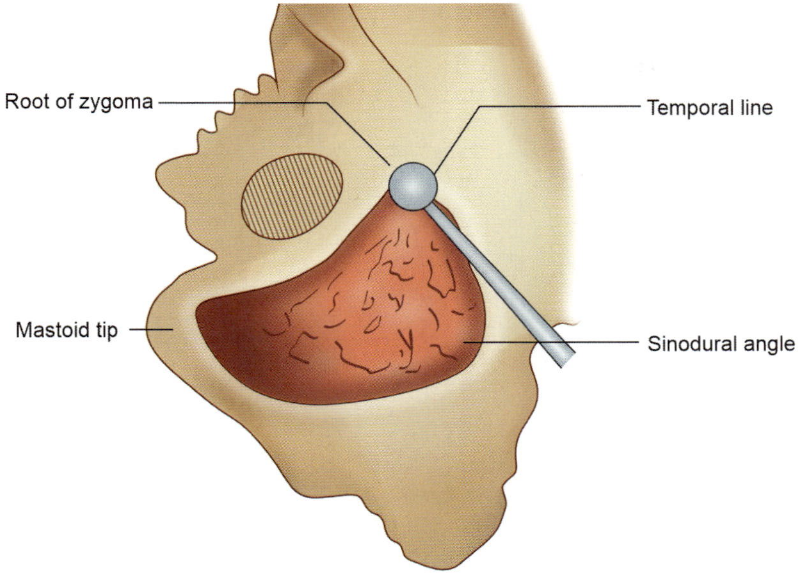

Fig. 6.1: Completed cortical mastoidectomy

Steps of Radical Mastoidectomy

1. Exposure of the mastoid area
2. Identification of mastoid antrum and completion of basic mastoidectomy (Schwartz or cortical mastoidectomy)
3. **Atticotomy:** Outer attic wall is removed and atticotomy is completed, using a small cutting burr, as described earlier.
4. **Canal wall down:** This is done as in case of a modified radical mastoidectomy taking care that the facial ridge is adequately lowered along the line of the facial canal. Lowering of the facial ridge is done by working along the axis of the facial canal (vertical segment) until the pyramidal process is exposed. All the disease along the facial recess area can be cleared once this step is completed.

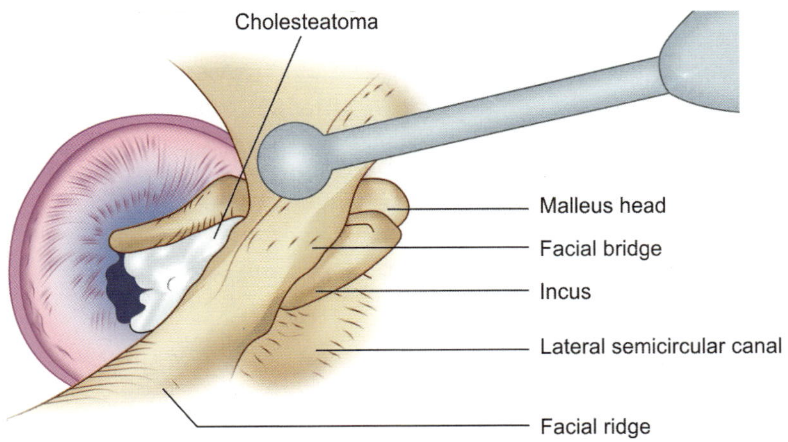

Fig. 6.2: Lowered facial ridge and removal of facial bridge

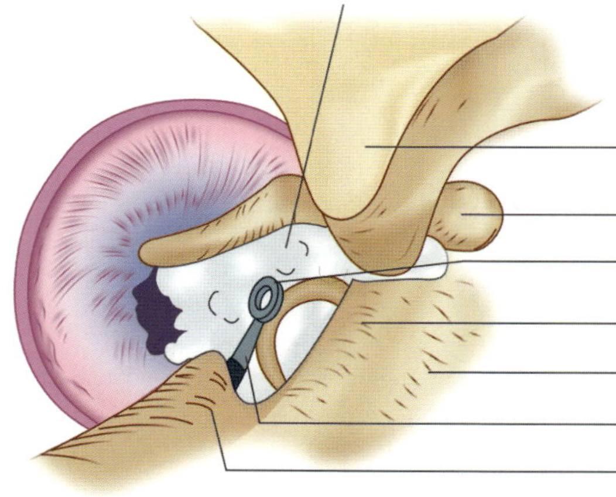

Fig. 6.3: Structures seen after removal of facial bridge and incus.

Meticulous clearance of cholesteatoma/disease from the sinus tympani may require removal of pyramid and bone anterior to the facial nerve, using of the diamond burr.

5. **Removal of middle ear contents:** This step marks the essential difference between radical mastoidectomy and modified radical mastoidectomy (in which healthy middle ear contents are preserved).

   Under magnification, following steps are done:

   i. The incudostapedial joint is separated
   ii. The tensor tympani muscle is cut just medial to malleus and it is pulled out from its semicircular canal
   iii. The cochleariform process is fractured and removed.
   iv. Ossicular chain is mobilized from attic space and they are removed using an alligator forceps. The stapes footplate is retained, if possible with its suprastructure (Fig. 6.5).

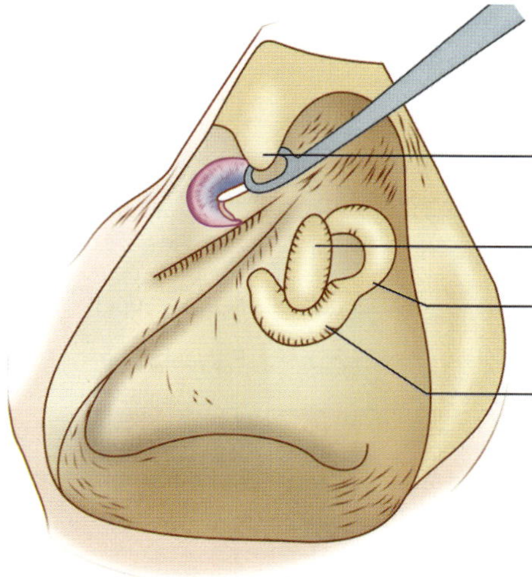

Fig. 6.4: Removal of anterior buttress. Note posterior buttress is already removed

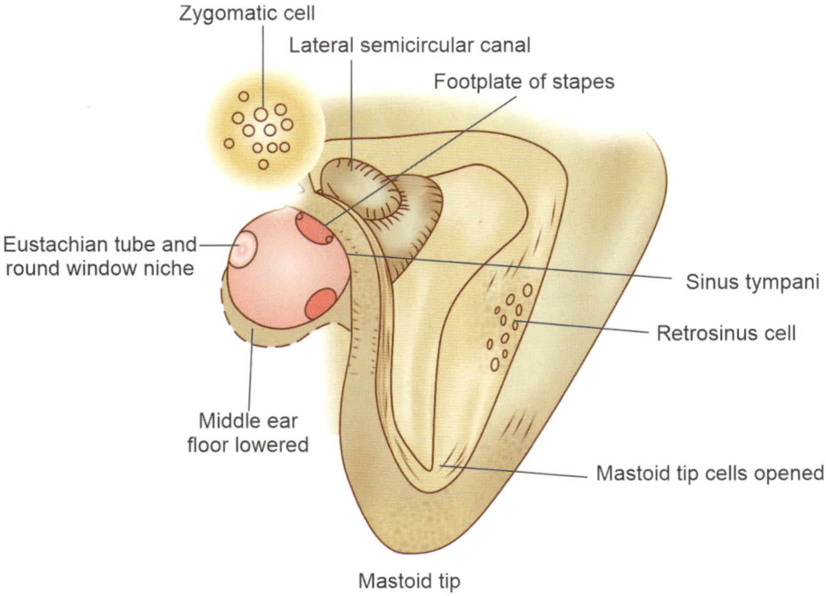

Fig. 6.5: Completed radical mastoidectomy

v. The tympanic membrane (with annulus) and all mucoperiosteal lining of the cavity are removed using a microelevator and cup forceps.

vi. The external auditory canal and the floor of hypotympanum is made level by removing the inferior bony annulus.

vii. Mucosa over the eustachian tubal orifices is curetted out and an attempt is made to seal the opening of eustachian tube by septal cartilage, ossicles, bone chips, muscle or fascia. This is to prevent future in growth of mucosa to middle ear space.

6. **Polishing (smoothening) of the cavity:** A large polishing burr is usually used for this purpose. This is done to avoid any pockets retaining pus or debris.

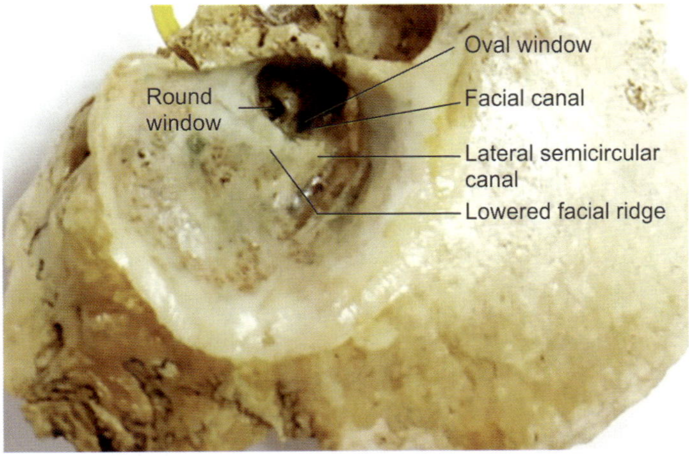

Fig. 6.6: Completed radical mastoidectomy in a cadaveric temporal bone

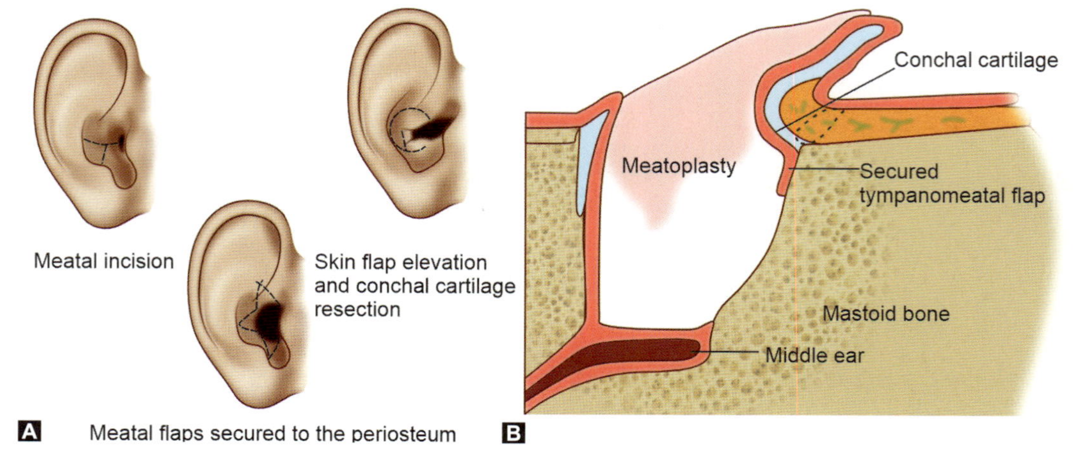

Fig. 6.7: (A) Steps of meatoplasty **(B)** after meatoplasty is completed

7. **Soft tissue meatoplasty/cavity obliteration:** These procedures may be needed during live operations as described under modified radical mastoidectomy. The size of the meatoplasty plays a crucial role in healing of mastoid bowl, where a large meatoplasty reduces its lateral surface, there by reduces the mastoid cavity besides giving easy access to mastoid bowl (Weiss et al, 1992).
8. Wound closure is done in layers—in live operation.

REFERENCES

1. Sheehy JL. Cholesteatoma surgery—Canal wall down procedure. *Ann Otol Rhinol Laryngol*, 1988; 97(1):30–5.
2. Syms CA, Syms MJ, Sheehy JL. Mastoidectomy—Intact Canal Wall Procedure. Brackmann DE, Shelton C, Arriaga MA eds. *Otologic Surgery*. 3. Saunders Elsevier; 2010. chap 16.
3. Sheehy J. Brackman DE, Graham MD. Cholesteatom surgery—Residual and Recurrence. Ann Otol Rhinol Laryngol, 1977; 86: 451–462
4. *Kuester, E.*: *On* the *principles of* the *treatment* of *suppuration* in *rigid-walled caves. German.Med. Wschr., 13: 254–257, 1889*
5. Von Bergmann E. Berl klin Wchnschr. 1888;36:1054.
6. Bento RF and de Oliveiria Fonseca AC. A brief history of mastoidectomy; Int Arch Otorhinolaryngol. 2013 Apr; 17(2): 168–178
7. Zaufal E. Technik der Trepanation des Proc. Mastoid. Nach Kuster'schen Grundsatzen. Arch Ohrenheilkd. 1890;30:291.
8. Cumming's Textbook of Otorhinolaryngology and Head and Neck Surgery, 2nd edition
9. Surgery of the Ear. Glasscock and Shambaugh. Chapter 10-Open cavity Mastoidectomy. 4th edition
10. Mawson's diseases of the ear, 5th edition. Chapter 18, Otitis Media
11. Learning Ear Surgery by Temporal Bone Dissection—KK Ramalingam
12. Weiss, *et al*. Surgery for recurrent and residual cholesteatoma. Laryngoscope 1992; 102:145–151.

Chapter 7

Combined Approach Tympanoplasty

Dipak Ranjan Nayak • Produl Hazarika • Asheesh Dora • Apoorva N Reddy

The eradication of disease and hearing restoration in most of the CSOM. Cases can be satisfactorily done by transmeatal or the transmastoid approach to the middle ear cavity. But in some cases, the disease because of its extent and activity is unable to be cleared out by these usual approaches and poses technical problems. It is here some surgeons resort to a more adventurous and difficult technique of combining the transmeatal and transmastoid routes known commonly as 'combined approach tympanoplasty' or canal up tympanoplasty and avoids the otherwise inevitable open cavity.

Historical Perspective

William House introduced access to the facial recess (posterior tympanotomy), by removing bone between the chorda tympani nerve and the facial, which led to tympano-ossicular reconstructions with mastoidectomy (the so-called closed-cavity mastoidectomy or tympanomastoidectomy or combined approach mastoidectomy) as well as the use of traditional mastoidectomy for the treatment of chronic suppurative and cholesteatomatous otitis (Bento and Fonseka, 2013). This lead to a revolution in mastoid surgery and tympano-ossicular reconstruction. This was subsequently developed and promoted by Sheey (1967), Jansen(1968). Combined approach tympanoplasty (CAT) aims at eliminating the disease with preservation of the bony meatal wall thus avoiding an exteriorized mastoid cavity, and reconstruction of a drum in the normal anatomical position.

The objectives of CAT are:

1. Production of a safe ear.
2. Production of a dry ear.
3. Production of a lasting hearing improvement.

CAT broadly consists of:

1. Simple mastoidectomy
2. Posterior tympanotomy
3. Anterior tympanotomy
4. Tympanoplasty

Simple mastoidectomy is done (Figs 7.1 and 7.2) by the postaural route, diseases if any are cleared, and sufficient room is made for subsequent instrumentation.

Posterior tympanotomy is the major and difficult part. It consists of opening the Facial Recess from its mastoid aspect and extending the exposure inferiorly to permit whatever access is necessary to the hypotympanum for the removal of diseased tissues. Anteriorly tympanotomy is done by the usual transmeatal approach, raising the tympanomeatal flap.

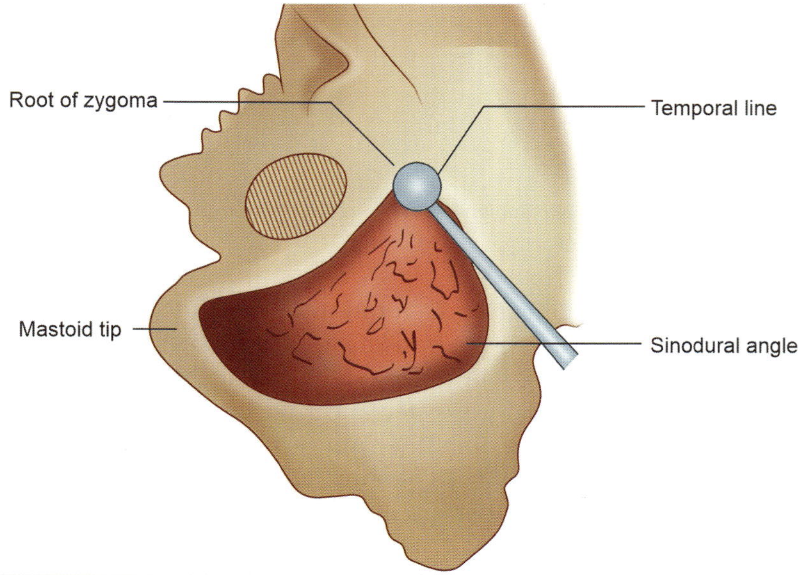

Fig. 7.1: Simple cortical mastoidectomy in progress

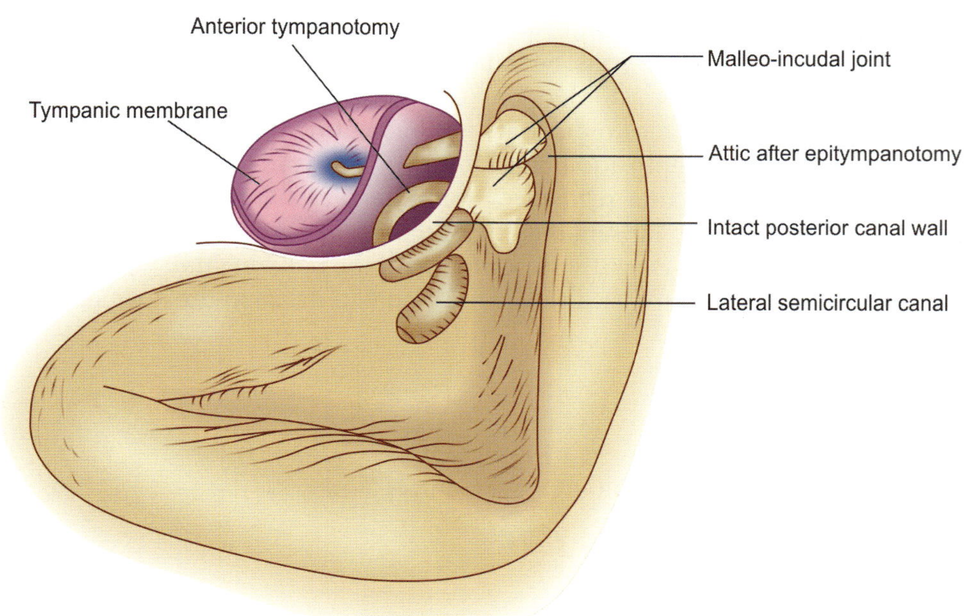

Fig. 7.2: Completed cortical mastoidectomy with epitympanotomy and anterior tympanotomy

Facial Recess Anatomy (Figs 7.3 and 7.4)

Facial recess is a collection of air cells in the posterior wall of the middle ear. It extends backwards and upwards in a conical fashion from the postsuperior quadrant of the mesotympanum. Laterally it is limited by the chorda tympani and the posterior superior quadrant of the annulus and medially the external genu of the upper descending part of the facial nerve. At the base of the conical space, lie the long process of the incus, the posterior crus of the stapes, the stapedius tendon and the pyramid. The apex of the recess extends into the bone deep to and below the fossa incudis for a varying distance. These form the landmark for the dissection.

To trace the facial nerve, trace digastrics ridge anteriorly to the stylomastoid foramen then trace up along the posterior end of horizontal semicircular canal on the posterior meatal wall. The nerve lies on the latter part.

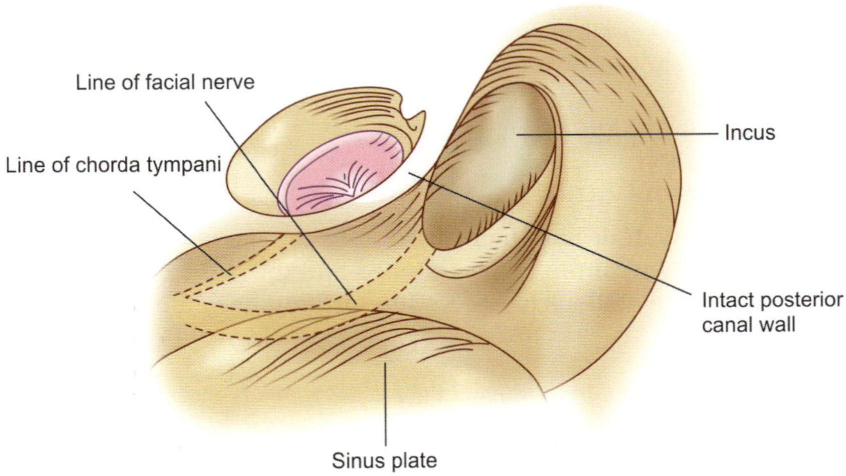

Fig. 7.3: Chorda-facial angle between the line of facial nerve and chorda tympani nerve

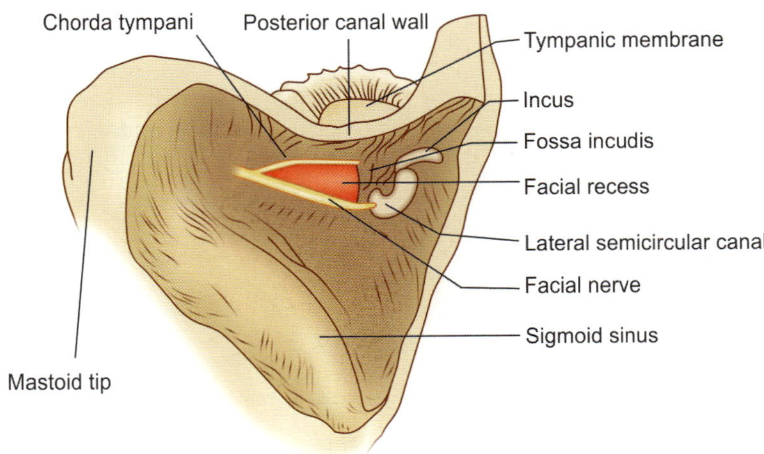

Fig. 7.4: Facial recess to open for posterior tympanotomy

Indications for CAT (Posterior Tympanotomy)

1. When trans canal technique cannot visualize the diseased areas completely.
2. Posterior superior quadrant retraction pocketing in to the facial recess and aditus.
3. Facial nerve decompression
4. An extended facial recess approach in the exposure of glomus tympanicum tumors, supralabrynthine tumors.
5. Route for insertion of cochlear implant
6. All cases of cholesterol granuloma

CAT is considered in a diploic/pneumatic bone in a reliable patient.

Contraindications

1. The only hearing ear—CAT is absolutely contraindicated as a means of treating dangerous disease.
2. Situations where preservation of canal wall prevents complete visualization of areas in which there was cholesteatoma.
3. Malignant tumors.
4. Intra cranial complications

1. Simple Mastoidectomy (Fig 7.2)

A simple mastoidectomy done and the mastoid cells are cleared of diseased mucosa and cholesteatoma. The epitympanum is then opened and the short process and body of the incus and the head of the malleus is exposed by drilling in to the root of the zygoma in an anterior direction.

2. Posterior Tympanotomy (Figs 7.4 and 7.5)

Now the posterior canal wall is thinned out superiorly and posteriorly from the cavity side. This thinning is done very meticulously following the canal wall contour.

There should not be any perforation or button holing of the canal wall. The thinning should be of very finite detail that some describe it as 'shell thin' or 'papery thin' enough to see the shadow of an instrument through it.

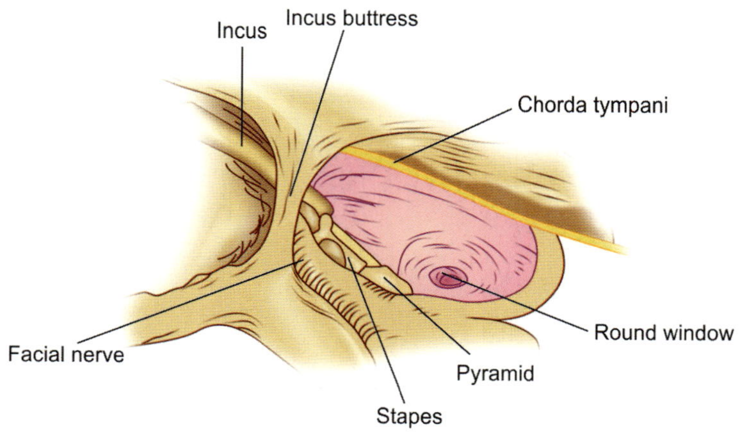

Fig. 7.5: Structures seen after posterior tympanotomy

The magnification of the microscope is changed from 6 to 10 and the facial recess area is properly focused. The landmarks here are the short process of the incus and the fossa incudis. A 2.5 mm burr is used and the bone lateral to the fossa incudis is removed as a trough. The direction of motion of the burr should be in an anteroinferior and medial direction. In case the ossicular chain is intact, care is taken not to allow the cutting burr come in contact with the incus, since sufficient acoustic energy may be transmitted to cause damage to cochlear function. A small buttress of bone is preserved between the short process of the incus and the facial recess to avoid this disruption of the ligaments to the short process of the incus and dislocation of the incudostapedial joint. If an intact incus makes the dissection difficult it should be removed.

Initially the trough should be about 2 mm wide and 2/3 rd of its width lies lateral to the tip of the short process of the incus.

Constant visual reference is made to the position of the horizontal portion of the facial nerve which lies medial to it. The color of the bone is seen and felt to change over the facial canal. It is ivory white and hard. Further dissection is done using a diamond burr. Smyth suggests that for adequate exposure the bone be removed until the sheaths of the nerves are clearly visible through the bone. The facial nerve in a living body appears 'pink' and in a preserved wet bone appears 'white'.

Once an entry is made in a recess, enlargement can be carried out in all directions but especially towards the hypotympanum so that a triangle is formed (Fig. 7.6).

In avoiding the facial nerve injury by dissecting laterally, the tendency to make a button hole in the postcanal wall should be prevented as this can later create a posterior retraction pocket extending into the mastoid and producing recurrent cholesteatoma years later.

During this dissection the surgeon should be very careful in not disrupting the chorda tympani nerve which runs laterally or the facial nerve medially or the fossa incudis and short process of the incus superiorly or transect the annulus laterally. A sound knowledge of their anatomy is warranted here. These are kept as the landmarks of the dissection.

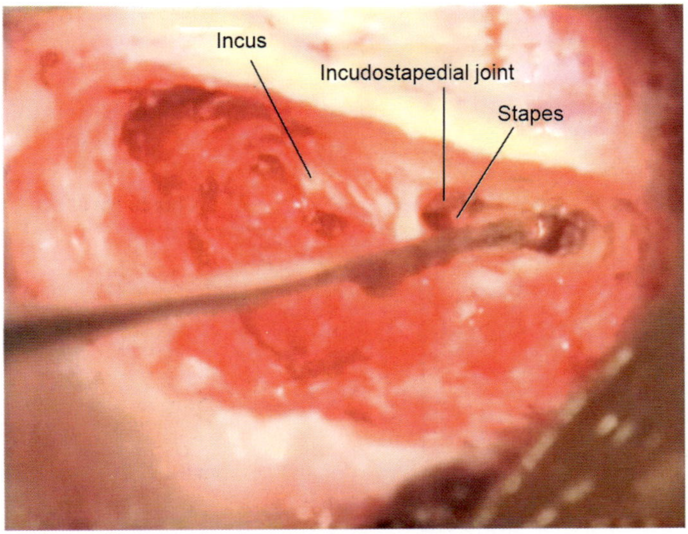

Fig. 7.6: Widening of posterior tympanotomy in progress

Once the facial recess is opened, the following structures are identified:

- Stapes
- Round window
- Pyramid
- Promontory
- Stapedius tendon

Further removal of the bone inferiorly helps to identify more structures namely stapedius tendon, hypotympanum and horizontal part of the facial nerve, and with the head tilted a little more anteriorly the eustachian tubal opening can also be made out.

Extending the Facial Recess

Facial recess extension provides necessary exposure to remove a small glomus tumor or extensive hypotympanic cholesteatoma. The dissection is extended inferiorly at the lateral aspect of the facial nerve. The chordo-facial angle is dissected and the chorda tympanic nerve is sacrificed. Dissection is done between the facial nerve medially and the annulus laterally. More bone can be removed inferiorly as the annulus turns anteriorly, moving away from the facial nerve in the hypotympanum. The jugular bulb is seen as it rises in to the hypotympanum, through the bone. The landmarks here are:

- Facial nerve
- Chorda tympani
- Annulus
- Tympanic membrane

In some cases there might be dehiscence of the bone and the jugular bulb lies on the floor of the canal. If so dissection should be done with utmost care.

If the dissection is further extended the bone of the inferior portion of the tympanic ring and mastoid tip may be removed lateral to facial nerve. This exposes the hypotympanum to the level of the eustachian tube.

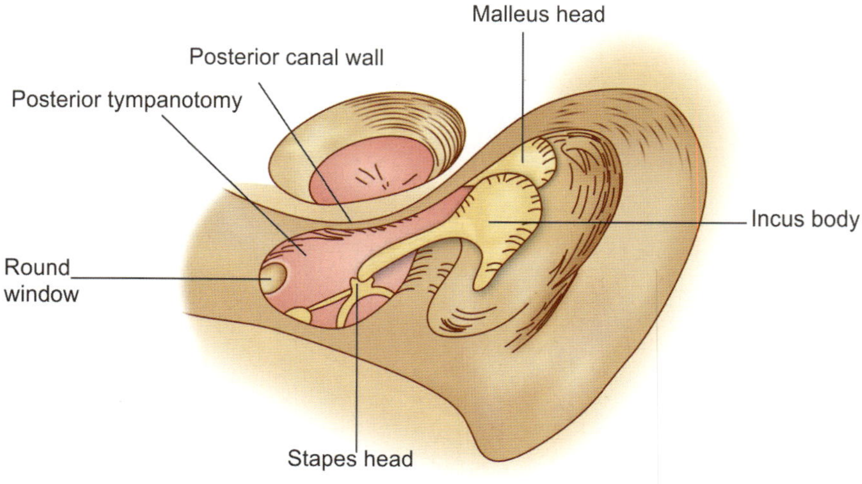

Fig. 7.7: Extended facial recess approach being completed by removal of bone overlying fossa incudis for complete exposure of incus and incudostapedial joint and round window niche

On removal of the retrofacial cells extending from mastoid into the middle ear, the sigmoid sinus can be followed in continuity with the jugular bulb. Dissecting more anteriorly, the carotid artery and the confluence of the two vessels leaving the carotid sheath and entering the base of the skull can be seen.

The bone occupying the part of the skull base where the artery turns anteriorly and the jugular vein turns posteriorly is called the jugulocarotid septum or the Crotch or vascular crest.

The jugular bulb can be opened (in wet temporal bone) and IX, X, XI cranial nerves are found in proximity to the multiple openings of the petrosal sinus.

Facial nerve, annulus, sigmoid sinus, jugular bulb, carotid artery are the landmarks to this dissection.

3. *Anterior Tympanotomy* (*Fig 7.8*)

Canal wall skin is elevated either by a microelevator or with Rosen's round knife. Elevation is continued up to the annulus and then the annulus is gently elevated, so that a tympanomeatal flap is obtained. Chorda tympani nerve is identified and is gently mobilized.

The tympanomeatal flap is pushed anteriorly and any canal overhang obscuring the view of the middle ear is either curetted out or drilled off to get a clear view. Structures in the middle ear are identified.

Handle of the malleus, long process of the incus, incudostapedial joint, stapes, stapedius tendon, round window, promontory, middle ear mucosa, etc. can be made out. This completes the anterior tympanotomy.

Thus the combined (anterior and posterior tympanotomy) approach enables the surgeon to see and clear diseased tissues from all the areas of the tympanomastoid cleft in spite of an intact canal wall (Fig. 7.9). Graft placement and ossicular reconstruction is possible for tympanoplasty (Fig. 7.10), discussed in details in Chapter 12.

The sinus tympani which lies medial to facial nerve and pyramid and posterior to the labyrinthian windows may be very difficult to reach as the facial nerve interferes with the posterior tympanotomy.

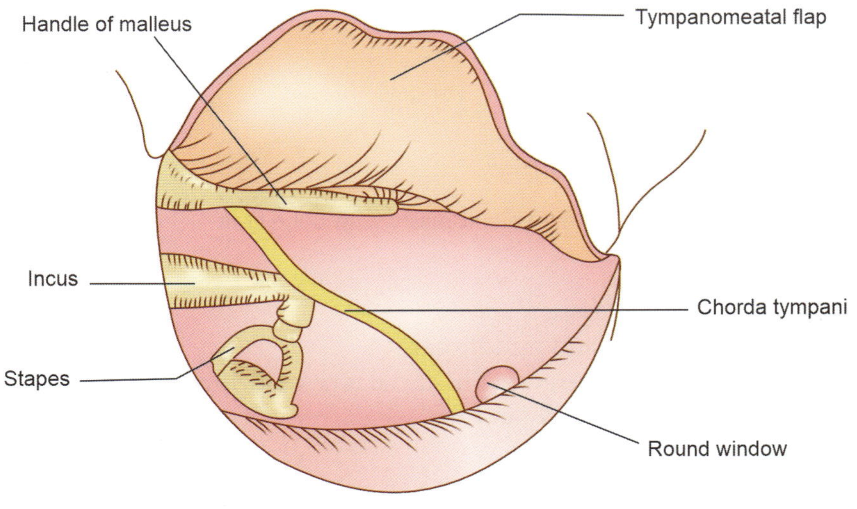

Fig. 7.8: Anterior tympanotomy exposure after elevation of tympanomeatal flap

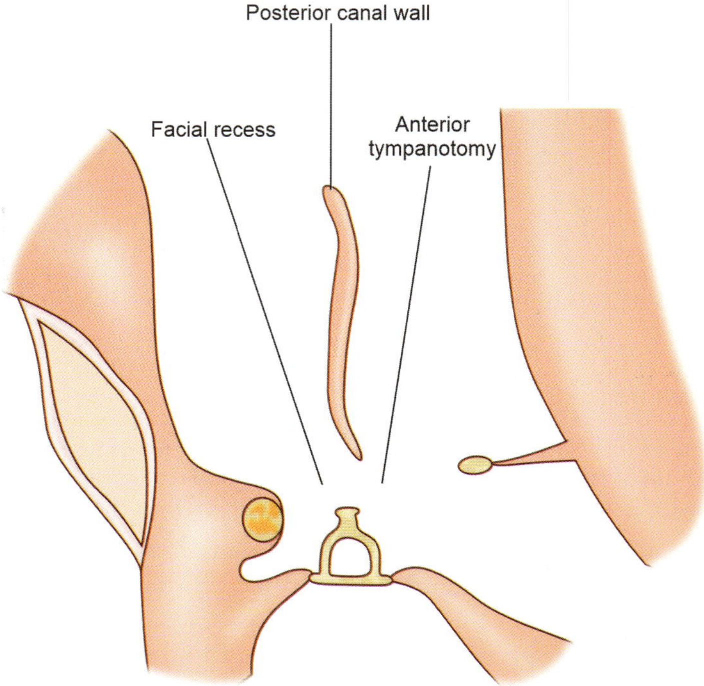

Fig. 7.9: Area of access through anterior and posterior tympanotomy in combined approach tympanoplasty

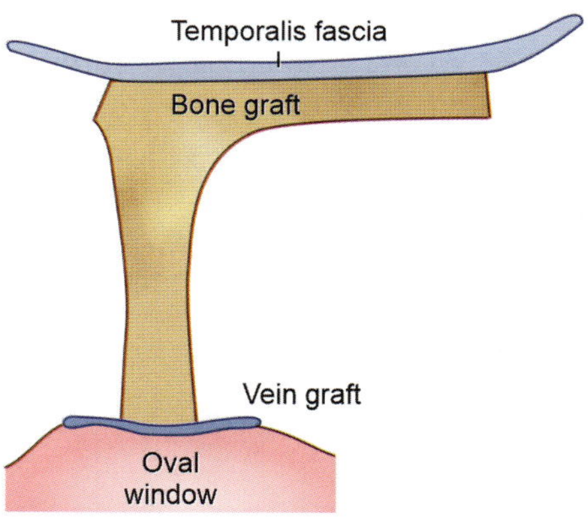

Fig. 7.10: Ossiculoplasty with bone graft

Advantages

1. Good exposure of mastoid and middle ear
2. Possibility of aeration after surgery. The facial recess opening ensures free ventilation of the whole cavity from eustachian tube.
3. Avoidance of an open mastoid cavity
4. Preservation of posterior meatal wall
5. Tympanoplasty with ossicular reconstruction can be done in the same sitting depending on the pathology.

Disadvantages

1. Approach of anterior attic disease through healthy bone.
2. Difficulty of the technique. Successful employment of this technique requires considerable experience in the management of CSOM and a high standard of technical competence.
3. Difficulty in removing cholesteatoma. O'Brien and Beales are of the view that it is impossible to be certain that the disease is removed completely by CAT, foolhardy and dangerous to reconstruct a closed tympanomastoid cavity that cannot be kept under observation.
4. Hidden recurrence of cholesteatoma in the tympanomastoid segment.
5. Regular follow up for a long period.

"In conclusion it is my opinion that CAT in the presence of cholesteatoma is not safe operation in the long term, but has certain real advantages over the older methods of tympanoplasty in improvement of function."

—Philip H. Beales

At society proceedings Royal Society of Medicine, Section on Otology.

REFERENCES AND FURTHER READING

1. Bento RF and de Oliveiria Fonseca AC. A brief history of mastoidectomy; Int Arch Otorhinolaryngol. 2013 Apr; 17(2): 168–78.
2. Sheehy JL, Patterson ME. Intact canal wall tympanoplasty with mastoidectomy. A review of eight years' experience; Laryngoscope. 1967 Aug;77(8):1502–42.
3. Jansen C. The combined approach for tympanoplasty. J Laryngol Otol. 1968;82(9):779–793.
4. Scott Brown-Diseases of Ear, Nose and Throat. 4th edition volume 2. The Ear pg. 296–303.
5. Paparella and Shumrick-*Otolaryngology* Volume 2 pg. 1519–21
6. Charles D Cummings. *Otolaryngology Head & Neck Surgery,* 2nd edition, volume 4, pg. 2992–93
7. Rob and Smith. *Operative surgery* 'CAT', pp. 89–99
8. K. J. Lee. *The surgical Atlas of Otology and Neuro-Otology,* pp. 158–60
9. *Journal of Otolaryngology* 81 Posterior Tympanotomy G. D. L. Smyth, pp. 69–73
10. *Journal of Otolaryngology 82* Society proceedings 'CAT' Philip H. Beales pg. 769 Jansen pg.779
11. *OCNA Surgical Technique in CAT* Feb 72 G. D. L. Smyth pg. 65
12. *Temporal bone dissection manual:* House Ear-Institute.
13. *Learning Ear Surgery by temporal bone dissection:* KK Ramalingam.
14. Beales pH. Combined Approach Tympanoplasty; The Journal of Laryngology and Otology, 82(8);1968:769–773.
15. O'Brien. Combined Approach Tympanoplasty; *The Journal of Largyngology and Otology,* Vol 85(9);1971:883–890.

Chapter

8

Endolymphatic Sac Decompression

Dipak Ranjan Nayak • Devaraj K • Sauvagini Acharya

Introduction

Operations of endolymphatic sac (ES) were first described in 1926–27 by George Portmann, but have been playing a significant role only since last 25 years.

The operations carried out on the ES are designed to create a permanent fistula in the ES or to ensure expansion of liquid when there is a crisis in Meniere's diseases (endolymphatic hydrops).

Historical Perspective

The first surgical attempt to endolymphatic sac was done by Portmann in 1927 when he made an incision over the endolymphatic sac to release endolymphatic pressure. In 1962 William House modified the Portmann's technique by communicating the sac opening to the aub-arachnoid space through subarachnoid shunt to drain endolymphatic hydrops. Shambaugh in 1966 described surgical decompression of endolymphatic sac without opening. Paparella (1976) emphasized the need of making a wide dural incision to expose and decompress the endolymphatic sac and duct completely, avoiding the posterior semicircular canal. Subsequently, open the sac and improve its drainage via a T-tube that served as an endolymphatic duct valve. Thomsen et al. (1981) performed a double-blind study, in which they treated patients with Ménière's disease either with endolymphatic sac decompression and shunting, or with a simple mastoidectomy as a control procedure.

Indications

The principle morphological change in Ménière's disease is an increase in volume of endolymphatic space (Hallpike and Cairns, 1938) mainly affecting cochlea and saccule and to a lesser extent utricle and least the semicircular canal (as their walls are thick).

ES is opened in well selected cases of Ménière's disease especially after the failure of medical or conservative treatment.

Case selection plays an important role.

Careful detailed history.
Tests of auditory function.
i. Pure tone audiometry: Unilateral low tone/SN loss
ii. Recruitment: +ve
iii. SISI: High score
iv. Bekesy audiometry: Type II
v. Good speech discrimination.

Electrocochleography: Broadening of SP/AP form.
Glycerol dehydration test, urea test, acetazolamide over hydration test.
Calorie test: Canal paresis/directional preponderance to normal side/both.

Possible explanation for benefits from SAC decompression surgeries are:

i. Endolymph can leak as it accumulates
ii. Inflammatory reaction to surgery increases blood flow and endolymph absorption
iii. Inflammation response causes increased endolymph absorption by osmosis.

Prognostic factors

a. Greater the preoperation SP → poorer the postoperative prognosis.
b. If no improvement in PTA and electrocochleography (SP/AP ratio) → poor prognosis postoperation.

Surgical Anatomy

ES is a pear shaped structure located in the thickened portion of posterior fossa dura medial to sigmoid sinus and inferior to postsemicircular canal.

The area of sac extends between posterior SSC, superiorly, medial aspect of sigmoid sinus posteriorly retrofacial area anteriorly and jugular bulb inferiorly.

According to Arenberg the location of sac depends to the amount of periaqueductal pneumatization. Sometimes it may occupy the medial wall of jugular bulb.

The exact position of the sac is identified by thickened white shiny double layered dura. Normally, the posterior fossa dura is dark and single layered. Sac can also be identified by presence of hypervascularity on the surface of the sac.

Donaldson's Line

It is an imaginary line drawn from horizontal SSC along its longitudinal axis bisecting the posterior semicircular canal passing up to the sigmoid sinus. The top of the sac is located here in the posterior fossa dura.

Technique

Simple Cortical Mastoidectomy Performed

- After completion of cortical mastoidectomy, using a large burr 1st landmark, **sigmoid sinus** is skeletonized, 2nd landmark, **mastoid antrum** is openened and widened. Retrofacial cells are exposed (Fig. 8.1).

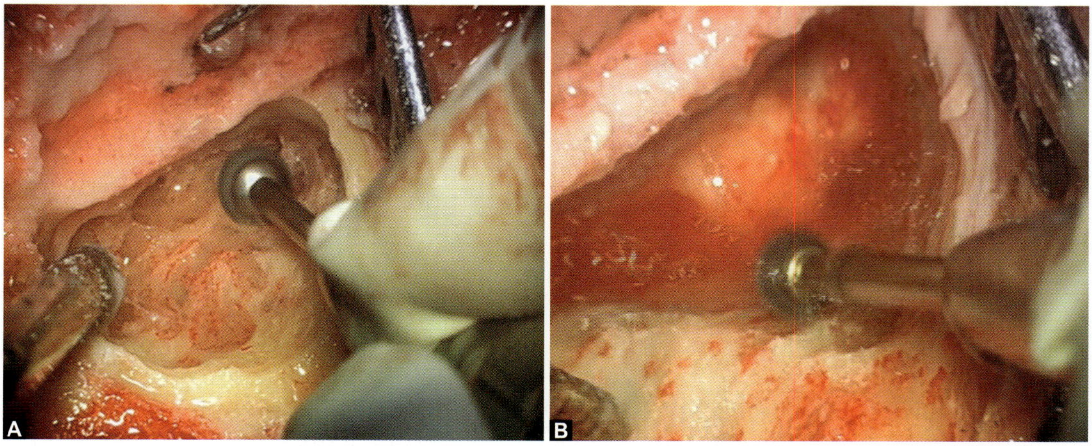

Fig. 8.1 A and B: Cortical mastoidectomy in progress while skeletonizing the sigmoid sinus

Exposure of Endolymphatic Sac (ES) (Figs 8.2 and 8.3)

- Antrum is enlarged further and aditus exposed
  - This exposes 3rd landmark → horizontal/lateral semicircular canal
  - By drilling deeper and post to it reach 4th landmark → posterior SSC
  - (Note: Do not open PSSC as it may cause total deafness in the living).
- Posterior fossa dura and particularly in the area just medical to sigmoid sinus and mastoid (descending portion) segment of facial nerve are skeletonized.

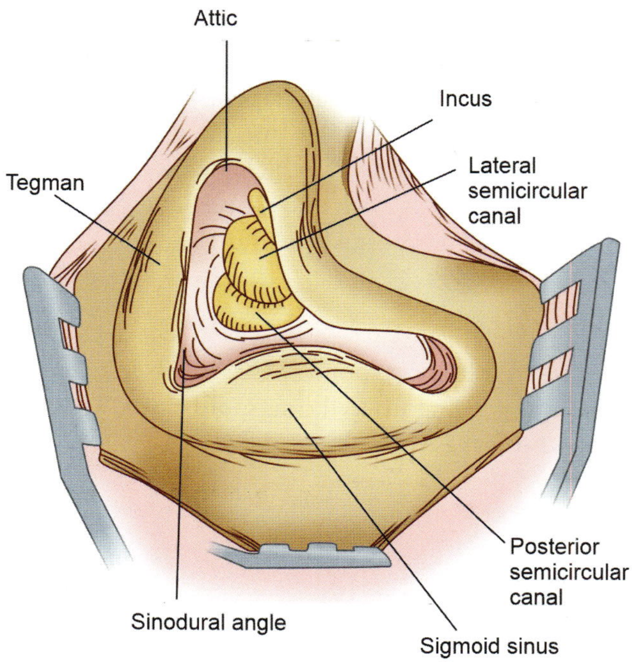

Fig. 8.2: Exposure of tegmen antri, sigmoid plate, lateral and posterior semicircular canals

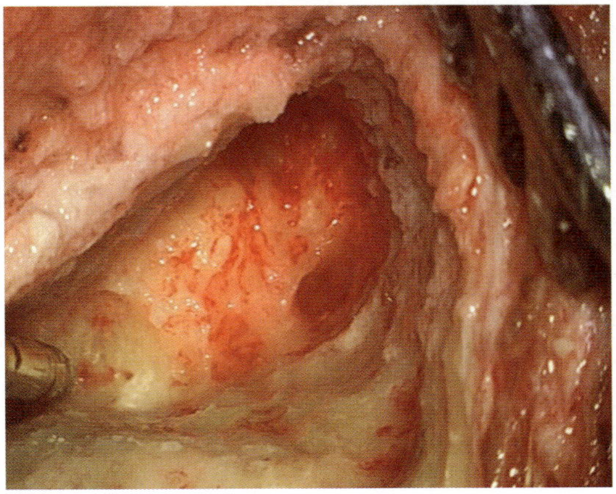

Fig. 8.3: Area to be drilled inferior to posterior semicircular canal for sac exposure

- Bone (dural plate over the sac) is removed in the area (2 cm high 1 cm wide)
  - Use small cutting burr.
  - When the cortex in the depth of petrous bone is reached it is replaced by a diamond burr.
  - Using constant irrigation posterior fossa dura is exposed.
- Landmarks of ES is identified:
  - ES lies in front of sigmoid sinus and behind the post SSC.
  - Position corresponds to A-P axis of HSSC or immediately below it.
  - Endolymphatic duct (which forms posterior superior boundary of ES) exits just medial of posterior semicircular canal. Endolymphatic sac lies deep and inferior to the posterior semicircular canal (Fig. 8.4).
  - Sac is identified by gently depressing the dura away from overlying bone of posterior canal and noting the spot at which dura is fixed to bone of canal by the duct.
- After the ES is exposed (appears white in color than the rest of dura which is grey).
  - Smooth glistening–moist in living.

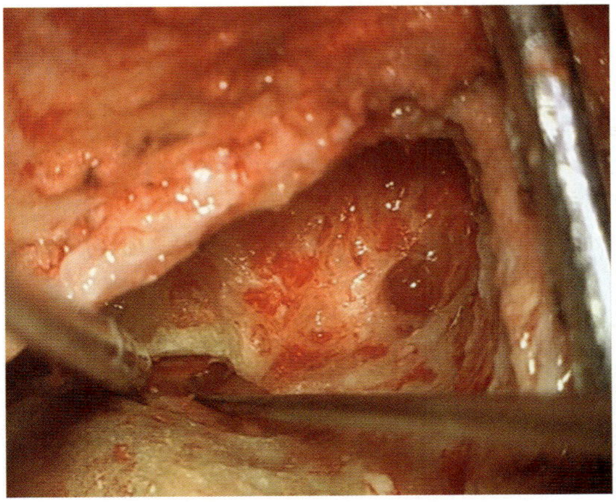

Fig. 8.4: Exposure of sac before further decompression

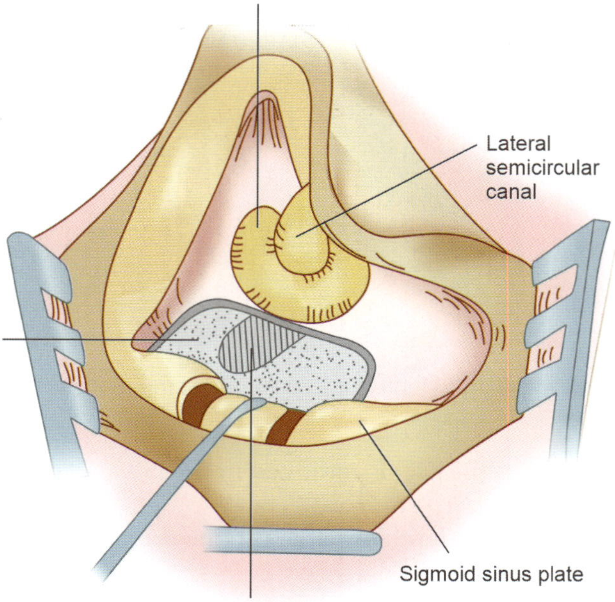

Fig. 8.5: Exposed sac and dura

- The superior and inferior limits of the ES is outlined with a blunt ended instrument (Fig. 8.5) (Note: Dimensions of the sac can be extremely variable—very large or very small).

- **Opening of ES:** Outer surface of dura incised from behind forward using ultrafine scalpel blade/sickle knife.
- **Closure:** A large piece of Gelfoam is placed in the depth of operative field and after placing a drain, wound is closed in layers.

Operative Problems

i. **Inability to expose presinus space corresponding to ES:** Using a very small burr, outer 1/3 of bony canal wall is removed.
ii. **Lack of space between sigmoid sinus and PSSC:** Commonly seen in small mastoids wherein SS is found projecting towards PSSC which can be taken care by using the smallest burr and extremely careful drilling.
iii. **Opening of sigmoid sinus:** Should be avoided by gradual thinning of bone over sigmoid sinus without exposing the sinus wall. If injured accidentally, can be controlled by placing Surgicel in the tear and reinforcement with a piece of muscle may be necessary.
iv. **Opening posterior semicircular canal:** Occurs if sigmoid sinus is very prominent or the otic capsule is placed very posteriorly (if it happens do NOT put the suction in

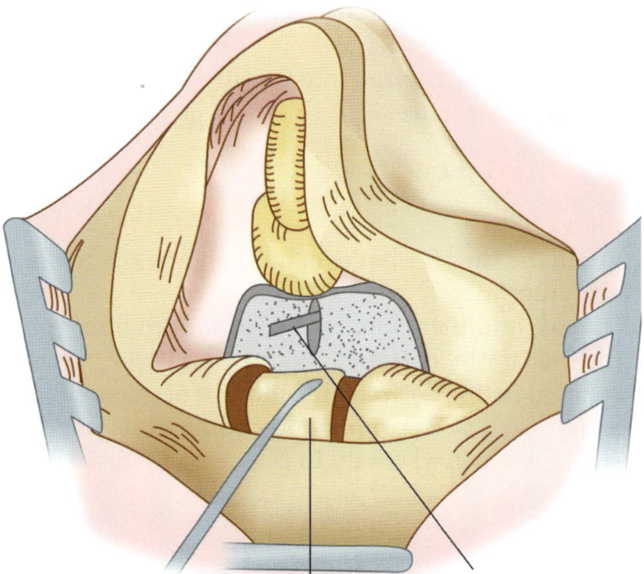

Fig. 8.6: T tube in place in the sac to create communication into mastoid

canal). Fistula is closed with a piece of conjunctiva / Gelfoam / muscle / vein graft. Then the area is covered with bone dust.

v. **Opening of dura:** Unusual, more in shunt operation. Closed with silk suture and covered with temporalis fascia graft maintained in place by Gelfoam / muscle (a persistent fistula → may cause meningitis.)

Modifications of Portmann's Technique

A. Subarachnoid Shunt (House), 1964

Technique similar to Portmann's except:

- Inner wall of sac also incised producing a dark bubble thus, joining endolymphatic space with subarachnoid space
- A small flanged Teflon / silastic shunt tube with an acute angle between flange and tube of 30–45° is bluntly inserted through the 'arachnoid bubble' in subarachnoid space. Tip of tube should be directed anterosuperiorly to avoid injury to cerebellum (inferiorly) or any adjacent vessel.
- **Secure flange within the lumen:** A vein graft or Gelfoam or piece of temporalis muscle used to cover this to prevent CSF fistula.
- The opening is maintained by placing a fragment of Gelfoam in the incision line.

B. Mastoid Shunt (Arenberg, Morrison, and Shea), 1979

- ES is exposed as in Portmann's technique
- External dural covering is incised and drainage is established into the mastoid cavity.
- Shea used Teflon film extending from endolymphatic space into the mastoid cavity.

- Arenberg used a one way valve into endolymphatic duct and a silastic sheet extending into mastoid.
- Morrison used a capillary tube inserted into the duct and connecting to a silastic sponge brought out into the mastoid space.

C. Modification by Hasegawa and Naito

- ES is exposed as above
- An incision is made in the dura—above, behind and below the endolymphatic sac.
- This flap is reflected anteriorly
- The subarachnoid space and the inner surface of sac are thus exposed.
- Sac is opened to the interior by cutting a window on inner surface of sac.
- This creates a permanent fistula between the interior of the sac and subarachnoid space.
- The original flap is returned to its original position and its dura is sutured behind.
- Gelfoam/muscle fills the mastoid cavity to prevent CSF fistula.

D. Decompression without Opening SAC (Shambaugh Jr.), 1966

- According to him, exposed sac is ischemic
- He places a piece of temporalis muscle on its (sac's) external surface to encourage revascularization.

Postoperative Care

1. Antibiotics and anti-inflammatory drugs
2. Patient not to move his head suddenly/excessively.
3. Bedrest—3 to 4 days
4. Vestibular exercises (if postoperative vertigo)
5. Remove silk sutures and external canal packing on 8th POD
6. Repeat audiogram and electrocochleography (after 7th POD, 6th month and 1 year later)

Complications

a. Mainly—sensorineural deafness (if posterior semicircular canal damaged).
b. Bleeding—if adjacent vessel damaged.
c. CSF fistula—meningitis

Conclusions

It is hoped that, by dealing fundamentally with the main functional defect of the disorder, the natural history of the disease may be altered, with preservation of hearing otherwise doomed to inexcoriable deterioration, this in addition to elimination or diminishing the attacks of vertigo and reducing tinnitus.

REFERENCES AND FURTHER READING

1. Portmann G. The saccus endolymphaticus and an operation for draining the same for the relief of vertigo. *J Laryngol Otol.* 1927;42(12):809–17.

2. House WF. Subarachnoid shunt for drainage of endolymphatic hydrops. A preliminary report. *Laryngoscope* 1962;72:713–29.
3. Shambaugh GE. Jr. Surgery of endolymphatic sac. Arch Otol 1966; 83: 305–10.
4. Paparella MM, Hanson DG. Endolymphatic sac drainage for intractable vertigo (method and experiences). *Laryngoscope* 1976; 86(05):697–703.
5. Thomsen J, Bretlau P, Tos M, Johnsen N J. Placebo effect in surgery for Ménière's disease. A double-blind, placebo-controlled study on endolymphatic sac shunt surgery. *Arch Otolaryngol.* 1981;107(05):271–7.
6. Shambaugh GE. Jr. Effect of endolymphatic sac decompression on fluctuating hearingloss. *Otolaryngol Clin of North Am.* 1975; 8:573.
7. KY Lee. The Surgical Atlas of Otology and Neuro-Otology, 1984; pg 309–16.
8. Anson, B.J. Surgical Anatomy of Endolymphatic Sac and Perilymphatic duct-. *Laryngoscope,* 1964; 74: 480.
9. House W. Subarachnoid Shunt for drainage of hydrops—The laryngoscope, 1964; 72: 713.
10. Ralph A. Nelson. Temporal Bone Dissection Manual, 1988.
11. Shambaugh and Glasscock. Surgery of Ear-4th edition, pg 486.
12. Paparella and Saunders. Atlas of Ear Surgery (1986).
13. Harold L. Mawson's Diseases of ear: Textbook of Otology, 5th edition, 1988; pg 628.

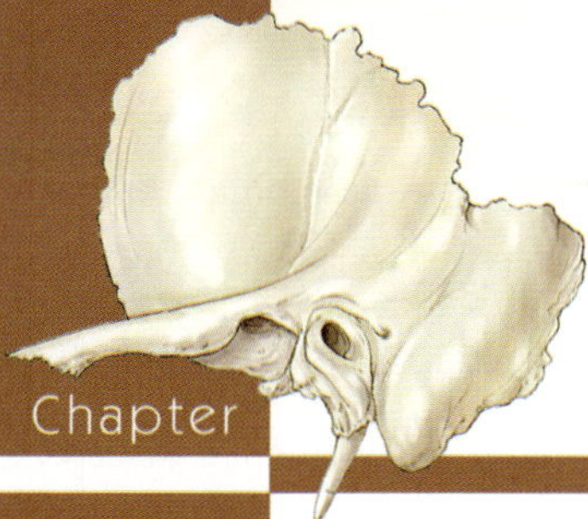

Chapter

9

Facial Nerve Decompression

Dipak Ranjan Nayak • Sampath Chandra Prasad Rao • Produl Hazarika • Santosh Pani

Introduction

The management of facial paralysis continues to evolve. Understanding the facial nerve anatomy and the different methods of evaluating the degree of facial nerve injury are crucial for successful management (Gordin et al, 2014). Following Bell's palsy, temporal bone trauma is the second most common cause of FN paralysis in adults (17%) and the most common cause in children (30%). Decompression of facial nerve is a procedure, where abnormal compression of facial nerve is relieved by surgical intervention (Angeli and Chiossone, 1997). It may be done from the internal auditory meatus up to the stylomastoid foramen, aims at adequate exposure of facial nerve at any point in its course with preservation of hearing and vestibular function, without further injury to the facial nerve.

Historical Perspective

Although the procedure was first suggested in 1923 (Adour and Diamond, 1982) but not performed until 1931 when Martin published the 1st intratemporal suturing. Most of the decompression surgery is done for temporal bone fracture (Kim et al, 2015). The current technique for exposure through the mastoid, middle cranial fossa and retrolabyrinthine combined approaches are described for total facial nerve decompression. This technique, properly performed, is a valuable treatment for facial nerve lesions (Pulec, 1996). The classical middle fossa approach was described by William House in 1961 to approach the contents of the internal auditory canal. The transmastoid approach is an effective treatment option that allows sufficient access to the facial nerve with low complication rates (Yanagihara et al, 1979, 2001).

Etiology

1. **Bell's palsy:** Idiopathic facial nerve paralysis.

2. **Trauma**
   i. Fracture of temporal bone in accidental trauma. It is of two types:
      a. Longitudinal
      b. Transverse always results in severely damaged or severed nerve.
   ii. Iatrogenic-injury to facial nerve during surgery.
3. **Tumors:** Progressive paralysis beyond 3 weeks following onset associated with no return of function by 6 months.
   a. Benign lesions (compress facial nerve):
      i. Neurilemmomas and neurofibromas commonly called facial nerve neuromas.
      ii. Glomus tumors—glomus tympanicum and glomus jugular.
      iii. Hemangiomas.
      iv. Primary cholesteatoma.
      v. Others—giant cell tumors, osteoblastomas, lipomas and adenomas.
   b. Malignant tumors (they invade facial nerve):
      i. Squamous cell cancer.
      ii. Adenocarcinoma.
      iii. Basal cell carcinoma of auricle.
      iv. Sarcomas.

Indications

- More than 90% difference between the affected side and the normal side in electroneurography.
- Complete facial nerve paralysis.
- Absence of voluntary compound muscle action potential in voluntary electromyography.
- Progressive deafness and vertigo.
- Presentation within 14 days of onset of complete paralysis.
- Patient desires operative intervention.

Contraindications

- Non-functional motor endplate muscle unit associated with fibrosis and muscle atrophy following long-standing facial palsy.
- Patient more than 65 years of age has less chance of recovery.

Principles of Facial Nerve Surgery

1. **Knowledge of anatomy:** A sound knowledge of the facial nerve anatomical course throughout its intratemporal course (Fig. 9.1) through extensive study and dissection of the cadaveric temporal bone.
2. **Facility and familiarity with microscopic and drill techniques:** Magnification as provided by Zeiss Surgical Microscope is a must while working within the confines of the temporal bone. Experience with various drills and knowledge of hazards and advantages of cutting and diamond drills is necessary.

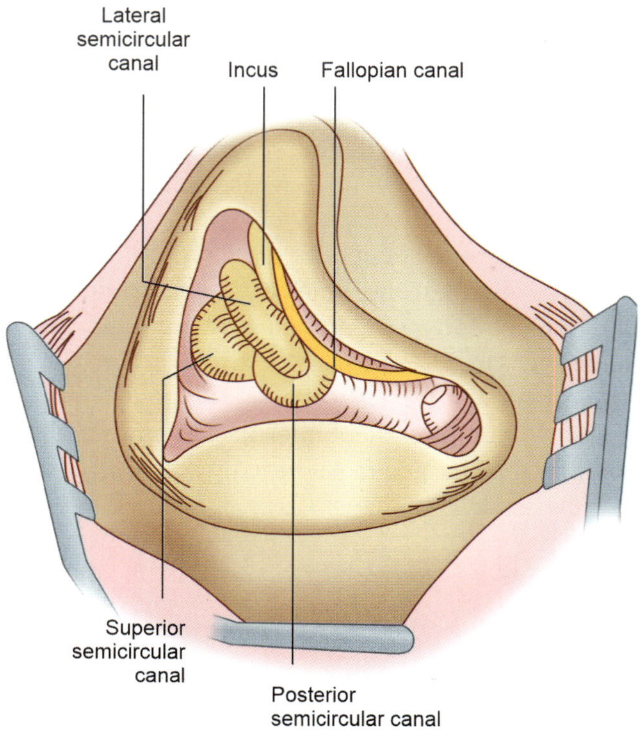

Fig. 9.1: Position of the facial canal in relations to lateral semicircular canal

3. **Suction irrigation:** Continuous suction irrigation is essential not only for cleansing of operative field of blood, bone chips and bone dust but also to keep the operative field cool and thereby protect the facial nerve and vital structures of labyrinth from heat damage.
4. **Experience in intracranial neuro-otologic surgery:** Detailed knowledge of the anatomy of the middle fossa is imperative during the middle fossa approach.

Transmastoid Approach

Exposure of facial nerve in its entire horizontal (tympanic) and vertical (mastoid) portion, i.e. from the geniculate ganglion up to the stylomastoid foramen.

Steps

1. A complete simple mastoidectomy is performed, the horizontal and posterior semicircular canals, digastrics ridge, middle fossa dural plate, sigmoid sinus and fossa incudis being identified.
2. **Skeletonizing the descending portion** (Fig. 9.2)**:** During complete simple mastoidectomy, most of the facial nerve has been well delineated. The nerve is followed from the exposed external genu and mastoid segment to stylomastoid foramen. In another method the digastric muscle is used as a landmark to find the facial nerve at the stylomastoid foramen. The nerve is then followed superiorly back to external genu and facial recess. The bone over the descending portion is thinned using a diamond burr.

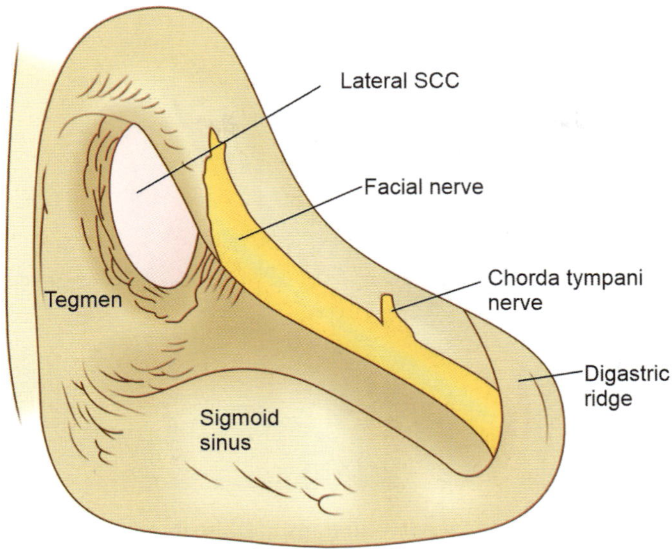

Fig. 9.2: Skeletonization of the descending portion of the facial nerve

3. **The horizontal portion:** The posterior bone canal wall is thinned down and the facial recess developed triangular area of bone bordered externally by chorda tympani nerve, medially by upper half of descending portion of facial nerve and superiorly by the short process of incus. When this recess has been opened up sufficiently it is possible to see the pyramidal eminence, the oval and round windows, the promontory, the stapes, incudostapedial joint and the horizontal portion of facial nerve as far anteriorly as the cochleariform process.
4. **Bone thinning for bone removal:** Performed in a barber pole fashion, i.e.
   i. Descending portion unroofed on post aspect,
   ii. External genu and facial recess portion on its lateral aspect, and

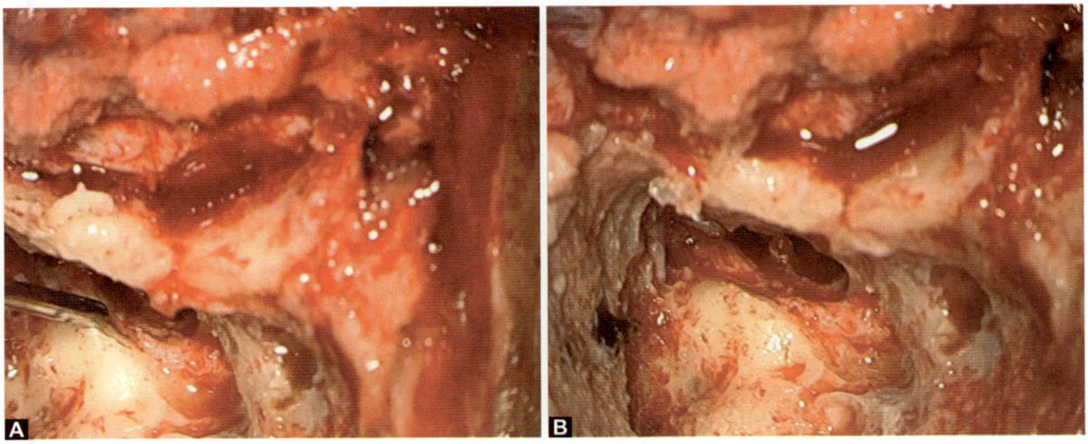

Fig. 9.3 A and B: Tympanic and mastoid segment of facial nerve decompression in longitudinal fracture of temporal bone

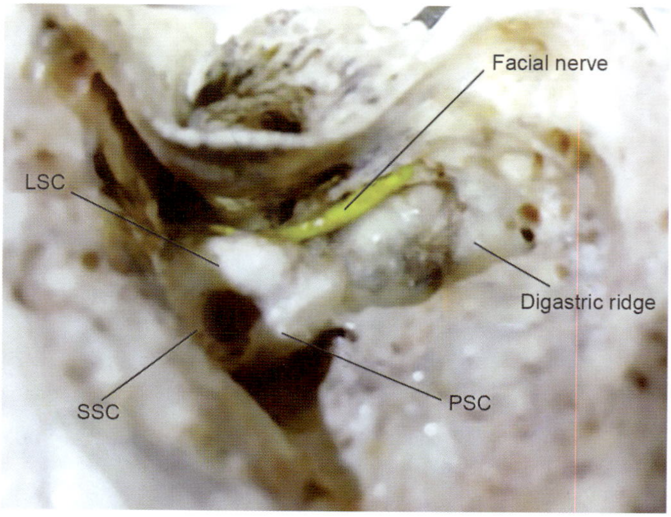

Fig. 9.4: Dissected facial nerve in transmastoid approach in a cadaver

iii. Horizontal segment along its inferior along inferior border to the level of cochleariform process.

This is done using a diamond burr with adequate irrigation and suctioning. In the descending portion decompression on lateral side will result in sacrifice of chorda tympani.

At external genu removal of bone on post side may damage the horizontal SCC.

Burring superiorly in the horizontal segment will also damage the horizontal SCC.

5. A straight micro raspatory is used to remove the final bony shell over the nerve.
6. After complete unroofing of facial nerve from the geniculate ganglion to stylomastoid foramen, a von Grafe cystotome knife is used to open the descending portion and a Ziegler needle knife to open the sheath of horizontal and labyrinthine portion. The post auricular wound is then closed in layers without drainage.

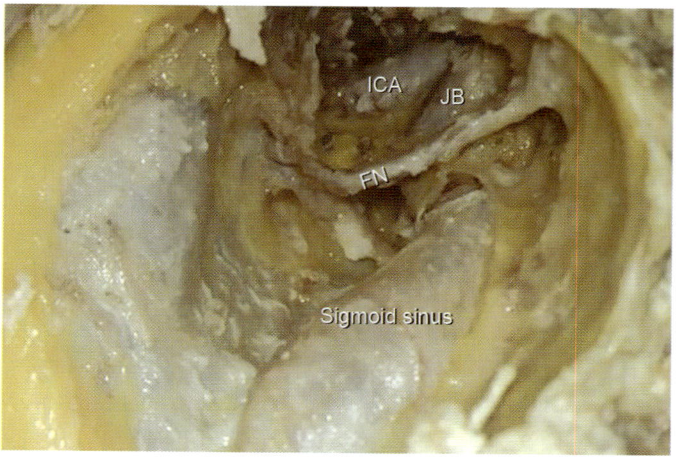

Fig. 9.5: Dissected facial nerve in cadaveric temporal bone through transmastoid and translabyrinthine approach

Middle Cranial Fossa Approach (Figs 9.6 and 9.7)

The classical approach described by House, follows the GSPN to geniculate ganglion and then approaches to labyrinthine segment of the facial nerve into the fundus of the internal auditory canal (Sameshima, 2019). This is indicated for exposure of facial nerve in its course through the internal auditory canal and labyrinthine portion of facial nerve and also for approaching the small intracanalicular acoustic neuroma to preserve hearing.

Steps

1. The point lies in supine position with the involved ear up. The surgeon sits at head end of table. An incision is made 1 cm anterior to tragus and carried through skin and subcutaneous tissue superiorly for about 6 cm after infiltrating the skin with 1% xylocaine with epinephrine.
2. The temporalis muscle is exposed and incised and displaced using an articulated temporalis muscle retractor exposing the underlying squamous portion of temporal bone. A rectangular bone flap of 5 × 5 cm is removed using a cutting burr and suction

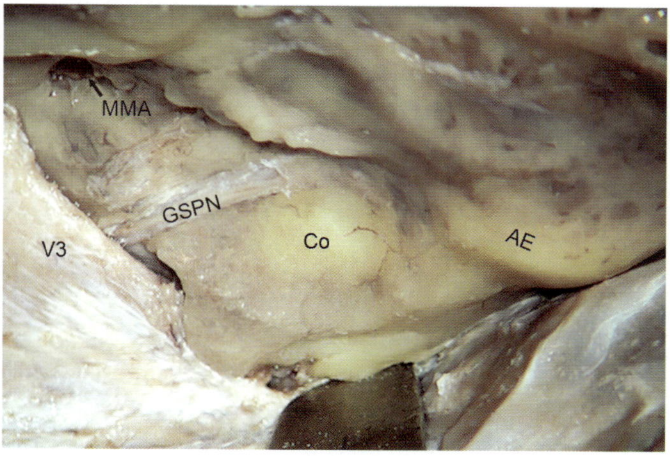

Fig. 9.6: Middle fossa exposure up to petrous apex. The structures that can be seen are middle meningeal artery (MMA), greater superficial petrosal nereve (GSPN), cochlea (Co), arcuate eminence (AE). Note 3rd division of Vth nerve (V3) at the petrous apex

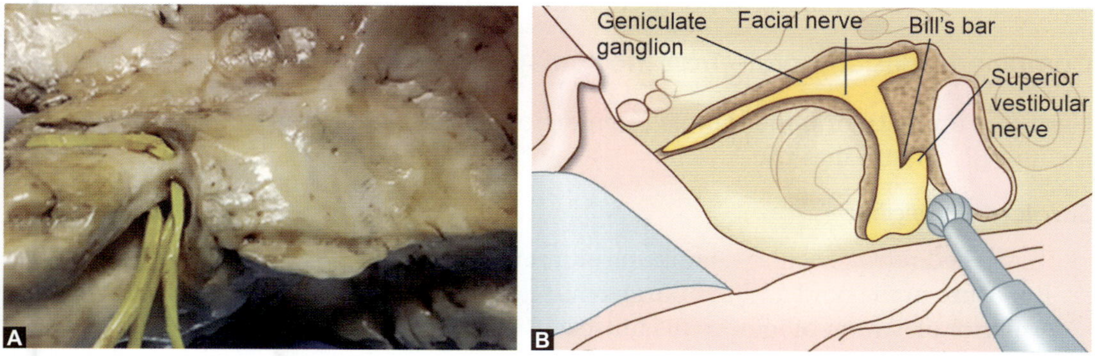

Fig. 9.7: Structure exposed in middle fossa approach in cadaveric bone **(A)** and in illustration **(B)**

irrigation. The base of the bone flap must approximate the level of the floor of middle cranial fossa. The anterior–posterior dimensions of the bone flap should lie 2/3 in front and 1/3 behind the EAC.

After the bleeding from the dura is controlled by electrocoagulation, the dura of temporal lobe of brain is elevated and held in place by a House-Urban self-retaining retractor. This exposes the floor of middle cranial fossa. The anterior limit of exposure is the foramen spinosum; posteriorly it is the arcuate eminence (corresponds to SC). The base of MCF reveals a number of landmarks:

i. Foramen spinosum
ii. Middle meningeal artery
iii. Arcuate eminence
iv. Greater superficial petrosal nerve
v. Tegmen tympani.

The middle meningeal artery is coagulated and divided. The dura covering the trigeminal nerve is carefully elevated from V3 using sharp dissector. After identifying the greater superficial petrosal nerve, a diamond burr is used to follow the nerve posteriorly to the geniculate ganglion. The geniculate ganglion will be superficial and hence a minimum of bone should be removed. At the geniculate ganglion the nerve turns laterally, posteriorly and inferiorly and is exposed up to the cochleariform process. From the geniculate ganglion, the labyrinthine portion of the nerve is followed posteriorly, medially and inferiorly up to lateral extent of internal auditory canal. In this portion the nerve is displaced posteriorly by the basal turn of cochlea.

The bone is removed over the facial nerve. The dissection is carried medially toward the opening of internal auditory canal into the posterior fossa. The exposure may be widened as the posterior fossa is approached. Once the dura is exposed, Bill's bar separating the anterior superior facial nerve compartment is identified. The dura is incised posteriorly over the superior vertibular nerve in order to make an incision away from the facial nerve and to leave an anteriorly based dural flap over facial nerve to protect the structure.

The blade of the dural retractor is now placed medial to the geniculate ganglion and as near to the superior petrosal sinus as possible.

Upon completion of the procedure all bleeding points are controlled. A plug of free temporal muscle is placed over the internal auditory canal to prevent postoperative CSF leakage. The dural elevators are removed and the temporal lobe is allowed to re-expand in its nerve portion in middle cranial fossa. The temporal bone flap and skin are brought together in layers. Drainage is not used. A dry sterile dressing is placed over the wound.

Combined Transtemporal—Transmastoid Approach

Used for supralabyrinthine tumors (hemangiomas, facial nerve neuromas) extending to the middle ear and mastoid.

Surgical Highlights

1. 'S' shaped retroauricular—temporal skin incision.
2. Exposure of mastoid and temporalis muscle.
3. Anterior elevation of temporalis muscle.
4. Mastoidectomy and exposure of mastoid and tympanic segments of facial nerve through a posterior tympanotomy.

5. 2 × 3 cm temporal craniotomy.
6. Exposure of meatal plane, superior semicircular canal and internal auditory canal.
7. Transtemporal exposure of nerve from meatal foramen to cochleariform process.
8. Wound closure.

Skin Incision and Mastoid Temporal Exposure

1. An 'S' shaped postauricular incision extends from the upper border of the temporalis muscle to the tip of the mastoid.
2. Exposure of the mastoid and temporalis muscle. The skin is reflected anteriorly. An anteriorly based periosteal flap is developed over the mastoid. The posterior and superior margins of the temporalis muscle are incised with electro cautery.
3. Exposure of temporal squama. Temporalis muscle is elevated with a bone raspatory and reflected forward up to the root of the zygomatic process to expose the temporal squama.

Transmastoid Approach

Mastoidectomy, posterior tympanotomy and exposure of mastoid and tympanic segments of facial nerve (refer to back)

Exposure of middle cranial fossa dura in the tegmen tympani a small hole is made in the tegmen tympani exposing the middle cranial fossa dura just anterior to the superior ampulla.

This opening will serve as a landmark when searching for the through the middle cranial fossa.

2 × 3 cm craniotomy and elevation of middle cranial fossa dura is done as mentioned previously.

The upper edge of mastoidectomy must be low enough to allow the inferior extension of the craniotomy. The middle cranial fossa retractor is introduced medial to the area where arcuate eminence is expected.

The reference opening in the tegmen tympani can be seen in the floor of middle cranial fossa.

Identification of Bony Superior Semicircular Canal (Fig. 9.6)

Anterior elevation of the dura towards the petrosal sulcus for the purpose of identification of meatal plane would require too much retraction of temporal lobe.

The blade of the middle fossa retractor is placed medial to the expected position of the superior semicircular canal (arcuate eminence) as indicated by the reference hold. The bony semicircular canal is then identified through the pneumatic cells behind the reference opening with a diamond burr.

Exposure of Meatal Plane (Fig. 9.6)

Elevation of the dura towards the petrosal sulcus needs excessive retraction of the temporal lobe. It would also mean working blindly as the dura is covered by the over-hanging bone.

This is solved by lowering the floor of the middle cranial fossa up to the level of the blue line of the superior semicircular canal and then progressively removing the anterior overhanging of the bone.

The excess of bone over the meatal plane is removed and the dura is elevated under the direct vision for 1 cm anterior to the superior semicircular canal with a curved suction and angled micro ear rasparatory elevator. The retractor is advanced simultaneously.

The blade of the middle fossa retractor is now anterior and medial to the blue line of the superior semicircular canal. Using the 60° angle the blue area of internal auditory canal is identified. No other landmarks (petrosal nerve, middle meningeal artery) are needed.

Exposure of Geniculum and Ossicles

The reference opening in the tegmen is enlarged to expose the ossicles, the geniculate ganglion and the tympanic segment of the facial nerve.

Exposure of the Facial Nerve in its Labyrinthine Part and up to the Internal Auditory Meatus is done as Mentioned Previously

For better exposure of the nerve, the head of malleus and the body of the incus may be removed. This is performed through transmastoid approach. The incudostapedial joint is separated and incus removed with a biopsy forceps.

The head of malleus is removed with a micro nipper. The incus can later be interposed between stapes and malleus handle.

A free muscle graft is placed over the internal auditory canal. The tegmen defect in the floor of the middle cranial fossa is reconstructed with a piece of craniotomy flap.

Structures at Risk

1. **Auditory system:** Ossicles intimately related to the tympanic portion of the facial nerve may be dislocated or traumatized and exposing the facial recess or during actual decompression of the facial nerve. Significant and irreversible sensory neural hearing loss result if the drill comes into contact with the ossicular chain.
2. **Vestibular system:** Cochlea, vestibule or the semicircular canals may be damaged due to instrumentation resulting in sensory neural hearing loss.
3. **Jugular bulb:** May ascend high and medial to facial nerve occasionally up to the level of inferior crus of posterior semicircular canal or even directly underneath internal auditory canal. If injured, leads to a profuse venous bleeding.
4. **Sigmoid sinus:** It may show variation in its location. May be superficial under the mastoid cortex or deep or may lie very anteriorly almost adjacent to posterior wall of EAC.
5. **Dura:** Cutting drill may tear the dura and may result in CSF leak and prolapse or herniation of cerebellum or temporal lobe which is avoided by using a diamond drill with a constant suction irrigation.

REFERENCES

1. Gordin E, Lee ST,Ducic Y, *et al*. Facial nerve trauma-Evaluation and considerations in management. *Craniomaxillofac Trauma Reconstr.* 2015 Mar; 8(1): 1–13.
2. Adour KK and Diamond C. Decompression of facial nerve in Bell's palsy-A historical review. *Otolaryngol Head Neck Surg*, 1982;90(4):453–60.
3. Angeli SI, Chiossone E. Surgical treatment of the facial nerve in facial paralysis. *Otolaryngol Clin North Am* 1997;30:683–700.

4. Martin, RC. Intratemporal suture of the facial nerve. *Arch Otolaryngol* 1931; 13: 259–64.
5. Kim SH, *et al*. Delayed facial nerve decompression for Bell's palsy. *European Archives of Oto-Rhino-Laryngology*, 2016; **273**, 1755–60.
6. Pulec JL. Total facial nerve decompression: technique to avoid complications. *Ear Nose Throat J*. 1996;75(7):410–5.
7. House WF. Surgical exposure of the internal auditory canal and its contents through middle fossa approach. *Laryngoscope*, 1961;71(11):1363–85.
8. Sameshima T. (2019) Dissection of Extended Middle Fossa and Anterior Petrosectomy Approach. In: July J., Wahjoepramono E. (eds) Neurovascular Surgery. Springer, Singapore.
9. Yanagihara N, Gyo K, Yumoto E, Tamaki M. Transmastoid decompression of the facial nerve in Bell's palsy. *Arch Otolaryngol*. 1979;105(9):530–4.
10. Yanagihara N, Hato N, Murakami S, Honda N. Transmastoid decompression as a treatment of bell palsy. *Otolaryngol Head Neck Surg*. 2001;124(3):282–6.
11. Surgery of ear-Michael E. Glasscock and George E. Shambaugh 1990.
12. Atlas of Ear surgery: Andrew W. Miglets, Michael M. Paparella and William H. Saunders 1990.
13. Operative surgery: Ear 2nd edition, Rob and Smith 1986.
14. Manual of temporal Bone Dissection: Nelson R, De la cruz A, Fayad J, House Ear Institute.

Chapter 10

Stapedectomy

Dipak Ranjan Nayak • Produl Hazarika • Rajalaxmi Panigrahi

Introduction

Otosclerosis is a disease of the otic capsule where the normal endochondral bone is replaced with spongy vascular bone formation leading to fixation of the stapes. Treatment of otosclerosis has been largely restricted to surgical efforts. Various surgical procedures have been adopted in the past until the development of stapedectomy as a standard procedure with insertion of a piston to connect the incus and oval window to bypass the stapes foot plate to transmit the sound wave.

Historical Perspective

It was in 1842, Meniere reported a case where the hearing was improved by tapping the stapes, which could be the first case of stapes mobilization. Kessel (1876) is the first person to do stapes surgery by doing mobilization or removal of stapes. It was Miot, however, who did the most consistent study of the subject. He reported a series of 200 such operations—through an incision in the drum head-in 1890. In 1892, Blake and Jack reported their experiences with extraction of the stapes for otosclerotic deafness. Jenkins in 1913 describes fenestration of lateral semicircular canal to improve hearing. Lempert (1938) standardized one stage fenestration surgery. In 1952, Rosen found hearing improvement after accidental stapes mobilization, which he standardized later (Rosen 1960). In 1954, Shambaugh who was using the microscope for fenestration operation, applied it to stapes mobilization. This made possible the development of anterior crurotomy mobilization and revival of stapedectomy by Shea in 1956. The first operation of stapedectomy, probably, was carried out by Jack of Boston, Massachusetts in 1891. Shea revived it and described it and though years have passed since the introduction of stapedectomy (Shea 2003). The basis of this procedure is to create a patent oval window, seal it with a membrane of either natural or an artificial material and provide connection between the incus and the neomembrane cover of the oval window. In doing this either all or a part of the stapes footplate is removed, the oval window is covered with vein, mucous membrane connective tissue, fat, gelfoam or collagen membrane; and sound transmission is reestablished with a stapes crus, polyethylene or Teflon tubing, a Teflon or stainless piston, stainless steel or tantalum wire, a platinum prosthesis, or a stapes carved from the patients mastoid cortex.

Evaluation and Case Selection for Stapes Surgery

The Pre and Per operative evaluations are extremely important in selection of the surgical technique. It is important to note the extent and type of otosclerosis; that is, the location and size of otosclerotic foci as well as the amount of foot plate invasion. Depending on the amount of otosclerotic bone deposition in the region of the footplate of stapes, they are divided into (Fig. 10.1):

- **Type I:** Less than half of the footplate is involved and normal thin bluish appearance of the footplate is retained.
- **Type II:** More than half of the footplate is involved with thickening of the footplate.
- **Type III:** Whole of the footplate is involved and appears thickened. The margin of the footplate can be identified.
- **Type IV:** Otosclerotic bone is deposited in the entire footplate obliterating the oval and/or round window.

The technique varies based on the pathology:

- Obliteration of oval window with involvement of the crura dictates a piston technique.
- Total footplate invasion requires its removal

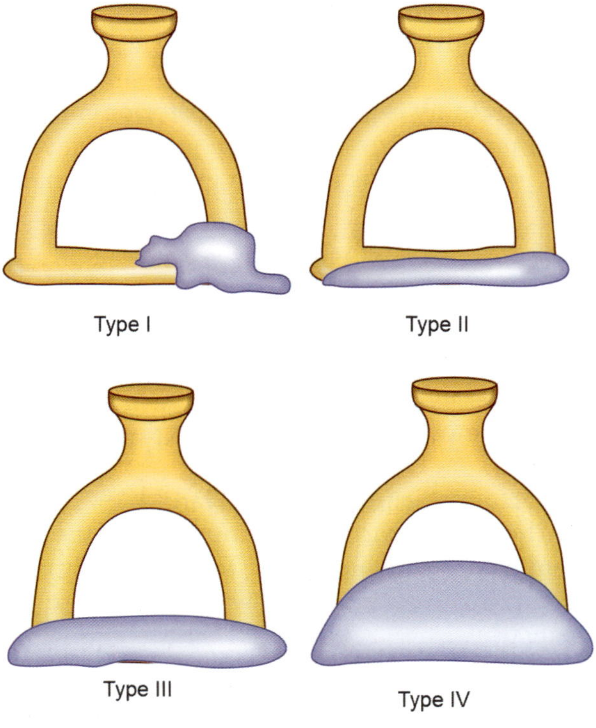

Fig. 10.1: Various types of footplates based on extent of the pathology

- If only a portion of footplate is involved, usually the anterior segment, the normal portion may be preserved
- Anatomic consideration like a narrow, deep oval window may require a thin prosthesis such as wire.

A prosthesis made from Teflon is the most widely employed. Some surgeons use a stainless steel/titanium piston, while others wire prosthesis—the 'Schuknecht Method'. A few surgeons avoid the use of prosthesis by using the crura of the stapes which remain after the footplate has been removed or fenestrated. This method is not always technically possible and long term results are not as satisfactory as those obtained by the use of prosthesis. In recent years it has been shown that the risks of damage to the internal ear at operation and the long term risk of perilymph fistula is less if a small fenestra is made in the posterior part of the footplate.

Various modifications of stapes surgery

i. **The interposition operation:** Portmann (1959) described interposition in stapes surgery. Here a 'platinectomy' or 'basectomy' or footplate excision is performed with preservation of the head, neck and crura and the entire stapes footplate is removed followed by replacement with vein graft. The stapedial tendon is thus preserved and integrity of incudostapedial joint is preserved. The medial end of the crura is reattached to the mobile vein graft.

ii. **Small fenestra stapedectomy (Marquette, 1965):** A calibrated hole in the centre of the footplate is made, the annular ligament is kept intact and prosthesis is placed from incus to the fenestra. The growth of the vestibular endothelium beneath the lower end of the prosthesis is rapid and is guided by the meniscus of the perilymph. The piston is firmly held in position at both ends.

iii. **Vein graft-Teflon interposition operation:** This is a combination of the vein graft stapedectomy and Teflon piston technique (Causse, 1965; Causse and Causse, 1984). A 0.8 mm stapedectomy is made at the posterior end of the footplate. Stapes supra-structure is removed. Large 6 mm vein graft is placed over the fenestrum and piston is placed between incus and vein graft, invaginating the graft into the fenestrum.

   Advantages are:
   - Immediate closure of oval window with little risk of piston being manipulated at the oval window or dropped into it.
   - Additional safeguard to the membranous structures of the vestibule.
   - Reduced tendency for perilymph fistula
   - Immediate sealing of the oval window makes it possible to monitor the progress more accurately.

iv. **Large fenestra stapedectomy** (Schuknecht and Harold, 1971). Schuknecht wire and fat graft stapedectomy. The greater part of the antiportion of the stapes footplate and the suprastructure are removed with a microhook. The previously prepared wire prosthesis with the fat graft is applied to seal the oval window and the wire is crimped on the terminal part of the incus.
   - Relatively easy to carry out
   - Immediate seal of the oval window obtained
   - Stainless steel wire prosthesis makes accurate placement of the graft. But,
   - More traumatic procedure

- Increased risk of damage to the underlying membranous structures in the vestibule.
- Incus is left bare with a diminished blood supply and greater risk of necrosis and if the wire is crimped too tightly, terminal portion of the long process may be damaged.

v. **Total stapedectomy (Ishiyama and Glasscock, 1998):** The essential feature is the total removal of the footplate. There is apparently little difference between the effectivity of acoustic energy, transmission between the intact 'super structure' of a stapes and an articulated prosthesis, with the exception of the unknown sequelae to the cochlea of deprivation of stapedius muscle-protection effect in the prosthetic case. The basic principles involve,
   - Gentle decompression of the perilymph space rather than violent 'uncorking'.
   - Careful removal of footplate fragments and bone dust
   - A blood free field and very delicate suction
   - Adequate, immediate sealing of oval window, preferably with a tissue transplant (vein graft/temporalis fascia).
   - Careful positioning of the strut to ensure its integration with newly created mobile membrane.

Total removal of footplate or oval window fenestration demands not only the utmost in microsurgical technique but a critical awareness of the problems inherent in exteriorization of the vestibule and the special demands placed upon the hydrodynamics of perilymph production and absorption. The ultimate fate of tissue grafts, gel foam and prosthesis is unknown. The status of the cochlea as a long range basis remains to be studied. The sequelae of deprivation of stapedius-muscle protection remain to be evaluated.

Special Problems during Stapedectomy

a. Abnormalities of the facial nerve. Dehiscence of facial nerve are not uncommon–about 0.5% of middle ears. The nerve bulges down and obscures the arch and the footplate. In most such cases, a hole can be made in the footplate, but if the surgery is likely to be blind it is safer to abandon, very rarely facial nerve takes an anomalous course, either splitting to surround the stapes or coursing inferior to the oval window. More difficult and dangerous problem arises when a revision is performed. Dehiscent nerve has become embedded and pulled down by fibrous tissue filling the oval window niche (Leek, 1974).
b. Persistent stapedial artery is seen in 0.2% cases.
c. **Floating footplate:** Potentially serious and may result in a dead ear if attempts are made to extract the footplate. A preliminary drill hole in the footplate or in the promontory margins helps in removing a floating footplate. The surgeon may sometimes elect to place a tissue graft and prosthesis and good results have been reported.
d. 'Biscuit footplate' is a thickened footplate with well defined margins produced by a primary focus in the footplate. With a Harrison knife or a tiny diamond drill, the footplate is cut across the centre, and the margins thinned until it can be extracted in two places. The tissue graft and prosthesis are applied.
e. Depressed footplate, submerged footplate. The footplate may totally submerge and this is caused by trying to remove a floating or the posterior part may become submerged when the fixation is confined to the anterior part. No attempts should be made to retrieve

the footplate by instruments as this may cause severe cochlear damage. Wayoff, Moeller and Roche (1971) describe method to deal the situation. Drops of blood are poured laterally to vestibule and when a clot forms it is removed by a lateral application of the sucker bringing the footplate to the surface.

f. Damage to the chorda tympani especially in bilateral operations. If the nerve is cut it will produce permanent loss of sensation of taste in the anterior two-thirds of the tongue on the same side.
g. **Obliterative otosclerosis:** Here a drill out is required since the oval window is obliterated. The approximate location of the oval window is obliterated. The approximate location of the oval window is established by the crura and fallopian canal. With a small diamond burr the bone in the oval window is thinned down until a blue area appears. Stapedectomy is done and tissue graft prosthesis placed.
h. Tympanic membrane tear
i. **Fixed malleus:** Ankylosis of malleus head to the attic wall can occur by itself or in combination with otospongiotic stapes ankylosis. A sharp blow against a micro-chisel applied to the neck of malleus may free it. Or the head should be amputated, using an endoaural or endomeatal atticotomy.
j. Round window closure. Involvement of the margin of the round window niche by Otospongiosis is very common, next in frequency to oval window involvement, but there is no effect on hearing until the niche is solidly closed, complete bone closure is rare stapedectomy in such a case results in some but not a great improvement in hearing. Attempts to open the round window have been disappointing.
k. Fracture of long process of incus. Rarely an unusually delicate and fragile long process may fracture while crimping the prosthesis. In such cases a pathway is made between tympanic membrane and the manubrium to receive a malleus to oval window prosthesis.
l. **Perilymph gusher:** A rare, alarming, serious problem of stapes surgery is profuse flow of perilymph the moment the vestibule is opened, owing to abnormal patency of cochlear duct. Elevation of head end of the table to reduce CSF pressure, sealing of the opening with tissue graft held in place with the prosthesis, followed by bedrest postoperatively with 30° elevation of the head of the bed are advised.

The Operation

Stapedectomy depends on six basic steps.

1. Obtaining the tissue graft: Temporalis fascia, perichondrium, vein, fat, clotted blood, etc.
2. Exposure of the oval window.
3. Removal of stapes suprastructure.
4. Footplate removal and creation of fenestra.
5. Tissue seal of the fenestra.
6. Prosthesis placement.

After preparation of the canal wall, the endaural speculum in place infiltration with xylocaine adrenalin is given at four points. Then speculum may be used to dilate the ear canal. With a 27-gauge needle, its beveled edge against the bony canal, a minimal amount of additional injection causes blanching of the epithelium down to the annulus. A self retaining speculum holder can be used.

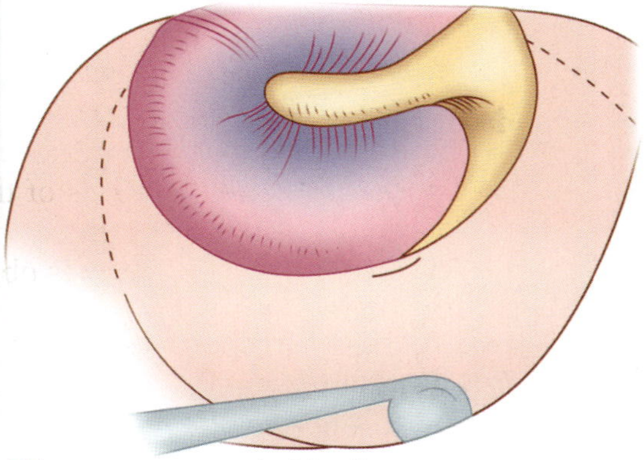

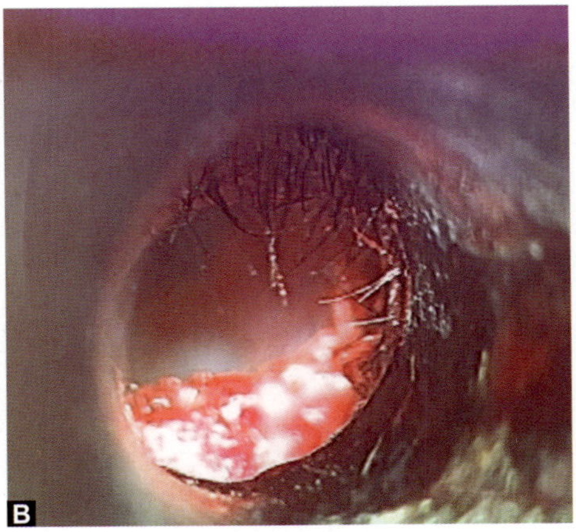

Fig. 10.2A and B: Transmeatal incision from 12 o' clock to 6 o'clock.

Under magnification of 6×, the middle ear is entered through a permeatal tympanotomy. The tympanomeatal flap is created by incision from the 6 o'clock position 2 mm away from the annulus outwards into the meatus to meet another incision from 12 o'clock position immediately above the short process of malleus curving outwards and then downwards, 6 mm away from the annulus at 9 o'clock position in either ear (Fig. 10.2). Elevation can be done by knife elevator or blunt elevator with simultaneous suctioning on a small cotton pledget in the plane (Fig. 10.3).

The fibrous annulus is identified and it is reflected out of the bony sulcus using a drum elevator, beginning at the posterosuperior angle. This exposes the chorda tympani nerve, running forwards lateral to the lower end of the long process of incus. The drum lead is folded forward exposing the middle ear (Fig. 10.4).

Usually the nerve can be reflected downwards with a curved Rosen needle, beyond the tip of the incus, without undue stretching (Fig. 10.5); but if this is not possible it is better to cut the nerve cleanly with crocodile micro-scissors. At this point, usually only the lenticular process and a small part of the stapes can be seen, the remainder of the oval window area being hidden by the bony canal. With a curette the bone is removed from the bony annulus overlying the oval window, from within outwards.

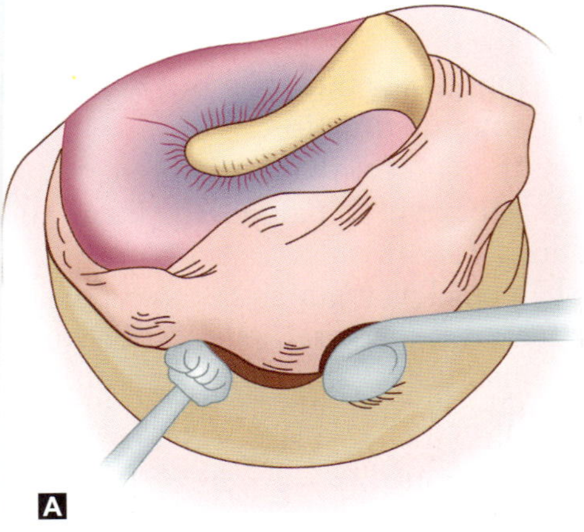

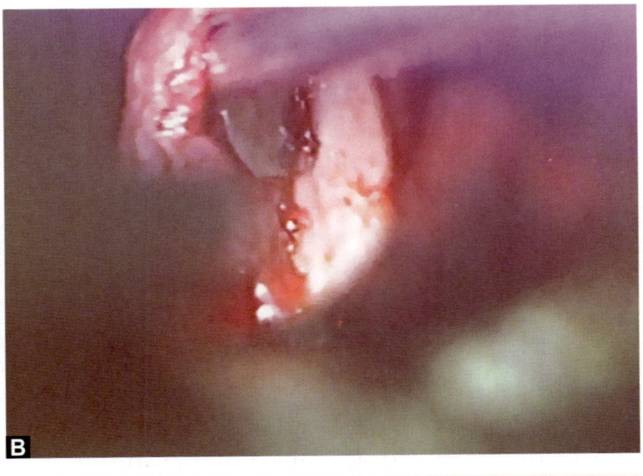

Fig. 10.3A and B: Elevation of tympanomeatal flap

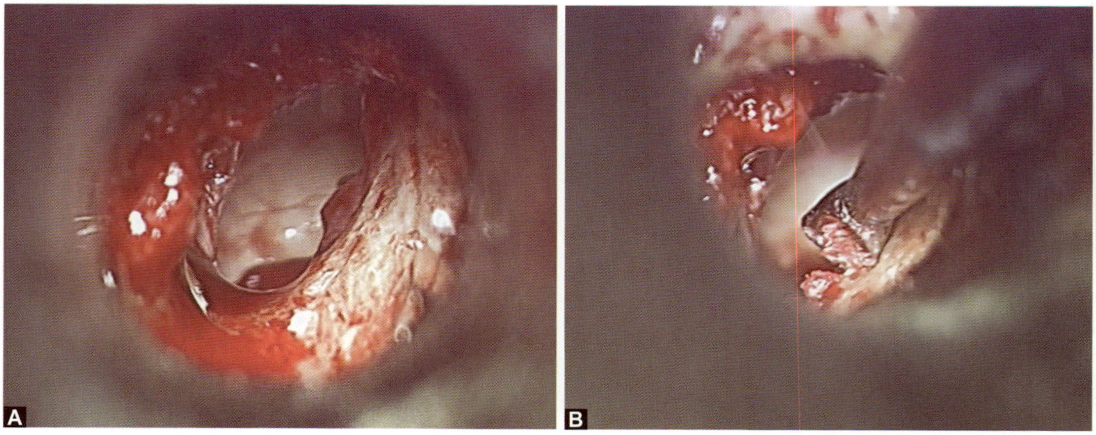

Fig. 10.4: (A) Tympanomeatal flap elevated with exposure of middle ear, (B) posterior over hanging meatal wall is curetted

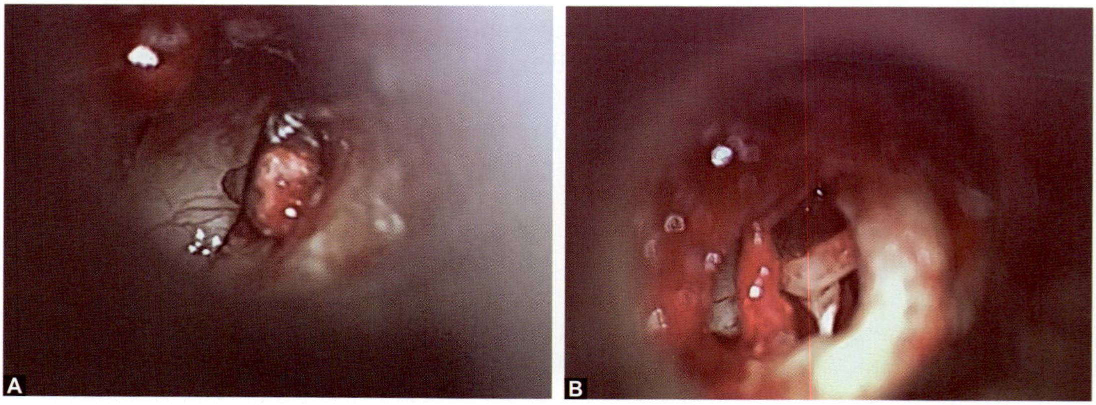

Fig. 10.5: (A) Long process of incus & chorda tympani exposed and (B) chorda has been retracted inferiorly to expose incudostapedial joint and stapedius tendon

Sufficient bone should be removed to expose the pyramid and stapedius tendon, the stapedial footplate and part of the horizontal portion of the bony fallopian canal (Fig. 10.6). Before approaching the stapes it is important to have complete hemostasis and to clear all bone chips from the middle ear and canal with a 20-gauge suction tip.

Now the head of the stapes is palpated to prove the clinical diagnosis of stapedial fixation. Look for the round window reflex. It is also important to palpate the incus and the malleus to rule out coexisting incudomalleolar ankylosis.

If any part of the stapes footplate is thin or bluish, a crack is made in the thin portion with a fine straight needle to allow introduction of a hook. The crack should be made before the removal of suprastructure to safeguard against the so-called floating footplate. The stapedius tendon is cut near its emergence from the pyramid (Fig. 10.7).

An incudostapedial joint knife separates the incus from the stapes. The suprastructure (head, neck and crura) of the stapes is then fractured by application of sidewise pressure to the head of the stapes using a Rosen's curved needle. At this point 10X magnification may be used. The stapes superstructure is removed using a fine alligator forceps.

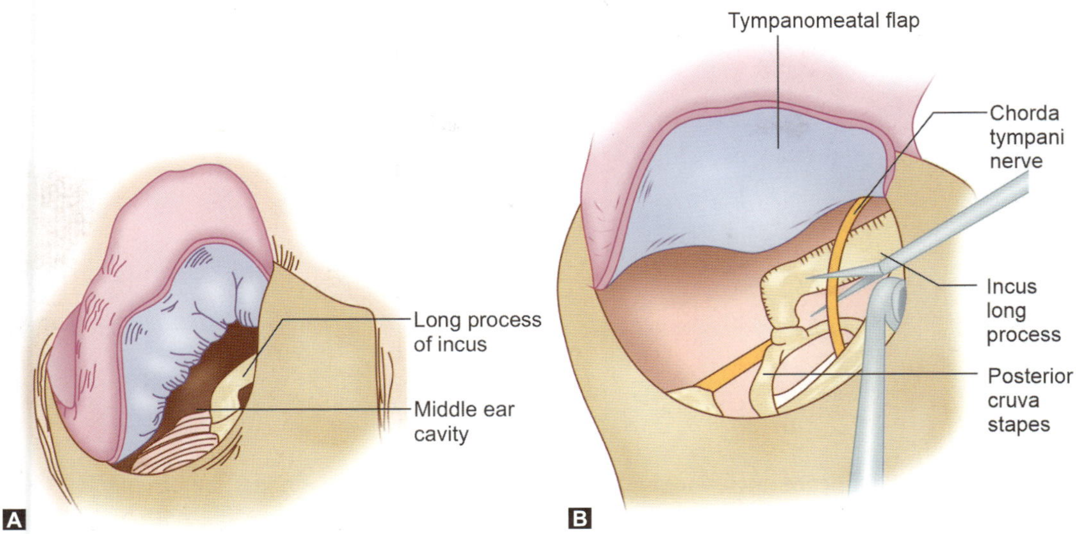

Fig. 10.6: (A) Exposure of incudostapedial joint, stapedius tendon, **(B)** Chorda is transected rarely if it prevent visualization of footplate

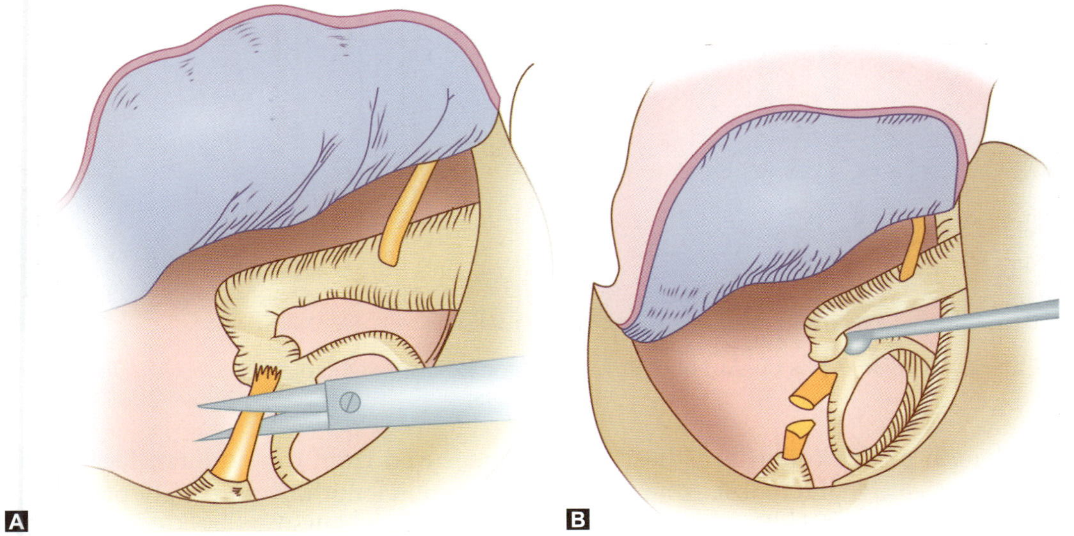

Fig. 10.7A and B: Transected chorda tympani nerve and stapedius tendon

It is best to leave the mucosa over the footplate intact to keep the fragments of the footplate in their original positions and thus prevent them from falling into the vestibule. A footplate 'hoe' or stapes hooks are often used to remove fragments of the footplate. The instrument tip should pass well under the footplate and catch only its edge.

A dry field is necessary in the oval window, careful suctioning with a 24 gauge suction tip is to be done. The tip should not be placed directly over the oval window. It is also important to decrease the force of suction. The stapedectomy is completed by total removal of the footplate which can be done with stapes hook. Sealing of the oval window is done now using temporalis fascia/vein graft (Fig. 10.8).

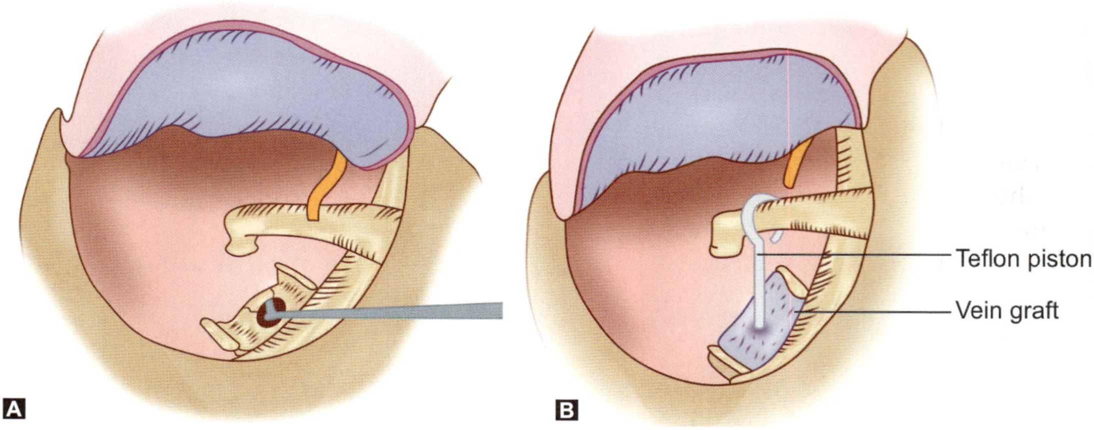

Fig. 10.8A and B: Stapedotomy window that has been covered with vein graft before placing the teflon piston

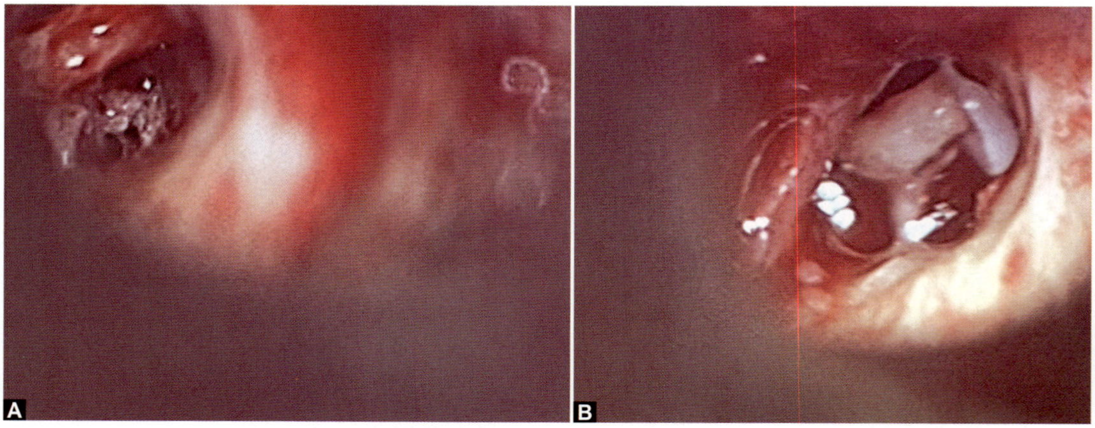

Fig. 10.9: (A) Footplate being opened and **(B)** Teflon piston *in situ* after footplate is covered with gelfoam

The length of the Teflon prosthesis is now measured from the undersurface of the lenticular process to the footplate and is usually 4 mm in length. Accordingly prosthesis is hooked on the long process of incus and placed on the oval window seal (Fig. 10.9). The teflon piston is crimped onto the long process of incus using a serrated crocodile forceps.

Stapedius tendon preservation technique and small fenestra stapedotomy: Here after exposure of incudostapedial joint stapes suprastructure and footplate, the posterior crura is drilled first, while preserving the incudostapedial joint and stapedius tendon. This exposes the posterior half of the footplate. A 7 mm skitter or regular drill is used to make a hole on the footplate. Finally anterior crura is removed while preserving the rest of the suprastructure, incudostapedial joint and the stapedius tendon.

Now the measurement is done between the footplate and long process of incus to determine the size of the prosthesis as described under stapedectomy. Teflon piston is resized as per the measurement, keeping 0.25 mm extra length. Then the piston is introduced and fixed as described under stapedectomy.

If the surgery is being done under the general anesthesia the use of nitrous oxide should be discontinued at this point as it may diffuse into the closed tympanic cavity after the tympanomeatal flap has been replaced. The tympanomeatal flap is replaced and three or four small gelatin sponge pieces are placed over the line of the incision. The meatus is being subsequently packed lightly with several large pieces of sponge.

When the stapes footplate is obliterated by dense over growth of otosclerotic bone this should be reduced with extreme care, by gentle anteroposterior strokes, with a slow rotation 1 mm cutting. The bone dust is removed periodically with suction irrigation. When the footplate has been thinned to a blue condition, it can be manually penetrated and partially removed, as in the standard procedure.

Laser Stapedectomy (Fig. 10.10)

Small fenestra stapedectomy surgery for fixation of the footplate is an operation that should be performed with laser. The concentrated heat energy produced by a laser can selectively vaporize unwanted tissue with minimal trauma in a virtually bloodless field (Perkins et al, 1992). There are currently two lasers approved by the Federal Drug Administration for otology surgery whose wave lengths fall in the visible electromagnetic spectrum. They are the argon laser (514 nm) and the KTP-532 laser (nm).

Risk Factors during Stapedectomy (Hammond, 1976)

1. **Age:** Young child with inherent risk for middle ear infection
2. **Occupation:** People working with environment of repeated barometric pressure changes.
3. **Noise exposure**
4. **Anesthetic risk**
5. **Second ear surgery:** Should be avoided after successful 1st ear surgery due to increase risk of late sensorineural hearing loss.
6. **Unilateral otosclerosis:** Serious disability in relation to individual's occupation
7. **Revision surgery:**
   a. In case of perilymph fistula
   b. Recurrence of conductive hearing loss

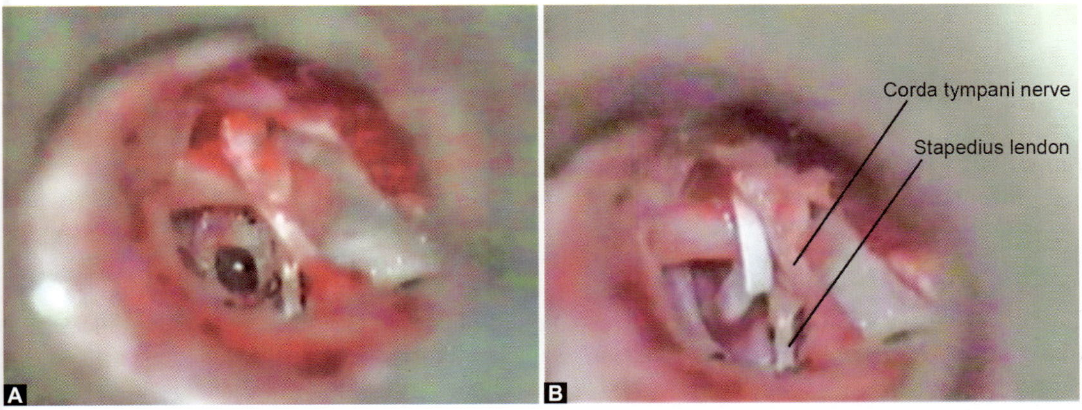

Fig. 10.10: Opening made in the footplate after vaporization of crura with laser. The teflon piston is inserted through the opening in the footplate and is fixed to the long process of the incus. Note the chorda and stapedius tendon have been preserved

Stapedectomy in the Temporal Bone

Practice in the temporal bone laboratory is a fundamental part of ontological training. Performing stapedectomy on a normal temporal bone is handicapped by the mobility of the footplate. A simple method of producing stapes footplate fixation in a normal temporal bone has been described by NJ Murrant and DJ Gatland (JLO Sep 1989). Here, using a large cutting burr, a superior labyrinthotomy is fashioned by drilling at a point where the line IAM bisects the line running back from GSPN to the AE. This allows entry to the vestibule via its roof, exposing the medial surface of the stapes footplate. The vestibule is sucked dry. A drop of superglue is placed on a fine piece of wire and then used to apply a fine coating of adhesive to the medial aspect of the vestibulostapedial joint. The mobility is rested and if need be further glue be applied. This produces a fixed footplate without disturbing the middle ear contents. The bone is repositioned and stapedectomy carried out in the normal fashion.

REFERENCES AND FURTHER READING

1. Menie`re P. De l'exploration de l'appareil auditif, ou recherches sur les moyens prospres a` conduir au diagnostic des maladies de l'oreille. Gaz Med Paris 1842;10:114–7. Surgery of the Ear, Michael E. Glasscock and George E. Shambaugh 1990.
2. Kessel J. U¨ ber die Durchschneidung des Steigbu¨gelmuskels beim Menschen und u¨ber die Extraction des Steigbu¨gels resp. der Columella bei Thieren. Arch Ohrenheilkd 1876;11:199–217.
3. Jenkins GJ. Otosclerosis: certain clinical features and experimental operative procedures. Trans XVIIth Inter Congr Med London 1913;16:609–18.
4. Lempert J. Improvement of hearing in cases of otosclerosis: a new one stage surgical technique. Arch Otolaryngol 1938;28:42–97.
5. Rosen S. Principle of stapes surgery. AMA Arch Otolaryngol. 1960;71(2):182–87.
6. Shea JJ, Shea PF, McKenna MJ. Stapedectomy for otosclerosis. In: Surgery of ear, Glasscock-Shambaugh. 5th edition. 2003. p. 547–75.
7. Bansal M. Teflon Vs Titanium implant in stapes surgery. Indian J Otolaryngol Head Neck Surg. 2016 Mar; 68(1): 16–19.
8. *Portmann*, M, and Claverie, G. "*Interposition*" in *Otosclerosis*, Otolaryngology 31:421–428, 1959.
9. Marquette J. Le syndrome de surdite du a une deficience de la prothese stapedienne: Comptesrendu s du Con gres de la Soci ete Francai se d'oto-rhino-laryngologie 1965:151–60.
10. Causse J.R.,: Present problems in the surgery of otosclerosis: The Journal of Laryng. Otol., 79/4: 265–199, 1965.
11. Causse J.B. and Causse J.R. (1984) Technique for otosclerosis. Am. J. Otol. 5, 392–96.
12. Schuknecht, Harold F. (1971): Stapedectomy. Little Brown and Company,Boston
13. Ishiyama A, Glasscock ME. Total stapedectomy. Operative Techniques in Otolaryngology-Head and Neck Surgery, 1998; 9:1, 3–7
14. Wayoff MR, Moeller RB, Roche R. A new and safe remomoval of stapes in dropped footplate. Eye Ear Nose Throat Mon 1971; Jul;50(7):246–8.
15. Leek JH: An anomalous facial nerve: The otologist's albatross. Laryngoscope 1974;84:1535–44.
16. Atlas of Ear Surgery, Andrew W. Miglets, Michael M. Paparella, William H. Saunders 1990.
17. Diseases of Nose, Throat, Ear, Head and Neck. 14th edition. John Jacob Ballenger.1991
18. Stapes surgery for Otosclerosis, Victor Goodhill. 1961
19. Hammond V. Indications for stapedectomy.The journal of Laryngology and Otology , Vol. 90, 23–30, Jan. 1976.
20. Perkins, *et al*. Laryngoscope 1992;102:1321–27.

Chapter

11

Myringoplasty

Suresh Pillai • Ajay Bhandarkar • Dipak Ranjan Nayak

Historical Perspective

Hippocrates, the father of medicine (450 BC), had observed that "pain around the ear with continued strong fever is to be dreaded for man may become delirious and die"[1]. So the importance of ear infections and their prompt treatment was known 2500 years ago.

The first attempt to close a perforated tympanic membrane was by Marcus Banzer[2] in 1640 when he used the pig's bladder for covering the defect. The next big development in myringoplasty occurred when Toynbee placed a rubber disc over a silver wire to cover a perforation which resulted in hearing improvement.[3] Then in 1853, William Wilde described the steps for a cortical mastoidectomy for ear sepsis and ear suppuration. The postauricular incision is named after him.

The first attempt at closure of a tympanic membrane perforation was by Berthold in 1878 when he de-epithelialized the outer layer of the tympanic membrane and grafted it with skin from the forearm.[4] He coined the term "myringoplasty" for this procedure.

The 20th century saw a sea of change in otology with the advent of antibiotics and the operating microscope and better designed instruments. Wullstein coined the term tympanoplasty in 1953, along with Zollner, for reconstructing the middle ear hearing mechanism using skin graft. But the disadvantages of the skin graft led to complications. Storrs publishing his study on the use of temporalis fascia in 1961. This was the culmination of 100 years of evolution of otologic surgery to tackle tympanic membrane perforations and hearing loss.

Various techniques of myringoplasty were described in order to improve the hearing results like overlay and underlay myringoplasty.[5–9] Both have their advantages and disadvantages.

Classification of Myringoplasty

Myringoplasty techniques are classified, based on placement of graft in relation to lamina propria of drum remnants and fibrous annulus, into the following types:

I. Overlay

Graft is placed over (lateral to) the annulus and medial to handle of malleus was popularized by Sheehy (1967)[7] (Fig. 11.1).

II. Underlay

Graft is placed below (medial to) the annulus (Fig. 11.2) (described originally by Shea and Tabb)[8,9]

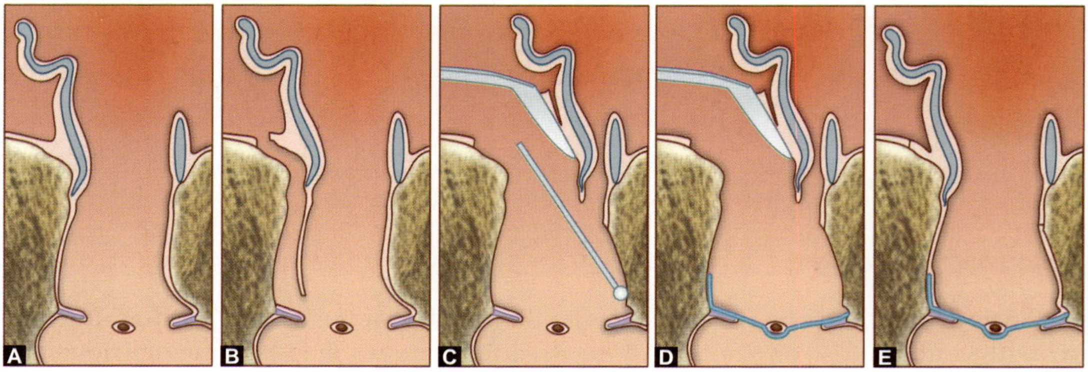

Fig. 11.1: Onlay technique of myringoplasty: **(A)** Perforation of the tympanic membrane; **(B)** Postauricular incision given and posterior canal wall skin (vascular strip) being raised and exposing posterior tympanic annulus; **(C)** Anterior canal skin being elevated and removed along with removal of skin over the entire annulus; **(D)** Graft placed over fibrotympanic annulus; **(E)** Placement of anterior canal wall skin and reposition of vascular strip over the graft (From original illustration done by Dipak R Nayak, Textbook of ENT)

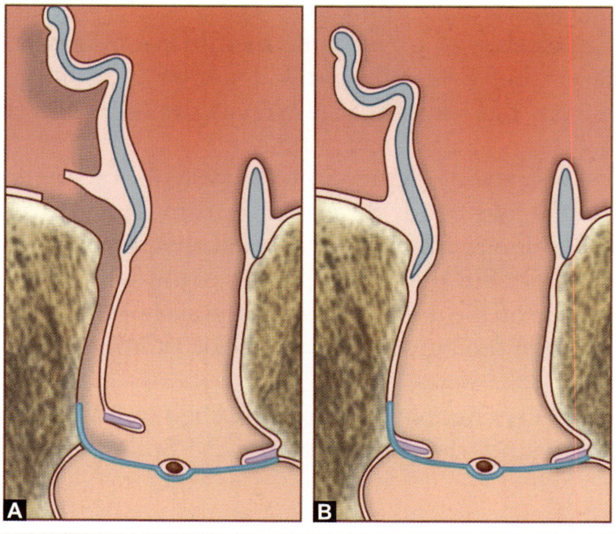

Fig. 11.2: **(A)** Tympanomeatal flap along with annulus elevated and mucosa underneath removed and the graft placed under tympanic annulus after raising tympanomeatal flap and **(B)** graft placed under tympanic annulus and tympanomeatal flap repositioned (from original illustration done by DRN, Textbook of ENT)

III. Interlay

This technique has been describe recently in early 90s. In interlay, the graft is placed between mucosa of the middle ear and annulus.[10,11]

This technique is very difficult technique to start and learn for a beginner. Hence one need to master underlay / onlay technique or both before starting with interlay technique. In this chapter the first two techniques will be described in details as follows.

1. Onlay Myringoplasty (Sheehy's Technique of Graft Plcement)[7]

Steps of Onlay Technique

- Infiltration of postauricular area and 4 quadrant infiltration in the ear canal with 2% lignocaine with 1:100000 adrenaline (Figs 11.3 and 11.4).
- Postauricular Wilde's incision 5 mm from postauricular groove with extension superiorly to take the graft (Fig. 11.5).
- **Temporalis fascia graft harvestation:** In cadaver the graft has to be harvested from the temporalis muscle before soft tissue from the temporal bone is removed (Fig. 11.6).

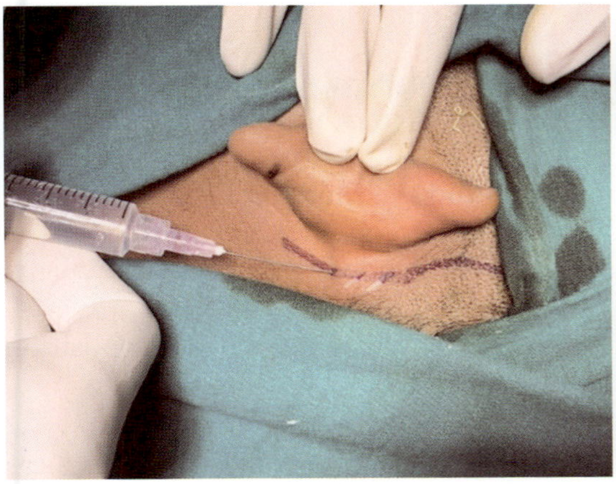

Fig. 11.3: Postauricular incision mark and infiltration

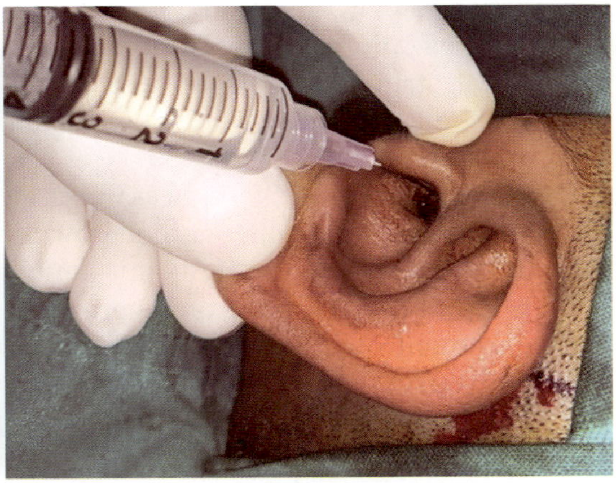

Fig. 11.4: Infiltration into anterior canal wall

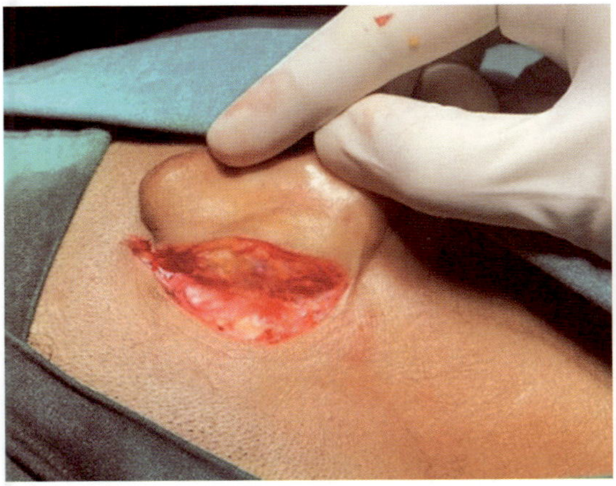

Fig. 11.5: Postauricular incision

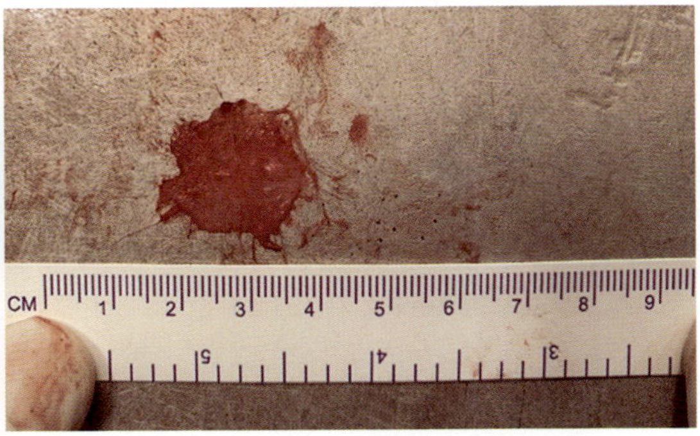

Fig. 11.6: Harvested temporalis fascia graft

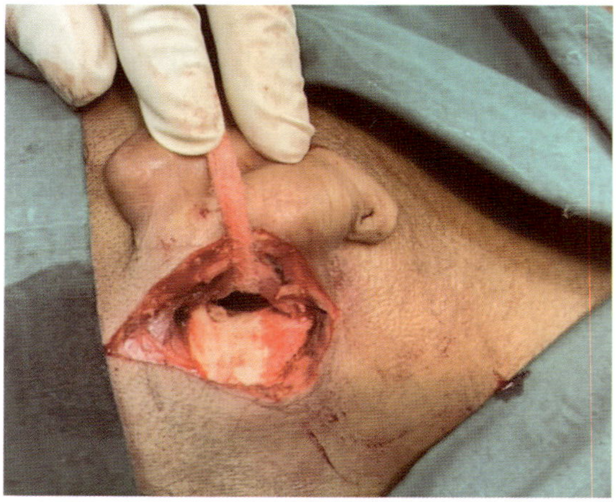

Fig. 11.7: Elevation of periosteal flap and securing of vascular strip

- Elevation of periosteal flap with anterior retraction of pinna (Fig. 11.7).
- De-epithelization of perforation margins.
- Vascular strip elevation, posterior canal wall skin between tympanosquamous to tympanomastoid suture line, which corresponds to 1 o' clock to 7o' clock position in right ear (Fig. 11.7).
- Removal of anterior canal skin as free graft (Figs 11.8 and 11.9) and reducing the anterior and posterior canal wall overhang by doing canalplasty (Fig. 11.10A and B).
- Graft placement on fibrotympanic annulus while tucking under the handle of malleus or its remnant depending on its presence (Fig. 11.11A).
- Replacement of free anterior meatal skin graft and vascular strip back in position (Fig. 11.11B).
- Packing of canal with gelfoam and umbilical tape. Then insertion of ear wick.
- Closure in three layers (periosteum, muscle with subcutaneous and skin), and application of mastoid dressing.

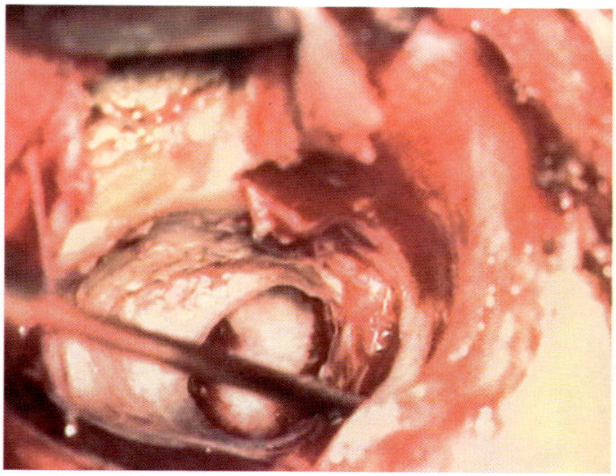

Fig. 11.8: Exposed posterior bony meatal wall after vascular strip have been secured between tympanomastoid suture line to tympanosquamous suture line

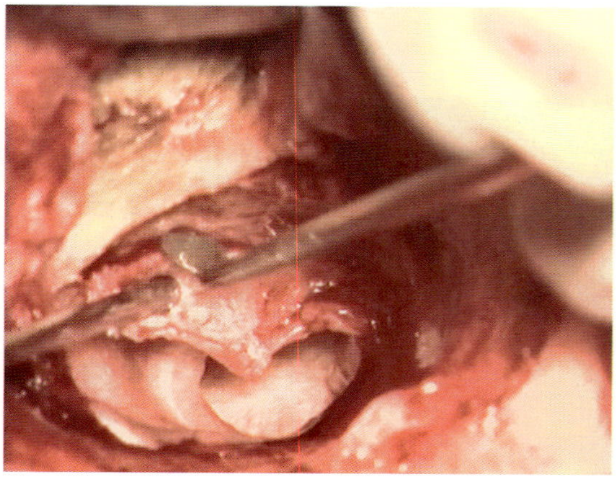

Fig. 11.9: Elevation of remaining anterior canal skin as a free graft from the annulus and anterior canal wall

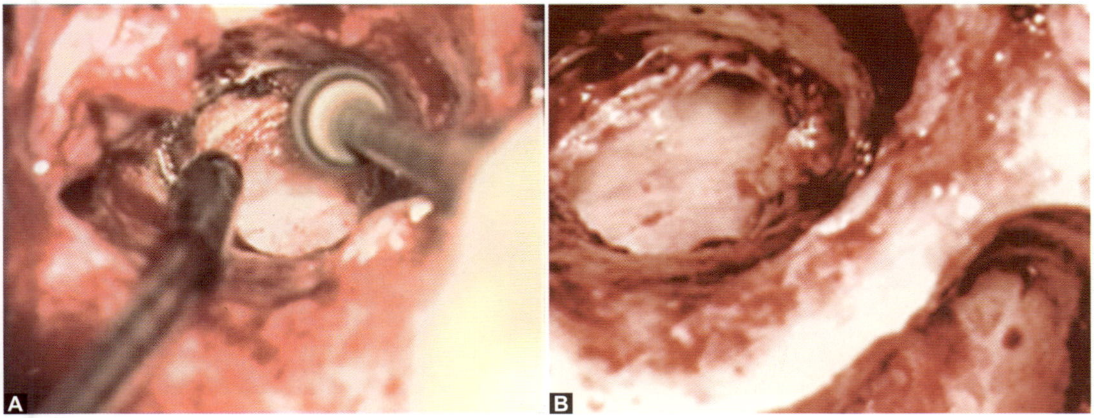

Fig. 11.10: **(A)** Canalplasty to remove anterior and posterior bony overhang and **(B)** clear view of entire annulus after canalplasty

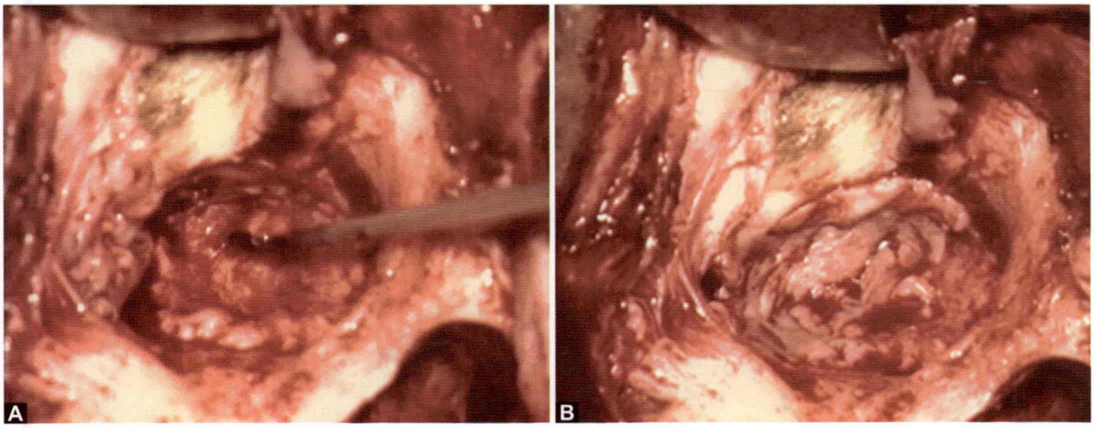

Fig. 11.11: **(A)** Graft placement done over tympanic annulus and underneath the malleus handle and **(B)** anterior canal wall skin replaced *in situ*

2. Underlay Myringoplasty (Shea, 1957 and 1960)

Steps of Underlay Technique

- Infiltration of xylocaine and adrenaline as in onlay technique
- Margins of tympanic membrane perforation are freshened.
- A circumferential incision is given on the posterior meatal wall from 6 to 12 o' clock position, 3 to 4 mm lateral to annulus (Fig. 11.12).
- Two lateral radial incisions given along tympanomastoid and tympanosquamous suture lines. This flap is elevated with a flap elevator and preserved as vascular strip (Fig. 11.12).
- Postauricular skin and periosteal incision given 5 mm posterior to postaural groove. Same incision can be extended upwards to procure the temporalis fascia graft.
- Anterior canal wall retractor is placed for reflecting the lateral posterior meatal wall skin as vascular strip and the periosteal flap (Fig. 11.13).
- Freshning of the edge of the perforation with a sickle knife/pick and scraping the mucosa from the under surface (Fig. 11.14)

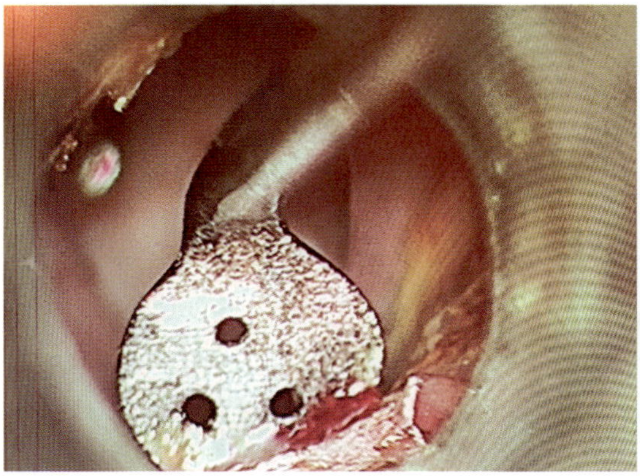

Fig. 11.12: Elevation of vascular strip with circular knife transmeatally

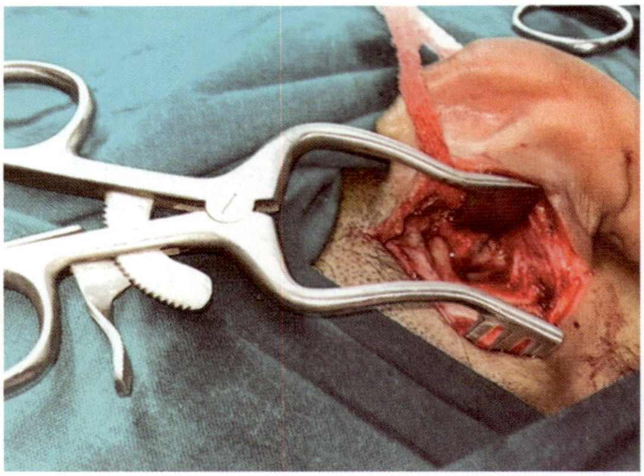

Fig. 11.13: Application of canal wall retractor after securing the vascular strip with a ribbon gauge

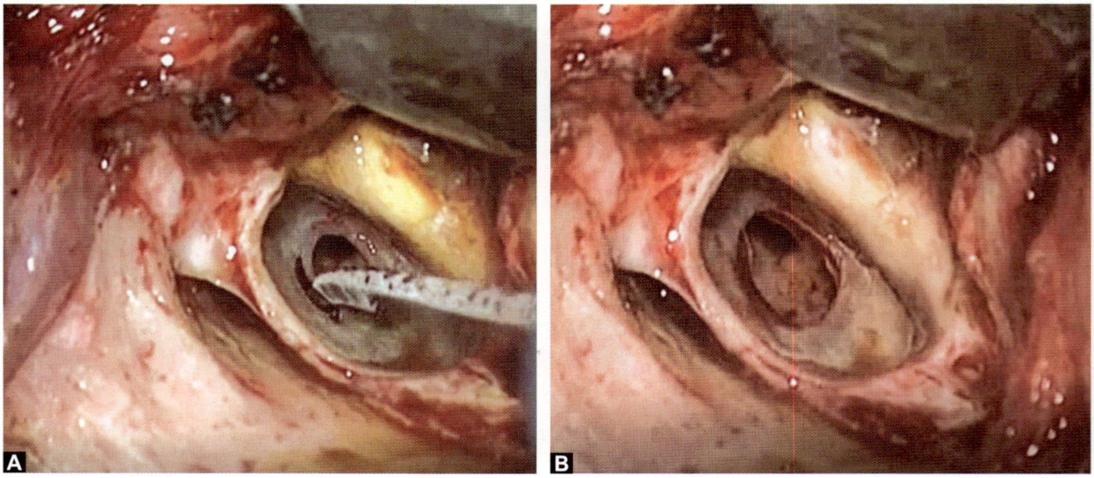

Fig. 11.14: **(A)** Perforation margin is freshened with a sickle knife by removing a cuff of epithelium and **(B)** After the perforation margin is freshened

- Tympanomeatal flap is elevated along with the annulus, taking care not to injure chorda tympani, long process of incus, handle of malleus. This elevation of meatal wall may requires two medial radial skin incisions (Figs 11.15 and 11.16).
- Temporalis fascia graft is placed medial to the handle of malleus covering the perforation. This requires support of graft by pieces of dry gel foam (Fig. 11.17)
- Tympanomeatal flap is repositioned on the graft (Fig. 11.18).
- Gelfoam is packed in deep meatus to support the tympanomeatal flap over the graft (Fig. 11.19).

3. Interlay Technique

- After the initial steps as in onlay and underlay technique, the tympanomeatal flap elevated up to the annulus, preserving the superior attachment near malleus head.

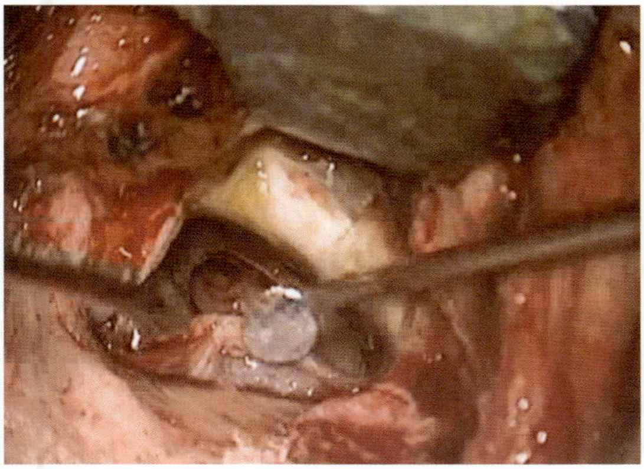

Fig. 11.15: Elevation of tympanomeatal flap

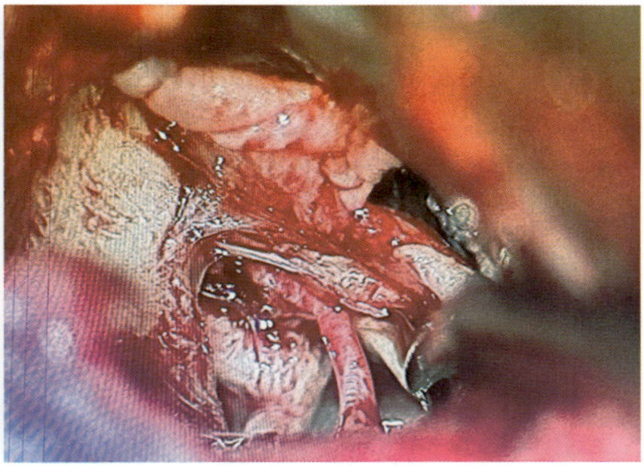

Fig. 11.16: Examination of mesotympanum and incudostapedial joint and separated chorda under magnification after reflection of the tympanomeatal flap

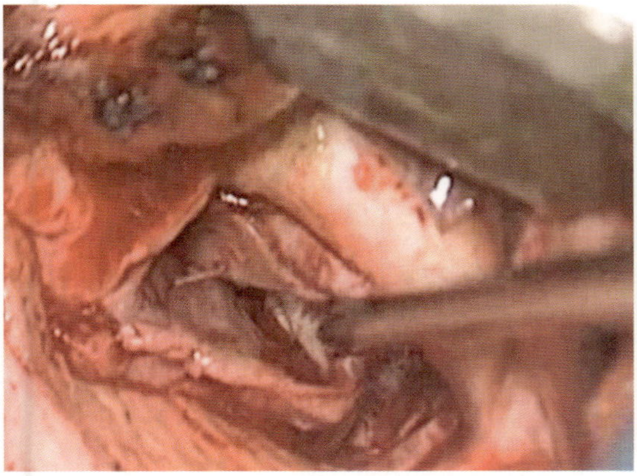

Fig. 11.17: Before the replacement of tympanomeatal flap the graft has been placed medial to handle of malleus and the annulus to cover the perforation

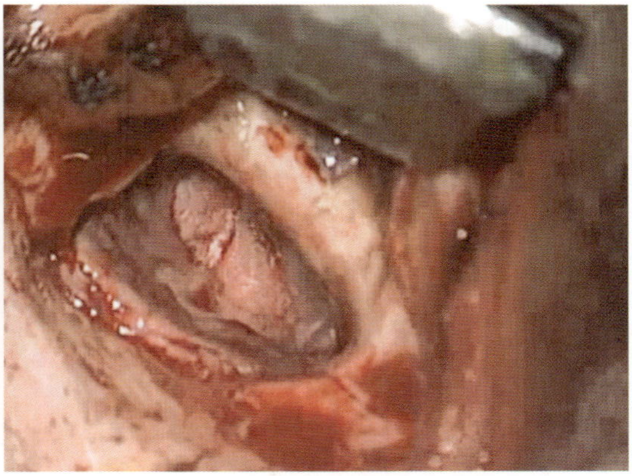

Fig. 11.18: Tympanomeatal flap returned back in place after graft placement

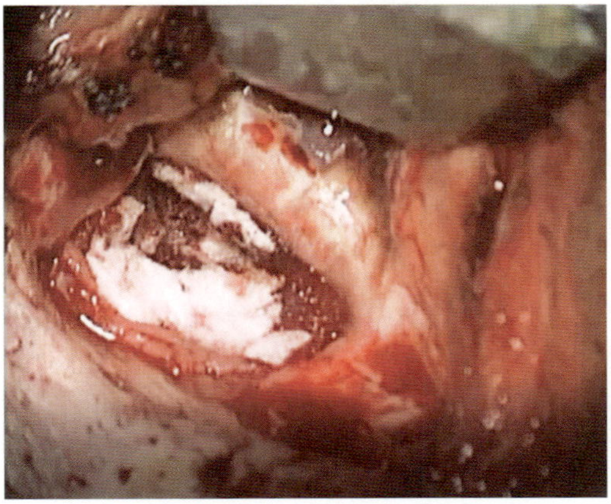

Fig. 11.19: Graft is secured with gelfoam

- Then the dissection starts at the annulus to separate from the bony sulcus and mucosa by separating it from the annulus by lifting the fibrous annulus and squamous epithelium and remnant tympanic membrane.
- Ossicular mobility and pathology checked
- Preserved temporalis fascia harvested at the beginning of surgery placed above the mucosal layer and underneath the annulus and remnant tympanic membrane (Fig. 11.20A and B).

Final Steps

This is common for all the three types of myringoplasty:

- **Lateral posterior** meatal wall flap (vascular strip) is replaced, canal is then packed with gelfoam and medicated umbilical tape/merocel wick (Fig. 11.21).
- Postauricular wound is closed in layers. Mastoid dressing is applied (Figs 11.22 to 11.24).

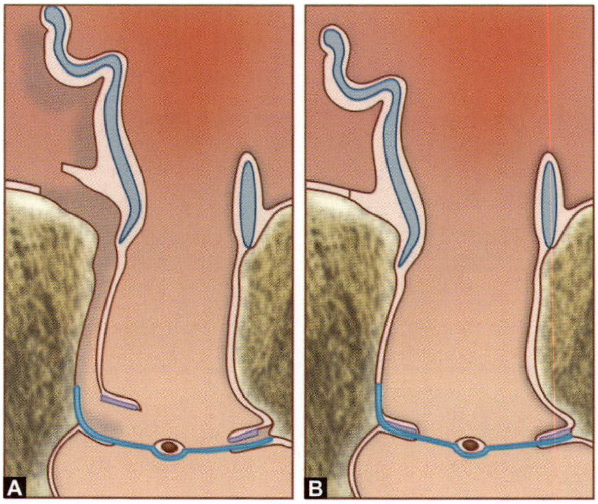

Fig. 11.20: (A) Tympanomeatal flap along with annulus elevated and mucosa underneath separated from the annulus preserved. **(B)** The graft placed over the preserved mucosa and the tympanic annulus with remnant tympanic membrane and tympanomeatal flap repositioned

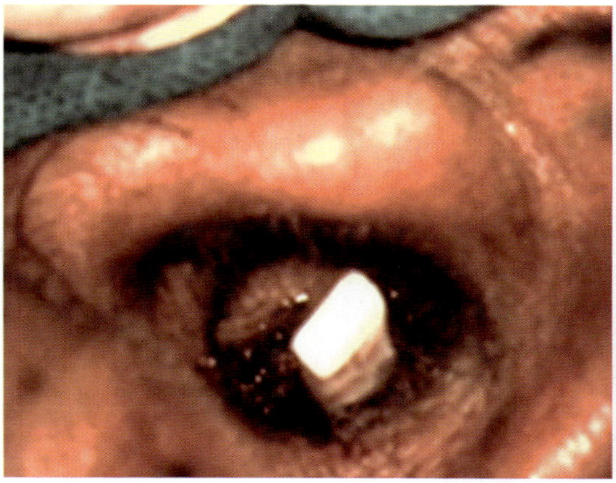

Fig. 11.21: Wick is placed in the external auditory canal

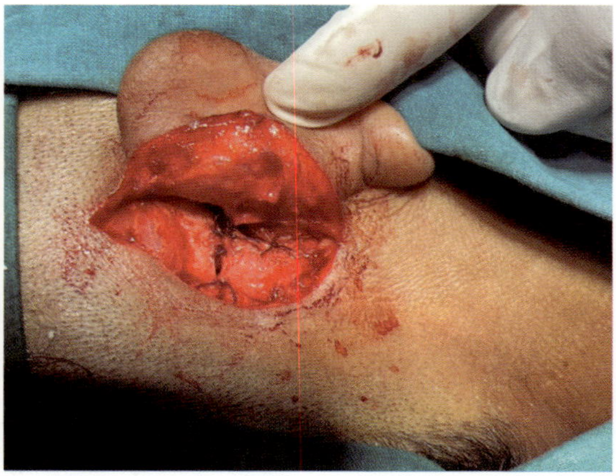

Fig. 11.22: Suturing periosteum

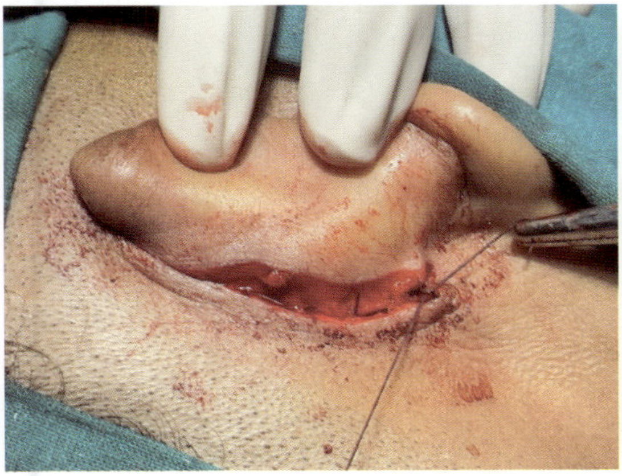

Fig. 11.23: Suturing subcutaneous and muscle layer

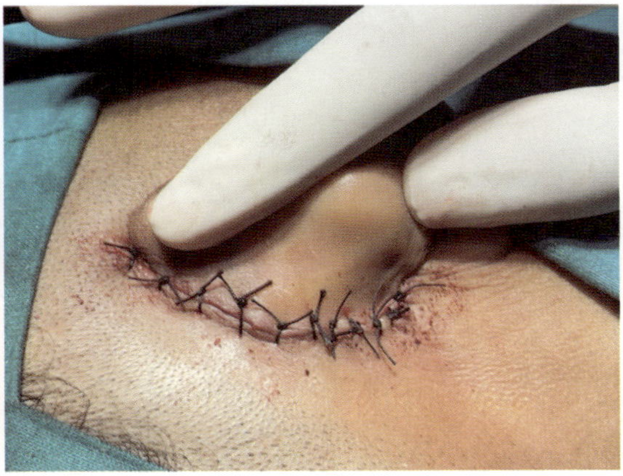

Fig. 11.24: Suturing skin

REFERENCES

1. Sarkar S. A review on the History of Tympanoplasty. *Indian J Otolaryngol Head Neck Surg.* 2013; 65: (suppl 3): 455–60.
2. Feenstra L, Kohn F E, Feyen J. The Concept of an Artificial Tympanic Membrane. *Clin Otolaryngol.* 1984; 9: 215–20.
3. Toynbee J. On the Use of an Artificial Membrana Tympani in Cases of Deafness Dependent Upon Perforation or Destruction of the Natural Organ. 1853. Churchill and Sons.
4. Berthold E. About myringoplasty. Wien Med Blatter. 1878; 26: 627–39.
5. House WF. Myringoplasty. *Arch Otolaryngol.* 1960;71:399–404.
6. House, WF, Sheehy, JL. Myringoplasty. Use of ear canal skin compared with other techniques. *Arch Otolaryngol* 1961; 73: 407–15.
7. Sheehy, JL, Glasscock, ME. Tympanic membrane grafting with temporalis fascia. *Arch Otolaryngol* 1967; 86: 391–402.
8. Shea JJ., Jr Vein graft closure of eardrum perforations. *J Laryngol Otol.* 1960;74:358–362. doi: 10.1017/S002221510005670X.
9. Tabb HG. Closure of perforations of the tympanic membrane by vein grafts. A preliminary report of twenty cases. *Laryngoscope.* 1960;70:271–86.
10. Komune S, Wakizono S, Hisashi K, Uemura T. Interlay Method For Myringoplasty. *Larynx Auris Nasus.* 1992;19(1):17–22.
11. Hay A, Blanshard j. The anterior interlay myringoplasty: outcome and hearing results in anterior and subtotal tympanic membrane perforations. *Otol Neurotol.* 2014 Oct;35(9):1569–76.

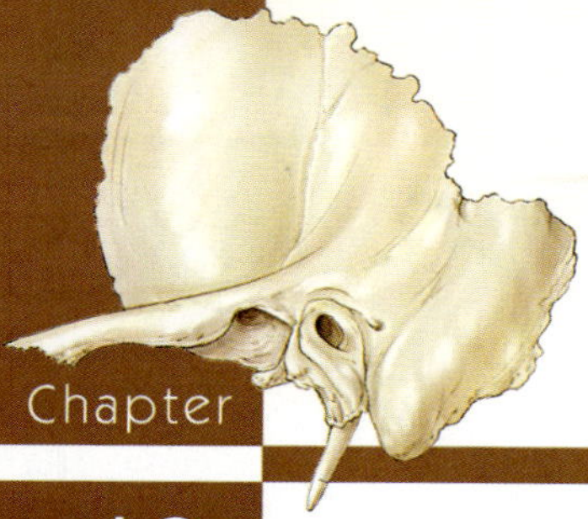

Chapter

12

Tympanoplasty and Ossiculoplasty

Produl Hazarika • P Satyanarayan Murty • Dipak Ranjan Nayak • Smruti Swain

Introduction

Tympanoplasty refers to the surgical procedure involving the reconstruction of the tympanic membrane and the ossicular chain. When the ossicular system pathology is addressed or is reconstructed alone, the term "Ossiculoplasty" is used. Chronic suppurative otitis media is one of the most prevalent diseases worldwide affecting the children with associated sequlae of hearing loss (Verhoef et al, 2006, Aarhaus et al, 2015). The main cause of hearing loss is due to perforation in the tympanic membrane. Ossicular pathology including discontinuity or both. Mucosal type of disease is frequently associated with drum perforation while squamous type of disease is commonly associated with ossicular pathology. Some author use the term 'mastoido-tympanoplasty' for intact canal wall mastoidectomy with tympanoplasty (Yang et al, 2010, Hazarika et al, 2018).

Historical Perspective

Banzer 1640 has first attempted at repair of a TM perforation using pigs bladder as a lateral graft with temporary improvement in hearing.[1] Berthold (1878) coined the term myringoplasty and placed cork plaster against TM to remove epithelium and then applied a full thickness skin graft. This procedure was popularized by Zollner and Wellston in 1956. Storrs in 1961 introduced the use of temporalis fascia grafting by underlay technique which was originally described by Shea in 1957 by using a vein graft. House1961, Glasscock and Sheehy, 1967 developed and refined techniques for lateral grafting (overlay). Tympanoplasty is a safe and effective procedure to treat diseases of the middle ear while restoring the hearing mechanism (Herhoeff, 2006). Ossiculoplasty was first described by Hall and Ryztner (1957) using autologous incus. The term 'Tympanoplasty' was first used in 1953 by Wullstein. This refers to any surgical procedure involving reconstruction of tympanic membrane/ossicular chain. The term 'Myringoplasty' is inter changeable with the term 'Tympanoplasty without ossicular reconstruction' and is described under chapter myringoplasty.

Physiologic Considerations

As sound waves travel from air to water/fluid medium 99% of energy is reflected at the air-water interface. This might be true in the case of ear also, if there was no middle ear ossicular chain. This prevents most of the sound energy being reflected. This transformer function of middle ear is accomplished primarily by the "Hydrolic Effect", which is the ratio between the area of tympanic membrane and the stapes footplate (17:1). The 17 to 1 hydraulic ratio times the 1.3 lever ratio yields a total increase of pressure level at the oval window 22 times. This is termed as sound pressure transformer ratio of normal human ear. The 22 times increase of pressure equals 26.8 dB. The "round window" function as a relief door which moves to and fro with the vibratory movement of cochlear fluid column.

A perforation of tympanic membrane removes the sound protection from the round window with a tendency for sound to reach both windows at nearly the same moment and thus cochlear fluid movements will be less.

A small perforation, for example, which still isolates round window from direct sound stimulation results in less than 30 dB conductive deficits. But a large perforation with no round window protection disrupts the hydraulic effect and a conductive deficit more than 30 dB is produced. In a total perforation there is loss of 40–45 dB, and in ossicular discontinuity or fixation behind an intact drum, up to 60 dB losses occur. The frequencies involved in the hearing loss are influenced by the perforation. In a small perforation low frequency loss occurs.

Tympanoplasty—Classification

Zollner (1955) and Wullstein (1956) classified tympanoplasty into five types (Fig. 12.1) and a sixth type was added later as describe by Gracia-Ibanez (1959). Thus the tympanoplasty types can be described as follows:

Type I

Perforated tympanic membrane with normal ossicular chain. The procedure includes inspection of the middle ear cleft with closure of the perforation (myringoplasty). The details of procedure have been described under.

Type II

Sound transmission through a functioning but deformed ossicular chain, e.g. erosion of the malleus.

Type II is modified to include any reformed mechanism joining the tympanic membrane with stapes footplate which retains a lever advantage. Thus there is type II a which is the original type II reconstruction. Type IIb is malleus stapes assembly or malleus footplate assembly. Type IIc is a new reconstruction independent of the malleus.

Type III

Destruction of the tympanic membrane and ossicular chain but intact and mobile stapes. Tympanic membrane graft is kept in contact with the stapes head. It also gives sound protection to the round window (columella tympanoplasty, Sheehy, 1987).

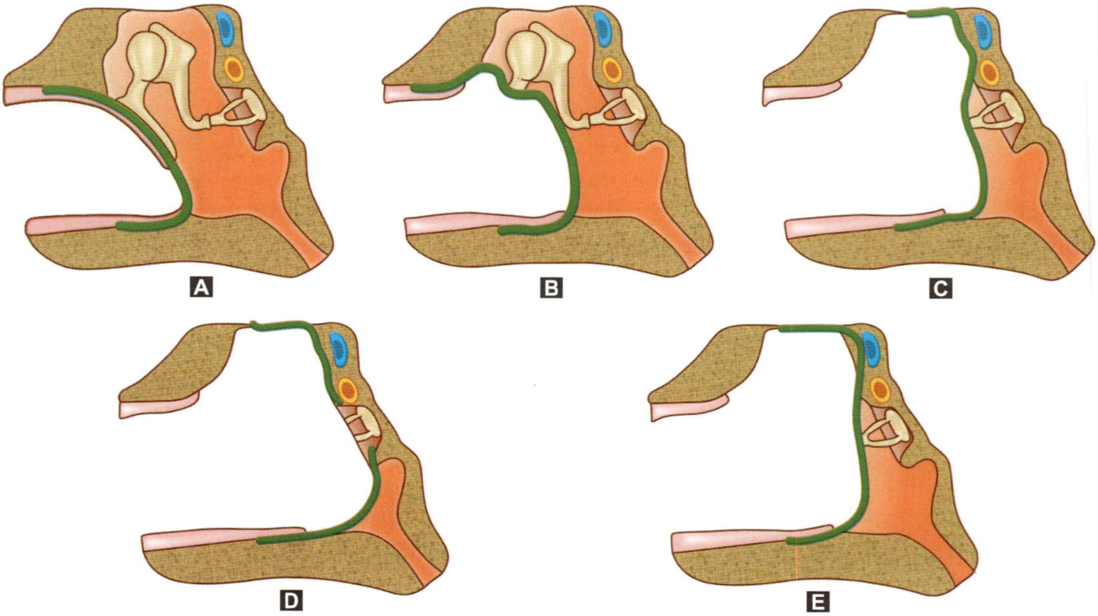

Fig. 12.1: Wullstein's tympanoplasty type: **(A)** Type I, **(B)** Type II, **(C)** Type III, **(D)** Type IV, **(E)** Type V

Type IV

Head, neck and crura of the stapes are missing; only a mobile footplate remains. Sound protection of the round window, is given by putting a graft from ET to round window, where mobile footplate of the stapes is left exposed. (Oval window or cavum minor tympanoplasty, Sheehy 1987).

Type V

Here the footplate is fixed. Fenestra is made to the horizontal semicircular canal. A graft seals off the middle ear to give sound protection to the round window.

Type VI

Sono Inversion

Here the round window is left exposed to the direct impact of sound waves. Mobile footplate is protected by a small tympanic air space in continuity with the eustachian tube.

Farrior's Classification of Ossiculoplasty

Farrior proposed the following type of tympanoplasty according to the basic pathologic anatomy at the completion of surgery rather than classifying them according to the method of reconstruction used.

- **Type I:** Reconstruction of a new eardrum. Ossicular chain is intact and mobile.
- **Type II:** Reconstruction of the new eardrum in its natural position.
- **Type III:** Reconstruction of the new eardrum on top of upright freely mobile stapes.
  - Type III: Classic.
  - Type III IG: Incus graft.

- Type III IGM: Incus graft to malleus
- Type III MG: Malleus head graft
- Type III BG: Bone graft
- Type III PORP: Partial ossicular replacement prosthesis

- **Type IV:** Reconstruction of a new eardrum and columella on footplate of stapes.
  - Type IV: Classic
  - Type IV IG: Incus graft
  - Type IV MG: Malleus graft
  - Type IV BG: bone graft
  - Type IV CG: Cartilage graft
  - Type IV TORP: Total ossicular replacement prosthesis
- **Type V:** Reconstruction of an eardrum either over a fistula in the horizontal semicircular canal or a new eardrum with a secondary fenestration of the horizontal semicircular canal. Saunders and Paparella (1973) modified the type V tympanoplasty and subdivided into:
  - Type Va: Fenestration of the horizontal semicircular canal
  - Type Vb: Stapedectomy in cases of tympanoplasty type IV with stapes fixation

Austin (1971) described the defects in ossicular chain and classified them based on anatomy:

Principle: Isolated loss of malleus handle (2% of ossicular defects) and isolated loss of stapes suprastructure 1.7% of ossicular defects were not classified because of their rarity.

Incus is absent in all cases and tympanic membrane repair required in all cases.

Common Ossicular Defects

Type a

When malleus handle and stapes suprastructure are present; after reconstructing the tympanic membrane defect, ossicular chain reconstruction is done from handle of malleus to stapes suprastructure with suitable cartilage, bone or partial ossicular replacement prosthesis.

Type b

Handle of malleus absent. Stapes suprastructure are present requiring reconstruction of the tympanic membrane, handle of malleus and incus.

Type c

Handle of malleus present. Stapes suprastructure absent, requiring reconstruction of the tympanic membrane and reconstruction of the ossicular chain from the handle of the malleus to stapes footplate.

Type d

Handle of malleus absent, stapes suprastructure absent requiring reconstruction of the tympanic membrane and handle of malleus, incus and stapes suprastructure.

Rare Ossicular Defects

Type e

Isolated loss of malleus handle requiring reconstruction of the tympanic membrane and malleus, removal of incus and its reconstruction

Type f

Isolated loss of stapes suprastructure requiring reconstruction of the tympanic membrane and stapes suprastructure

Type g

Malleus handle present. Incus and stapes fixed.

Type h

Malleus handle and incus absent and stapes fixed.

Procedure

It is important to learn mastoidectomy through temporal bone dissection as most of the pathologies are related to cholesteatoma. The details of the procedures are already described under cortical and modified/radical mastoidectomy. The steps have been highlighted below.

Important Landmark

Macewen's Triangle

This is a triangular area on the lateral surface of temporal bone. It is bounded above by superiorly—posterior root of zygoma (suprameatal crest), base is formed by posterosuperior margin of bony external auditory canal and posteriorly, the tangential line from posterior meatal wall, extending vertically upwards.

This area forms a cribriform appearance. The mastoid antrum lies about 15 mm from the surface (adult).

"Always proceed from one landmark to another".

- A straight cut is made along temporal line posteriorly with 6 mm cutting burr with constant irrigation and suction.
- A perpendicular cut to the first one outlining the bony posterior canal.
- Mastoid cortex removed in systematic saucerization method.
- The deepest penetration should be at the apex of first two cuts (Macewen's triangle) which leads to mastoid antrum.
- The horizontal semicircular canal is identified as the hard bone on the medial part. This gives a clue about further proceeding to fossa incudis, epitympanum anteriorly and superiorly. The external genu of facial nerve is anteroinferior to the lateral semicircular canal and while proceeding posteriorly, it stays close to the posterior semicircular canal (**described under cortical mastoidectomy**).
- Visualize incus. It stays superior and lateral to the facial recess. (Facial recess is a collection of air cells lying lateral to facial nerve at the external genu.)
- Landmark useful for exposing facial recess are external genu of facial nerve medially, fossa incudis superiorly, chorda tympani laterally

- With a diamond burr (2.5 mm) facial recess is thinned out. A small buttress of bone is left against the tip of incus.
- Identify chorda tympani and posterior aspect of facial nerve.
- Still smaller burr is used to open facial recess. Once it is opened, the mesotympanum is exposed. Pyramidal process, stapes suprastructure, incudostapedial joint, round window stapedius muscle are seen (**described under combined approach mastoidectomy**).
- Remove the buttress. It allows visualization of horizontal portion of facial nerve, tensor tympani, cochleariform process comes into the view. So also sinus tympani and subiculum (ridge of the bone separating sinus tympani from RW niche) can be seen. By extending the facial recess inferiorly hypotympanum, mesotympanum, etc. comes into better view.
- Exploring epitympanum: This discloses short process of incus, head of malleus, ossicular ligaments and horizontal portion of facial nerve. Anterior to head of malleus is epitympanic recess. It is common place for recurrent disease (cholesteatoma).
- Incudostapedial joint is now dislocated. Incus is removed. Head of the malleus is resected from the handle of malleus at its neck by using malleus nipper. The disease is now removed completely from the antrum, aditus, epitympanum, sinus tympanum and other areas of extension. Now various types of tympanoplasty can be performed based on the residual defect in the ossicular chain and the tympanic membrane.

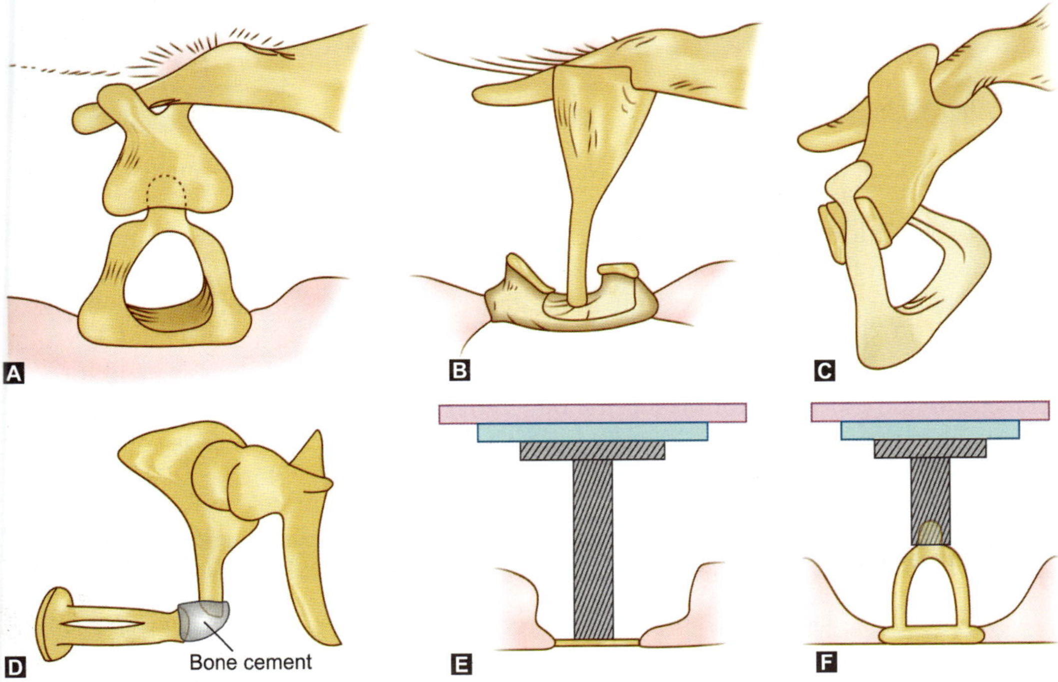

Fig. 12.2: Various types of ossiculoplasty: **(A)** Austin type A Incus transposition between malleus handle and stapes head, **(B)** Austin type between malleus handle and stapes footplate, **(C)** Incus transposition, **(D)** Reconstruction of eroded lenticular process with bone cement, **(E)** Total ossicular reconstruction prosthesis over stapes footplate, **(F)** Partial ossicular reconstruction prosthesis over stapes head

Ossicular Reconstruction

The following ossiculoplasty type can be practiced in a fresh cadaveric temporal bone. Incus transposition necessitate the removal of incus before reconstruction. The incus should be free from disease like cholesteatoma. Then it is sculptured with the help of a diamond drill as per requirement and then transposed between stapes head and malleus handle or stapes footplate and malleus handle depending on the status of ossicular chain. If remnant incus is not suitable, septal cartilage can be harvested for reconstruction.

Recently bone cement is being used for lenticular process erosion in the absence of cholesteatoma (mucosal type of disease). Advantages of using bone cement maintains normal anatomy while closing the air–bone gap. It is also easy to perform and is quite cost effectiveness (Babu and Siederman, 2004).

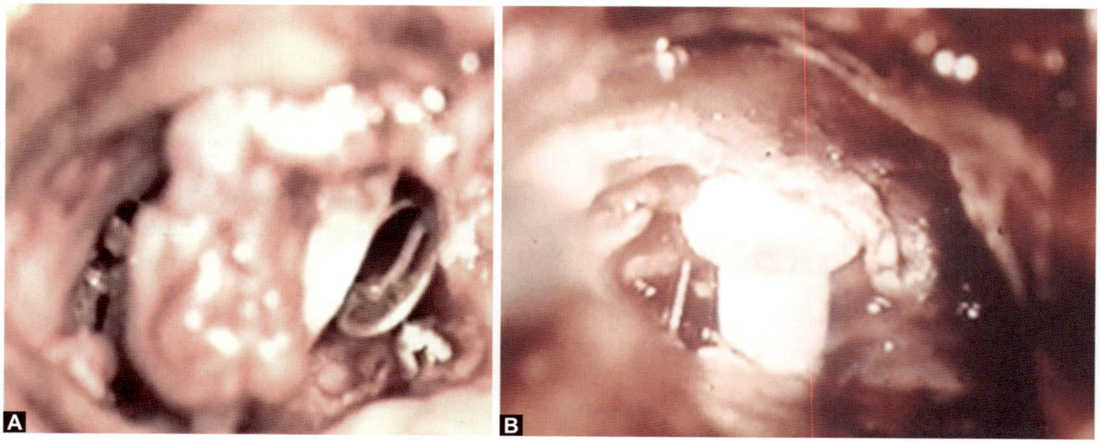

Fig. 12.3: Ossciculoplasty using **(A)** titanium PORP and **(B)** plastipore PORP

In case of canal down mastoidectomy for cholesteatoma surgery, both incus and malleus may needs to be removed. In such cases partial ossicular and total ossicular replacement prosthesis can be used with good air bone gap closure. Various materials including titanium (Fig. 12.3A), hydroxyapatite and plastipore (Fig. 12.3B) partial and total ossicular prosthesis are available. These prosthesis require additional cartilage augmentation to prevent extrusion especially for plastipore than hydroxyapatite (House and Teufert, 2001). Titanium is a satisfactory material for use in ossicular reconstruction because of its ease of insertion, tissue tolerance, and low rate of extrusion (Martin and Harner, 2004).

REFERENCES

1. Yang L, Jian-jun S, Dan-heng Z. The technique of mastoidotympanoplasty with epitympanoplasty in the treatment of cholesteatomatous otitis media,2010; 8 (3): 254–54.
2. Hazarika P, Punnose SE, Victor J, et al. Evaluation of the hearing results after mastoido-tympanoplasty operation with or without ossiculoplasty: A percentage change versus absolute change; a different methodology. *Ind J Otol* 2018; 24 (3): 148–56.
3. Aarhus L., Tambs K., Kvestad E., Engdahl B. (2015). Childhood otitis media: a cohort study with 30-year follow-up of hearing (The HUNT Study) Ear Hear, 2015; 36 302–08.
4. Verhoeff M., van der Veen E. L., Rovers M. M., Sanders E. A., Schilder A. G. Chronic suppurative otitis media: a review *Int J Pediatr Otorhinolaryngol*, 2006; 70, 1–12.

5. Sarkar S. A review on the History of Tympanoplasty. *Indian J Otolaryngol Head Neck Surg*. 2013; 65: (suppl 3): 455–60.
6. Berthold E. About myringoplasty. Wien Med Blatter. 1878; 26: 627–39.
7. Gracia-Ibanez L. [Mobilization, fenestration and a new audio surgical system: sonoinversion] *Arch Ital Otol Rinol Laringol*. 1959;70 (Suppl 40):68–81.
8. House WF. Myringoplasty. *Arch Otolaryngol*. 1960;71:399–404.
9. House, WF, Sheehy, JL. Myringoplasty. Use of ear canal skin compared with other techniques. *Arch Otolaryngol* 1961; 73: 407–15.
10. Sheehy, JL, Glasscock, ME. Tympanic membrane grafting with temporalis fascia. *Arch Otolaryngol* 1967; 86: 391–402.
11. Glasscock ME. Tympanic membrane grafting with fascia: overlay vs. undersurface technique. *Laryngoscope*. 1973;83:754–770. doi: 10.1288/00005537–197305000-00011.
12. Zollner F. The principles of plastic surgery of the sound-conducting apparatus. *J Laryngol Otol*. 1955;69:637. doi: 10.1017/S0022215100051240.
13. Wullstein H. Theory and practice of tympanoplasty. *Laryngoscope*. 1956; 66, 1076–93. doi: 10.1288/00005537–195608000-00008.
14. Verhoeff M. Chronic suppurative otitis media: A review. *Int J Ped Oto* .2006; 70(1): 1–12.
15. Atlas of ear Surgery-Andrew W. Miglets, Michael M. Paparella and W. H. Saunders IV edition
16. Scoty Brown's Otolaryngology: V Edition: Otology.
17. Surgery of the ear-Michael E. Glasscock; George E. Shambaugh. IV Edition.
18. Babu S and Siederman MD. Ossicular reconstruction using bone cement. *Otol Neurotol*. 2004 Mar; 25(2):98–101.
19. House JW, Teufert KB. Extrusion rates and hearing results in ossicular reconstruction. *Otolaryngol Head Neck Surg*. 2001; 125(3):135–41.
20. Martin AD, Harner SG. Ossicular reconstruction with titanium prosthesis. *Laryngoscope*, 2004; 114(1):61–4.

Chapter 13

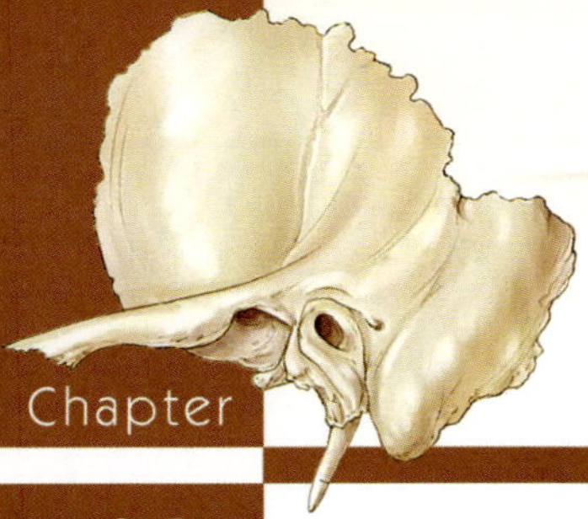

Historical Perspective and Principle of Cochlear Implant Surgery

Produl Hazarika • Dipak Ranjan Nayak • Manushrut

Introduction

A cochlear implant is a complex electronic device that facilitates severely or profoundly deaf patient to hear by receiving and processing sounds and speech. This achievement due to cochlear implantation with successful outcome is possible due to close cooperation between engineers and otologists who have developed this new technology to give hope and aspiration to the deaf child (Eshraghi et al., 2012).

Historical Perspective

Auditory perception from an electrical stimulation was first experienced in 1790 by Alessandro Volta, while passing current across his own head using batteries.[1] It was Djourno and Eyries whose study on auditory stimulation resulted in recognizing sound subsequent studies by Simmons with bipolar electrode stimulation producing sound with speech discrimination helped in establishing the foundation for Cochlear implant development in 1957. The cochlear implant was first introduced by William House initially in 1961 in two cases but discontinued because of infection (House, 1987). In 1976, William House reintroduced the cochlear implant in the same patient with a 4 channel one and later concentrated on developing a single channel cochlear implant device. In 1984, the 3M/House single channel cochlear implant had gained Food and Drug Administration approval. Graeme Clark and colleagues develop multi-channel prototype with an array of 20 electrodes, efforts that would later lead to the founding of Cochlear Ltd., a branch of Nucleus, manufacturer of heart pacemakers (Henkel, 2013). With development of multichannel device with multiple electrode implantation and better processing of signals it was possible to stimulate different parts of cochlea with better hearing outcome. A lot of evolution has taken place since then. Cochlear implant is an electronic device, which is used in profoundly deaf patients to electrically stimulate the cochlear nerve by placing single or multiple electrodes in the cochlea.

Cochlear implant is an electronic device, which is used in profoundly deaf patients to electrically stimulate the cochlear nerve.

There are single channel cochlear implants. Multiple electrode system is regarded to be better as it gives multichannel stimulation which provides more speech understanding.

Principle of Cochlear Implant Surgery

The cochlear implant can only be gained by the patients having loss of hair cell with residual viable auditory neurons. Patient those who have viable auditory neuron established by various auditory testing are good candidates for implant surgery (Brackmann, 1976). A cochlear implants have basically an external and internal part. The external part consists of a microphone, a speech processor and a transmitter coil. The internal part consists of a receiver stimulator. The microphone transmits the sound into voltage waveform. This voltage is applied to a speech processor which may be body worn or behind the ear via a small cable.

The speech processor filters the speech waveform into frequency bands. The output of the filters are referred to a map of the patient's electric current threshold and comfortable listening level for the individual electrode. Thus, a code is produced for the stimulus parameter. This code together with the power is transmitted to the implanted receiver stimulator by the external transmitter. This receiver stimulator directs current pulses to the appropriate electrode array lying close to the auditory fibers which lies close within the basal turn of cochlea. The current excites the auditory population of the auditory nerve fibers to stimulate the pattern of the auditory nerve activity in response to sound, thereby providing meaningful representation of speech and environmental sound.

How the Device Produce Hearing Sensation Step by Step

1. Sound is received by a microphone (1)
2. Sound is sent from microphone to speech processor(2)
3. Speech processor select and codes useful sounds
4. Code is sent to transmitter (3)
5. Transmitter sends code across skin to receiver (4)
6. Receiver stimulator converts code to electrical signals
7. Electrical signals are transmitted to electrodes array (5) to stimulate hearing nerve fibres
8. Signals are recognized as sounds by the brain, producing hearing sensation (6)

Hybrid Implants (Electroacoustic Stimulation)

The concept of hybrid implant or electroacoustic stimulation (EAS) was first described by Von Ilberg et al., 1999, attempt to preserve residual hearing in patients who had a stable, steeply sloping bilateral high frequency sensorineural hearing loss. These patients were not successful hearing aid users but at the same time, they did not qualify for a CI from an audiometric perspective. The EAS concept is characterized by insertion of a CI electrode into the basal turn of the cochlea, up to about the 1,000 Hz region at the maximum. The CI stimulates the high frequency region of the cochlea, while the built-in hearing aid stimulates the apical region using natural hearing, assuming residual hearing is preserved postoperatively.

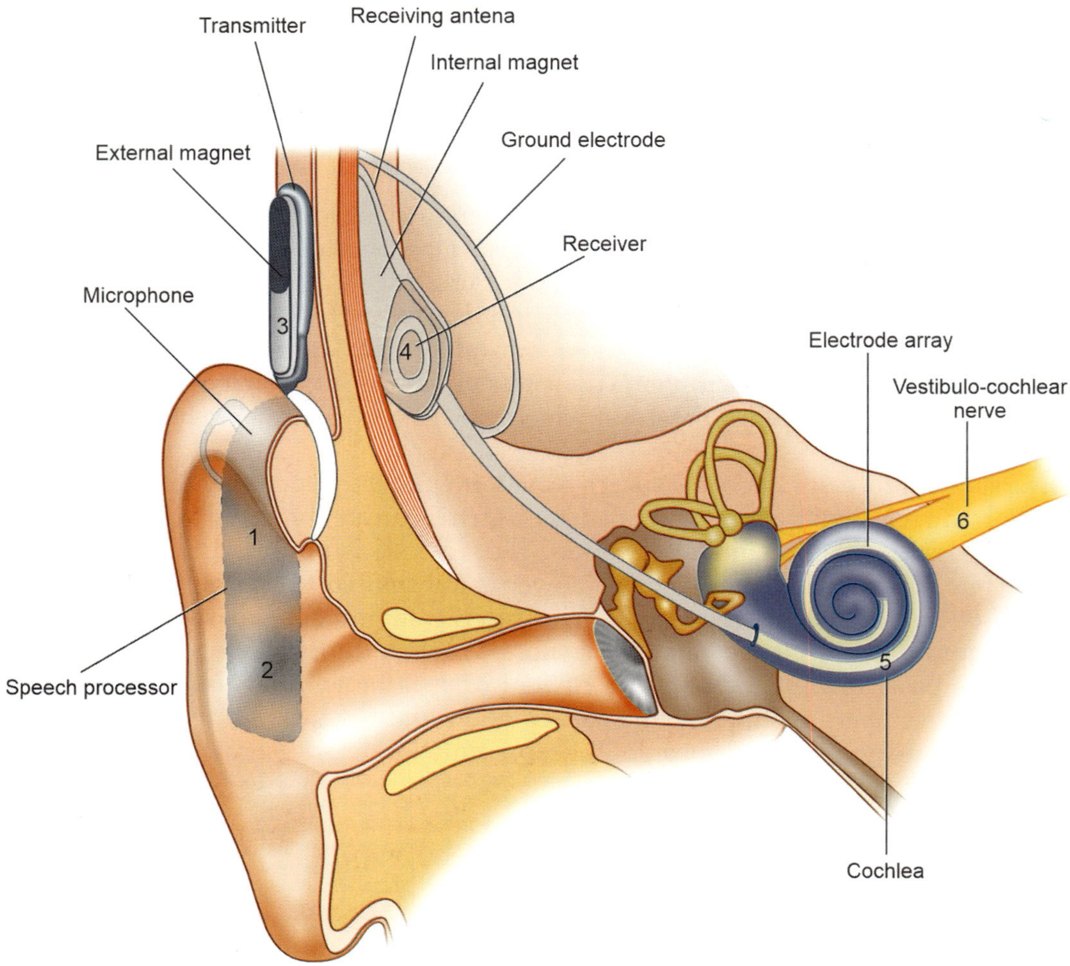

Fig. 13.1: Stepwise function of the cochlear implant device

Patient Selection

1. Congenital deafness
2. Acquired deaf adult patient with hearing loss of above 90 db that is postlingual deafness
3. Acquired profoundly deaf child with normal cochlear development. Implant between 2–4 years of age gives best result. Multichannel to be the best.
4. Postlingual profound deafness caused by meningitis is not a good candidate for cochlear implant. Meningitis initiates new bone formation leading to cochlear obliteration making insertion of electrode difficult.

Adults

a. **Acquired postlingually deaf:** This includes patients who became deaf after 12 years of age, when they have had the adequate experience to develop normal speech perception, speech productions and language skills. There is no age limit provided the selection criteria are met and patient's general condition permits an elective surgical procedure under GA.

b. **Acquired prelingually deaf and congenitally deaf:** 30% patients belong to this group. Patient is not accustomed to sound (promontory test useful) and has difficulty in understanding speech. Rehabilitation is very difficult and preoperative counseling of family members is very important.

Children

1. Age 1–17 years
2. Bilateral profound sensorineural deafness
3. None/little benefit from the conventional hearing aid
4. Psychologically appropriate
5. Adequate communication skills
6. Willingness of parents to participate in extensive rehabilitation program
7. Otologically stable

*US FDA has approved beginning of 12 months as eligible age for implant. Cochlea is adult sized at birth but only by 1 year are the mastoid antrum and facial recess, which provide access to middle ear for electrode implantation, is adequately developed.

Parental Counseling

1. To know the benefits, limitations and risks of implantation
2. Have realistic expectations for a given patient
3. To know the long term aspects including device failure/upgrade

Cochlear implantation is difficult to predict in children because:
- Takes long time for rehabilitation.
- Improvement in speech perception skills may not be obvious until they have been used for 1 year or more.
- Acquired postlingually deaf–commonest cause is meningitis. X-ray may show neo-osteogenesis is basal turn of cochlea.
- Congenitally deaf:
    - ***Acquired:*** Cochlea and auditory pathways normal, implant may not be a problem
    - ***Hereditary:*** Usually occurs during first trimester of pregnancy, abnormalities of otic capsule present, e.g. Mondini's—limited number of cochlear turns, Michel's–no development of cochlea

Evaluation, Assessment and Diagnosis

1. **Otological history:** To determine etiology of deafness
2. **Otological examination**
    - Congenital deformities to be ruled out
    - Ear must be free of infection/OME
    - Intact tympanic membrane
3. **Radiological examination**
    - High resolution, thin CT scan of cochlea:
        - Whether cochlea present or absent
        - Any congenital anomaly
        - Intracochlear neo-osteogenesis secondary to labyrinthitis
        - Any temporal bone fracture

- MRI
    - Clearly shows sclerosing labyrinthitis (loss of endo/perilymph signal)
    - Patency of cochlea

4. **Audiology**
    - Pure tone audiometry:
        - Profound SN loss >90 db at all frequencies
        - Inability to attain an aided (lip reading) speech detection threshold of 70 db SPL (53 db HL)
        - No speech recognition—speech score 0%
    - Other tests of sound recognition:
        - MAC (minimum auditory capabilities)
        - Speech discrimination test (poor score)
        - Evoked response audiometry (to make sure that no useful cochlear function exists)
        - Patient can also be compared to current implant users. Test scores of the best current implant subjects serve to establish upper performance limits
5. **Psychological**
    - To detect people with organic brain dysfunction, mental retardation, undetected psychosis or unrealistic expectations
    - Information regarding family dynamics and patient's milieu
6. **Other tests**
    a. ***Test for vision:*** Blindness severely affect the rehabilitation program
    b. ***Promontory stimulation test:*** On stimulation of promontory—patient fails to hear—(+) test. If test is positive—high chance of successful implantation
    Method:
        - Transtympanic, needle electrode kept on the promontory as close as possible to the round window membrane.
        - Reference electrode kept on the ear lobe/mastoid process.
        - DC current passed through a battery, optimum stimulus is a constant voltage/current, supplied in square wave bursts.
        - Subject hears the transition from anodal to cathodal current at the slower presentation rates.
        - BERA recording done (but problems such as massive artefacts and inconsistent responses occur).
    c. ***Round window stimulation test:***
        - Tympanotomy is performed and the active electrode is placed directly on the round window membrane.
        - BERA recording can be done simultaneously.
        - Useful in confirming the intactness of auditory pathways especially in prelingually deaf subjects.

Preoperative Counselling (to Correct Common Patient Misconceptions)

- Does implant provide recognizable speech? NO, sound is distorted and unlike their previous recollection of speech
- Does implant works better than a hearing aid in a noisy environment? NO
- Is implant less noticeable than a hearing aid? NO, speech processor looks like an old fashioned body worn hearing aid. However, recent speech processors are very small and attached with the microphone and similar to the hearing aid

- Is it true that once implant is fitted, no hospital visits are needed? NO, several visits are required to adjust the outputs to obtain the best speech processor setting/programs especially with multichannel devices. Maximum benefit is obtained after several visits. Any device breakages (broken leads, etc) requires revisiting the implant team at the hospital.

Surgical Implantation (For Details Discussed in Chapter 14)

1. Aim

- To embed the body of the implant in the skull
- To trail the electrodes via the mastoid through a posterior tympanotomy, to the round window and then to the cochlea.

2. Steps

Head is shaved in a wide margin around the intended incision

- **Incision:**
  - Aim is to provide coverage of the external portion of the implant package while preserving the vascular supply of the postauricular flap.
  - Although several types of incisions and periosteal flaps have been described in the past but have been discontinued due to associated complications. A lazy 'S' incision with elevation of skin and soft tissue posteriorly and creation of a superiorly based musculoperiosteal flap details described in Chapter 14.
- **Marking for the implant bed:** This is done and marked after initial marks done with the template (described in Chapter 14) and it varies with the type of implant used.
- **Cortical mastoidectomy:**
  - Edges overhang, not saucerized (so the electrode snugly fits)
  - Horizontal semicircular canal and fossa incudis with short process of incus identified
- **Posterior tympanotomy**
  - Facial recess exposed using fossa incudis as initial landmark (boundaries of facial recess superiorly fossa incudis anterolaterally-chorda tympani posteromedially—facial canal)
  - Facial canal is thinned down till facial nerve is seen through the bone (pink in live individuals, white in cadaver)
    - If the posterior tympanotomy is done too laterally annulus gets damaged, and betadine from external meatus appears (Betadine sign)
    - Various facial nerve anomalies should be kept in mind:
      i. *Dehiscence—Commonest (55%):* Majority in the tympanic segment (91%), where the commonest site is above the oval window (83%); and 9% in the mastoid segment. In 26% it protrudes from the canal, opens into the facial recess in 79% and in sinus tympani in 21%.
      ii. *Abnormal routing*
        - Overhangs oval window (narrow niche/conductive hearing loss) due to impingement on the stapes.
        - Passes through stapedial arch (confused with stapedial artery).
        - Passes between oval and round window.
        - Passes lateral to annulus (mastoid portion): <5%.
        - Passes over the promontory anterior to round window.

iii. *Branching of nerve/absence of nerve*
 - These anomalies are common in patients who have other congenital anomalies of temporal bone / external ear
 - Use of intraoperative facial nerve monitoring is ideal
 - Knowledge of known variations in facial nerve anatomy is very essential (Ogawa and Sando; Ann Otol Rhinol Laryngol 91: 33–60, 1982)

> Note: Round window niche is visualized through the facial recess, 2 mm inferior to the stapes. (Occasionally it is placed posteriorly, not visualized clearly).

 - Advantages of posterior tympanotomy approach:
   - Direct access aids surgeon in successful preparation of round window niche for electrode.
   - Allows surgeon to open the round window with limited damage to intracochlear tissues.
   - Surgeon's view through the opening in the facial recess provides an unobscured view down the scala tympani. This is particularly important in cases where neo-osteogenesis has occluded the scala. A small diamond burr can be used to drill an opening 6 mm diameter, down the scala tympani.

- **Cochleostomy**
  - Cochleostomy created anteroinferiorly to the annulus of round window membrane. A small fenestra, slightly larger than the electrode to be implanted is developed.
  - A small diamond burr is used to 'blue line' the endosteum of scala tympani and the endosteal membrane is removed with small pricks. (This approach by passes the hook area of the scala tympani, allowing direct insertion of active electrode array.)
  - After insertion of electrode, the round window area is sealed with small pieces of temporal fascia or fat.
- **Round window**
  - Can be confused with a hypotympanic cell. Niche is kidney shaped, lying mostly in a horizontal plane, anterior portion is more vertical.
  - Arises from a bony annulus, inferomedial portion of this annulus projects as the crista semilunaris (scutum).
  - Can be opened by a central cruciate incision and scutum has to be drilled to visualize the interior of cochlea. If any doubt concerning the location of the basal turn / its patency, drill anterior lip around window to visualize the interior of the cochlea.
- **Electrode insertion**
  - Done smoothly without force.
  - Caution: At 8–9 mm depth, tip of electrode contacts the spinal ligament as it rounds the first cochlear turn (Clifford and Gibson, 1987).
  - Undue force at this point may buckle the electrode / force the tip through the basilar membrane. So if the electrode halts at this point, gently rotate it and progress slowly (e.g. the nucleus electrode can be inserted approximately 20 mm, the depth of penetration is according to the number of stiffening rings left outside cochlea.)
- **Sitting the body of the implant**
  - A circular area of the bone is removed from the skull around the initial sitting mark. The implant should have the external edge approximately 5 mm above the surface of the skull to allow the patient to site the transmitter coil. When the skull is thin,

an outer circle should be drilled completely down to the dura leaving a thin bone in the centre.

- On pressing the implant into position, the dura can be safely moved medially averting the need to have the implant sited too externally causing an obvious postauricular hump.
- The trail of electrodes leaving the implant should be sited in a bony groove leading to the mastoid, as this avoids movement, on a temporalis muscle contraction, which could eventually break the electrode.
- Several holes are drilled about the bony groove and around the bony overhang of the mastoid cavity to provide a means of placing sutures to secure the implant.

➲ **Closure**

- Periosteal layer is sutured together as described earlier, stabilizing the electrode assembly
- Drain not inserted (increases chances of infection)
- Do not use monopolar diathermy for hemostasis after ear electrodes are inserted

3. *Postoperative Care*

➲ Prophylactic board spectrum antibiotics for 7 days
➲ Labyrinthine sedatives
➲ X-ray mastoid and temporal bone to check position of electrodes

4. *Complications*

➲ Uncommon
➲ Can be minimized by careful preoperative planning and meticulous surgical techniques divided into:

a. *Immediate (mostly flap related)*
- Hematoma under skin flap
- Postauricular flap necrosis (wise to keep flap limbs broad)
- CSF leak, meningitis (due to dural tear)
- Facial palsy
- Gusher (of perilymph on doing a cochleostomy in Mondini's deformity)

b. *Long term*
- Increasing tinnitus
- Rare-facial twitching, numbness, persistent giddiness, taste disturbances
- Persistent perilymph leaks (House, 1985)

c. *Implant problems*
- Device failure—breakage of leads
- Leakage of body fluids into implants
- Electrical interference from nearby electromagnetic fields (House sigma system)

Rehabilitation

➲ Primary aim—to help individuals overcome the handicap of profound deafness by improving their overall communication function

- For the surgery to be totally successful, individual communication needs must be fulfilled. To date no implant can restore hearing to a normal function. Three weeks after surgery, the scalp flap has healed sufficiently to allow the implant to be activated.

- With first switched 'on', the dynamic range is minute (i.e. little difference between just hearing the sound and the sound becoming uncomfortably loud)
- During initial postoperative sessions, the current level which is most comfortable is determined for each channel
- In single channel devices, output is filtered to provide an even sensation, throughout the frequency range of the device
- Multichannel devices are more complex to program as the output range for every channel has to be set individually
- Once set, the channel in some complex to program as the output range for every channel has to be set individually
- Once set, the channel in some complex devices (e.g. nucleus), are tested to determine the rank order of pitch sensation
- Ideally, most apical electrode gives lowest pitch sensation while most basal electrode gives highest pitch sensation. This is rare clinically. Often several electrodes give exactly same pitch sensation or inappropriate pitches are encountered. This is a result of damage to the spiral ganglion cells by the primary pathology or during insertion of electrodes.
- These inappropriate electrodes are rerecorded/switched off
- Gradually over the following weeks, the dynamic range increases
- The average patient requires 8 programs, set at weekly intervals, before a final program is reached, at least after 2 months

Note: A program can suddenly change even some months after implantation

Protocols for Rehabilitation

Speech Tracking (Defillipo and Scot, 1978)

- A passage is read using materials appropriate for patient's skill level. The patient is required to repeat the words. If the patient gives a wrong response, the word is repeated and then if necessary, careful hierarchies of clues are given. The tester cannot proceed until the patient has repeated the correct word.
- Performance is measured as the number of words repeated during the 10 minute segment (typical session is two-minute segments).
- Results are compared with lip reading alone, lip reading plus audition and audition alone. Progress in each condition is charted over a period of time
- This procedure was selected for use in rehabilitation as it closely simulates running speech and appears to have good validity as a measure of receptive communication function.

Measurement of Threshold of Hearing for Pure Tones

- Done using the usual setting of the device
- Shows how the device performs across the frequencies and indicates its frequency limits

Speech Prosody Tests

- Shows, if the gross features of speech are perceived, such as distinguishing one versus two syllables, a male or female speaker, a stressed word in a sentence, etc.

Vowel and Consonant Recognition Tests

- Patient is given number of vowels or consonants by listening alone. He / she attempts to identity each sound which is charted, each response against the vowel or consonant given
- It gives indication of how many vowel / consonants can be detected using implants as also an indication of where the main error exists.

Closed Set Discrimination Tests

- Patient is given a list of alternative choices and the patient to distinguished between hood, heed, hide and hud; there is a 1 / 5 possibilty of guessing correctly or chance level is 20%

Open Set Discrimination Tests

- Open set means that the patient has no hope of guessing the answer, so the chance level is 0%
- Patient understands words / sentences without multiple answer formats / lip reading
- No contextural clues should be given
- True open-set speech discrimination (OSD) tests are:
  i. CID (Standard central institute of deaf) sentences and everyday open set sounds (e.g. dog barking, telephone ringing)
  ii. Monosyllable words and spondee recognition tests—these are the most difficult OSD tests.

Other Tests

a. Minimum auditory capabilities (MAC) battery
   - Vowel recognition
   - Familiar sounds
   - Spondee recognition
   - Monosyllabic word identification
   - Lip-reading testing
   - Monosyllabic trochee-spondee (MTS) test

b. 4-Choice spondee

c. NU-6

d. Iowa medical consonant and vowel recognition tests

e. Tests to know the hearing handicap
   - Denver scale of communication functions
   - McCarthy-Alpiner scale

Various Preliminary Cochlear Implant Programs

1. **University of California, San Francisco/Storz CI Program (1974):** Thirteen patients have been implanted with a four channel implant device, in a clinic trial sponsored by the Storz Instrument Company, of which ten patients have been fitted with external speech processor and transmitter. Eight have some OSD understanding and all ten demonstrate significant improvement in lip-reading with their device. UCSF also developed 16-channel CI with Clarion and electrode insertion tool for safe placement of eletrode.

2. **Vienna/Hochmair CI Program (1977–78):** Fifty six postlingually deaf patients have received either an intracochlear or an extracochlear CI (multichannel), that employee's broadband stimulation. 65% of users showed substantial improvement in aided speech understanding v/s lip-reading alone. 60% of postlingually deaf patients have achieved some open set understanding without lip-reading. (Founding of MED-EL)
3. **University of Melbourne/Cochlear Corp. (Nucleus) CI Program (1978):** The nucleus multichannel cochlear prosthesis has been implanted in over 100 patients. Speech discrimination improved greatly in most patients. Overall results are satisfactory (G. M. Clark)

REFERENCES AND FURTHER READING

1. Eshraghi AA, Gupta C, Ozdamar O, et al. Biomedical engineering principle of modern cochlear implant. The anatomical record, 2012; 295:1957–66.
2. Volta A. Asimov's Biographical Encyclopedia of Science and Technology. Doubleday & amp; Company; Garden City, New York: 1982. Historical records documenting the first galvanic battery, "*The Volta Column*." Circa 1800.
3. Djourno A, Eyries C. Auditory prosthesis by means of a distant electrical stimulation of the sensory nerve with the use of an indwelt coiling. *Presse Med.* 31. 1957;65(63):1417.
4. House LR. Cochlear implant: the beginning. *Laryngoscope*. 1987;97(8, pt 1):996–9973302573
5. House WF. Cochlear implants. *Ann Otol Rhinol Laryngol*. 1976;85(3, pt 2):(suppl 27) 1–93779582
6. Henkel G. History of cochlear implnt. ENT Today 2013. Retrieved from https://www.enttoday.org/article/history-of-the-cochlear-implant/
7. House WF (2011). The Struggles of a Medical Innovator: Cochlear Implants and Other Ear Surgeries: a Memoir; Better Hearing Institute
8. Brackmann DE. Cochlear implant: Basic principles. *Laryngoscope*, 1976; 86(3):373–88.
9. Von Ilberg C, Kiefer J, Tillen J, et al. Electrical-acoustic stimulation of auditory syatem. ORL, 1099; 61:334–340
10. De Filippo CL, Scott BL. A method for training and evaluating the reception of ongoing speech, *J Acoust Soc Am.* 1978 Apr;63(4):1186–92.
11. Ogawa A, Sando I. Spatial Occupancy of vessels and facial nerve in the facial canal. Annal Otal Rhinol Laryngol. 1982;91(14–57).

Chapter

14

Cochlear Implantation: An Overview

Shankar B Medikeri • Madhuri Gore • Rashmi A Deshpande

Introduction

A cochlear implant (CI) or bionic ear is a device, that is, surgically implanted in the cochlea. The implant bypasses the inner ear hair cells and stimulates the 8th nerve endings electrically. Due to the invasive nature of the implant, the considerable variability of performance of recipients, the high cost of the device, selection criteria for the cochlear implant is designed to identify and predict those that would benefit or have *favourable outcomes*. Over the years, improvements in implant technology, surgical techniques and (re) habilitation methods coupled with a greater understanding of hearing loss and related issues have led to an increase in recommendation of bilateral implantation and inclusion of those with multiple associated issues for implantation.

Appropriate selection is half the battle won, and thus all candidates must be carefully selected. A child or adult with hearing loss has other conditions related to structure and function, e.g. cochlear anomalies, facial paresis, visual impairments, sensory integration issues, autism, and related issues such as poor family support that impact outcomes. Hence all assessments are done by a team of professionals.

The following questions are asked during the selection process:

- What is the audiological status (sensitivity and perception)?
- Is the perception commensurate with the degree of hearing loss?
- Do electrophysiological tests tally with behavioural findings?
- What are the speech, language and communication skills?
- Are there any associated issues?
- What can be the expectations?
- What is the commitment from parents/family/spouse/caregiver?

Audiological assessment forms the basis to determine candidacy. The aim is to obtain a profile of peripheral and central abilities. Behavioural, physiological and electrophysiological tests are carried out to do the same. This information along with radiological evaluation helps to select the ear to be implanted (in case of unilateral implantation).

- **Status of hearing sensitivity and perception:** Basic audiological tests such as pure tone audiometry and speech perception tests give the degree and type of hearing loss and an understanding of the communication difficulties faced by the adults with hearing loss. Careful and meticulous assessment of the pure tone thresholds and recording speech perception scores help to choose the better ear to implant. These are especially important in the case of cochlear anomalies. Typically, candidates are those with severe to profound degree of hearing loss receiving inadequate benefit from hearing aids as recorded with low speech perception scores or inadequate language skills. Presence of tinnitus must be noted. Tinnitus may disappear after implantation or may continue. This factor must be discussed.
- **Is the perception commensurate with the degree of hearing loss?** Speech perception scores reveal the extent to which the candidate relies on hearing to process speech. Even with a profound degree of hearing loss, the ability to perceive temporal aspects of speech/sound will help the individual to speech read. Obtaining speech perception scores separately in auditory and audiovisual modes will give an understanding of auditory visual integration of patient. The ability to utilize acoustic and visual cues synergistically also depends partly on the consistent use of hearing aids. Hence, the use of a hearing aid is recorded as in hours of daily use and long-term use. Regular use of hearing aids indicates better neural preservation and is an indicator of family commitment. Aided audiogram and aided speech perception scores *separately* for each ear enable the appropriate ear to be selected. Audiologists pay special attention to aided threshold at 2 kHz. Insufficient amplification at 2 kHz, despite the presence of thresholds well within the speech spectrum in lower frequencies prevents the audibility of consonants and will cause a delay in speech and language acquisition, since meaning in speech is derived primarily from consonants. The benefit of hearing aids can thus be quantified in terms of thresholds and speech perception scores. A candidate with word perception score less than 40% is generally recommended for implantation if speech perception test can be administered.
- **Do objective tests tally with behavioural findings?** Objective measures are recorded through physiological and electrophysiological tests that help to diagnose auditory neuropathy spectrum disorder or confirm the degree of hearing loss in others. Physiological tests such as the immittance test indicate the status of the middle ear and the reflex pathway. Otoacoustic emissions indicate the status of outer hair cells in the cochlea. The use of auditory Brainstem response (ABR) with clicks and tone bursts or auditory steady state response (ASSR) confirms the configuration and degree of hearing loss. These tests are necessary given that implantation can be carried out on infants as young as 12 months.

The conduction of all these tests is a requirement for diagnosis and appropriate management. The presence of OAEs, ringing pattern of cochlear microphonics in ABR, enable identification of auditory neuropathy spectrum disorder (ANSD). Literature reports of variable outcomes in persons with ANSD with CI (Teagle, Roush, Woodard, Hatch, Zdanski, Buss, Buchman (2010). It is the presence of long latency responses (LLR) from the auditory cortex that confirm the signal reaches higher centers and establish candidacy for CI in these cases. Electrically evoked auditory brainstem response (EABR) or even the behavioural promontory test is indicated not only in ANSD, but in a few patients of long-standing deafness without intervention, as well as in cases of cochlear nerve deficiency (Dutt and Kumar, 2019).

- **Speech language and communication skills:** A comprehensive oromotor assessment is required. Children with sensorineural hearing loss may have associated structural defects such as cleft lip and palate, facial paresis that may be associated with dysphagia impacting outcomes. Speech of the child is an important indicator of hearing or the lack thereof. Speech quality reflects what the child hears. Quality of voice, vocalization, and communication are assessed formally or informally during play or therapy. A child who uses voice but has no consonants in repertoire often has an insufficient hearing in the high frequencies with hearing aid and would need an implant to allow greater access to sound. Congenitally deaf adults with intelligible or better quality of speech, typically have better hearing skills leading to better outcomes even though implanted late.

  The level of language in the components of expression, reception, and pragmatics are assessed using multiple tests. In the case of very young children, non-verbal communication, gestures used are described and assessed. The language tests typically used are language and age specific such as test for assessment of Syntax in Kannada (Basavaraj 1981) or specifically for deaf children such as Scales of Early Communication Skills for Hearing-Impaired Children (Moog and Geers, 1975). Norm referenced scales such as REELS, or criterion and norm referenced scales such as ALD (Lakkanna, Venkatesh, and Bhat, 2008), are language independent and can thus be used irrespective of language spoken at home. Significant delays in language age as compared to chronological age is a factor to recommend for CI.

  Speech-language assessment in adults is sometimes required. In the case of cross over older candidates or adults with congenital hearing loss, the clarity of speech is a prognostic factor and helps to set expectations. Increased preimplant clarity of speech is associated with better outcomes.
- **Associated problems:** Associated problems such as autism spectrum disorder, cleft palate and cognitive deficits have been observed in children with hearing loss. Screening for autism spectrum disorder (ASD) has thus become mandatory. In young children, MChat-R (Robins, Casagrande, Barton, Chen, Dumont-Mathieu, and Fein 2014) and the Communication DEALL Developmental Check list (Karanth, 2007), a criterion referenced list are useful to screen for ASD. Cognition, social behavior, form perception, and sensory integration are variables that influence a general trend of learning from sensory inputs. Inputs from the psychologist, occupational therapist and physiotherapist are mandatory as well as inputs from the teacher, if child is going to school. A more recent addition to the test battery is documenting vestibular function.
- **Medical and radiological assessment:** All children should undergo complete ear, nose and throat examination to identify any debris or wax in the external ear, middle ear infection or any associated issues. If wax is present, ears must be cleaned and middle ear infections to be treated before submitting the child for further audiological evaluations. Medical assessment by the paediatrician or physician is typically carried out for other disorders based on signs and symptoms. Vision defects associated with high risk births, Usher's syndrome, cardiac issues (Jervell Lange syndrome), epilepsy or intellectual disability/cognitive deficits may have concerns for CI surgery and outcomes. Thus, the cardiologist, neurologist and psychologist should also be part of the team in the decision making for CI.

The radiological evaluation of sensorineural hearing loss:

1. **HRCT of temporal bones (Fig. 14.1):** Both axial and coronal cuts should be taken to study the anatomy of the cochlea for its malformations, pneumatisation of the mastoid,

course of the facial nerve, high jugular bulb, enlarged vestibular and cochlear aqueducts. The presence of any infection of the middle ear and mastoid, abnormalities of middle ear ossicles will be assessed. With 3D reconstruction, the cochlear duct length can be measured which will be of help in selecting the electrodes for implantation. HRCT temporal bones can also show a narrow internal auditory canal or double internal auditory canals in some cases.

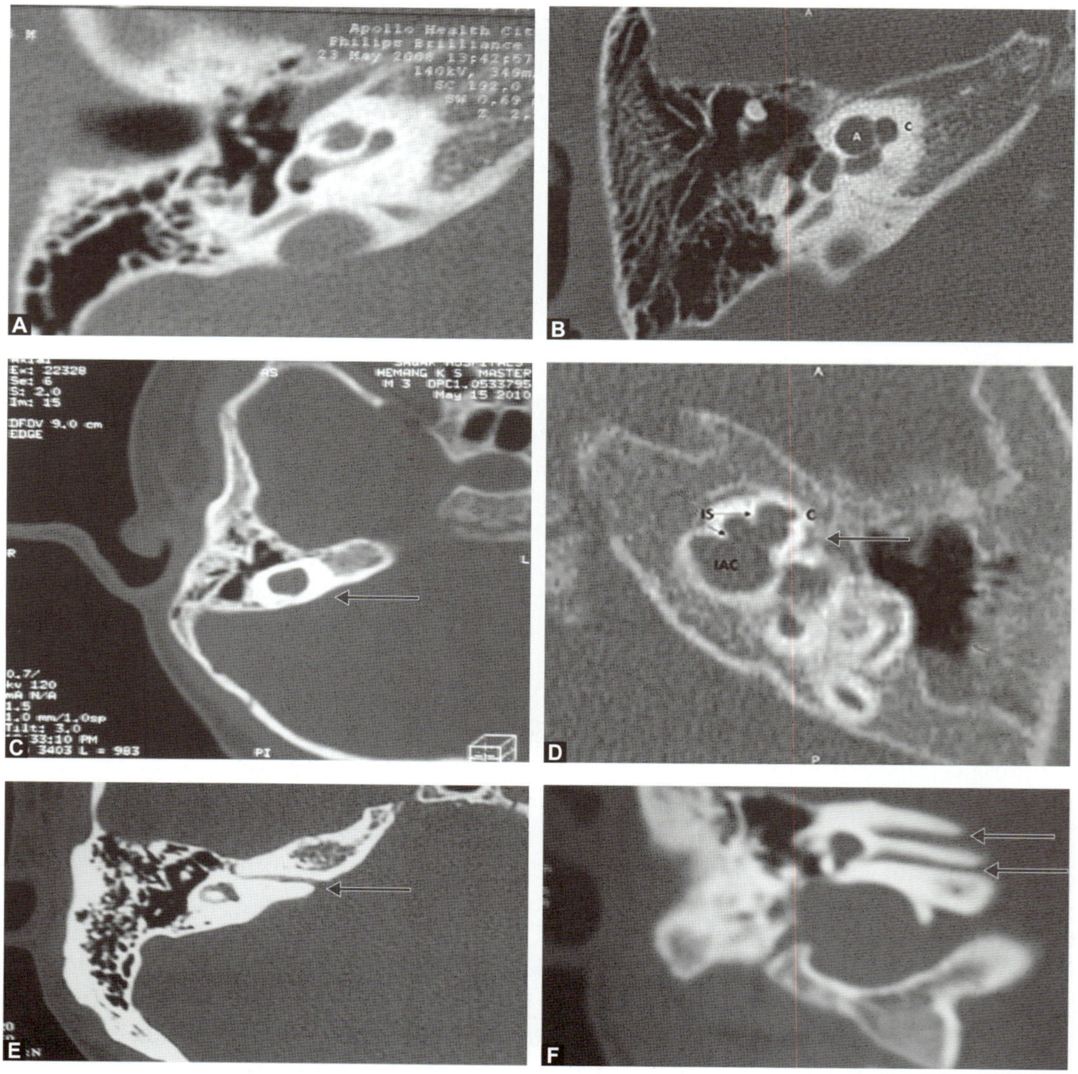

Fig. 14.1: Cochlear anomalies: **(A)** Normal cochlea with high jugular bulb, **(B)** IP Type II partition (mondini deformity), **(C)** Common cavity, **(D)** Incomplete partition type III, **(E)** Narrow internal auditory canal, **(F)** Double internal auditory canals

2. **MRI brain and internal auditory canal** (Fig. 14.2) will help to know in detail about the cochlear nerve, vestibular nerves, vestibulocochlear nerve and the facial nerve. Whether these nerves are present or absent, and if present, whether they are of normal size or hypo-plastic. In a given individual, if the size of the cochlear nerve is same as

that of facial nerve, then it is normal. If it is smaller than the facial nerve, it is called hypo-plastic. The MRI also gives information about any abnormal changes in the brain itself.

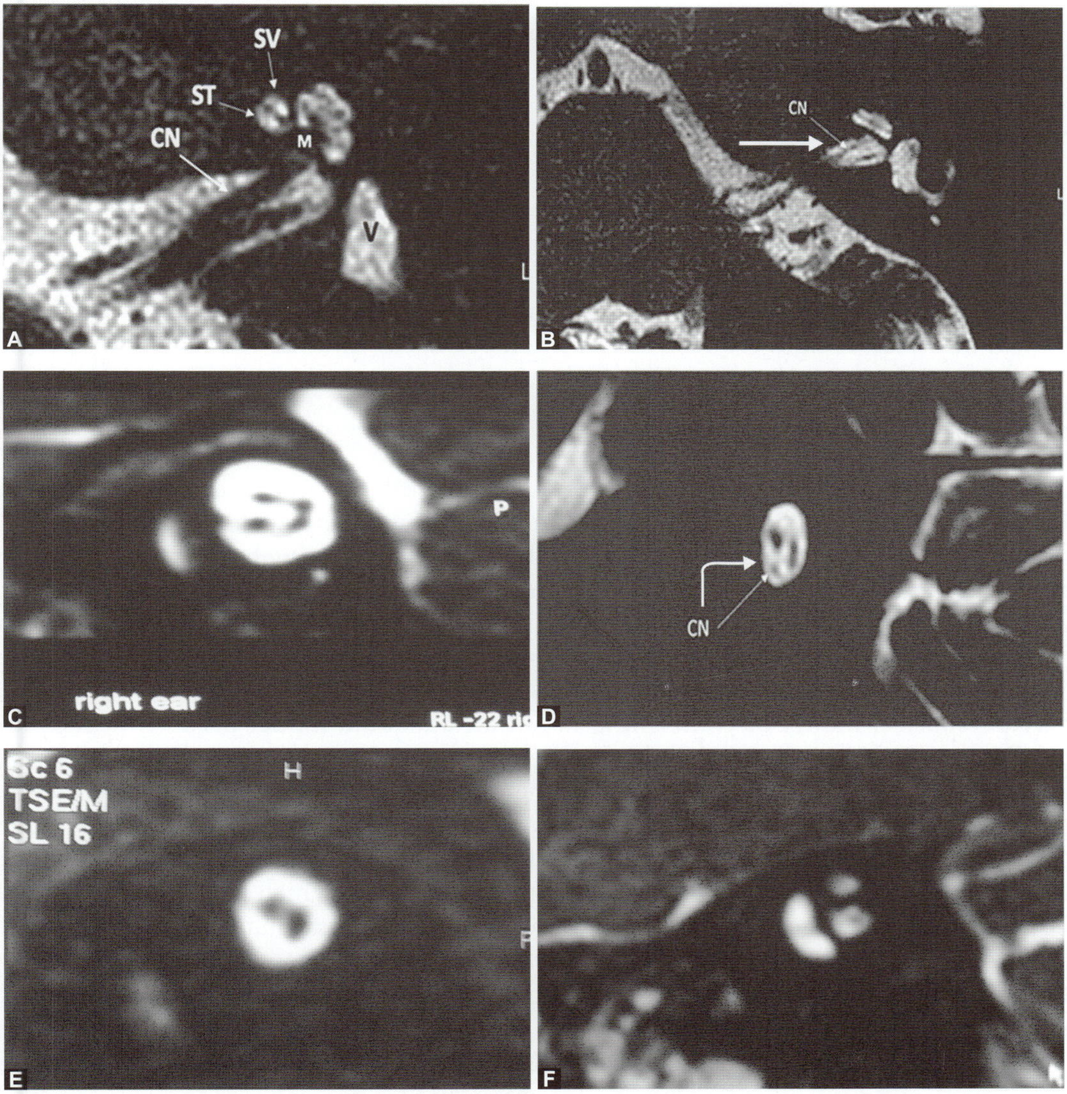

Fig. 14.2: Cochlear nerve details—MRI scan with axial cuts and oblique sagittal cuts: **(A)** Normal cochlear nerve; **(B)** Thin cochlear nerve; **(C)** IAC showing 4 nerve bundles, i.e. facial nerve, cochlear nerve, superior vestibular nerve and inferior vestibular nerve; **(D)** Thin cochlear nerve in IAC; **(E)** IAC showing 2 nerve bundles, i.e. facial nerve and vestibular nerve; **(F)** IAC showing single nerve

3. **MR cochleogram** helps to study the cochlear anomalies in detail and the fluid signals in the normal cochlea and obliteration of the cochlea due to postmeningitis fibrosis or ossification.

Classification of cochlear anomalies (Sennaroglu and Bajin, 2017)

a. Michel deformity
b. Rudimentary otocyst

c. Cochlear aplasia
d. Common cavity
e. Cochlear hypoplasia—CH-I, CH-II, CH-III and CH-IV
f. Incomplete partition
   - IP–I (cystic cochleovestibular malformation)
   - IP–II (Mondini deformity)
   - IP–III (X linked deafness)
g. Enlarged vestibular aqueduct
h. Cochlear aperture abnormalities

4. **Postimplantation studies** like intraoperative C-arm picture will help us to know the position of the electrode on the table. Postoperative digital X-ray of the mastoid-modified Stenver's view or Transorbital view (specially in bilateral cases) will clearly delineate the position of the electrode in the cochlea. Postoperative CT scan picture will throw more light on the exact position of the electrode array within the cochlea, whether it in the scala tympani or scala vestibuli.

Pre-implant Counselling

During counselling, parents/caregivers/family members/and in case of teenagers/adults the candidates themselves get an understanding of the evaluations done. When they hear about cochlear implants as one of the options for hearing impairment, they may be already grappling with information about hearing loss and hearing aids. Now they must assimilate complex information regarding surgery, technology, and (re)habilitation. Parents/caregivers/candidates may perceive cochlear implants as a cure and not as a (re) habilitation approach.

A persuasion model of counselling is not an adequate model because it does not provide ownership of decision to the families (Luterman, 2003). Information counselling involves technological information about the implant, processor and surgery. Parents/caregivers, immediate family members in case of babies and young children need to be counselled about cochlear implant surgery along with postoperative care. Teenagers and adult candidates themselves may have many questions which need to be answered. Counselling is an ongoing process and families will need informational counselling as well as adjustment counselling (ASHA, 2008). The role of siblings and extended family members must be extolled during counselling. They can become a part of the entire process and help achieve better outcomes.

There are several other contentions like does the child need cochlear implant or will he/she do well with hearing aids? How early can the surgery be done for the child? Whether unilateral or bilateral implantation or bimodal? Which system? Cost factor? What is the benefit that can be achieved postimplantation? How long will they have to undergo postoperative (re) habilitation. Here information counselling becomes very significant to make an informed decision. Some children derive more benefit from a cochlear implant than other children do.

During the candidacy process, parents should be counselled regarding potential outcomes pertaining to their child's development of auditory verbal/oral communication. The multidisciplinary CI team members must assess the abilities, motivation, and level of involvement of the family and child/teenager/adult including whether the family has a realistic view of the child's/candidate's potential to benefit from a cochlear implant. An expectation questionnaire can be used as a part of the counselling process. The families should be encouraged to meet the other cochlear implant recipients and their families who have undergone cochlear implantation and (re) habilitation program.

The parents need to be cautioned about the importance of postimplant (re) habilitation process. The family and caregivers need to understand the importance of therapy and mapping postimplantation. Adolescents and adults need to be explained about the changes that would take place regarding hearing postcochlear implantation, the adjustments that would be required. Counselling in adults would have to focus on realistic expectations concerning hearing, and their outcomes are also dependent on the individual personality, and his/her attitude towards the problem, and its solution.

Surgical Technique of Cochlear Implantation

There are various techniques of surgery in cochlear implantation:

1. Mastoidectomy with posterior tympanotomy technique
2. Suprameatal approach (SMA)
3. Middle fossa approach
4. Transcanal wall technique (Veria technique)
5. Pericanal electrode insertion technique
6. Trans-aditus technique

In this chapter we are describing the mastoidectomy with posterior tympanotomy technique that is most accepted and practiced by majority of CI surgeons. For insertion of electrode one can either use round window/extended round window or cochleostomy depending on the accessibility of the round window in any given case. In this book the mastoidectomy and posterior tympanotomy technique with all the three electrode insertion options are described.

Preoperative Vaccination: All children for cochlear implantation are vaccinated for *H. influenzae* and pneumococci 4 weeks prior to surgery (Table 14.1).

Table 14.1: Vaccination schedule: CDC and prevention advisory committee pneumococcal vaccine

Age at cochlear implantation	*Primary immunization*	*Immunization before cochlear implantation*
2 to 6 years	○ No primary immunization ○ 4 doses of PCV 7series	○ Receive 2 doses of PCV13 ○ Only one dose of PCV13
6 to 18 years	○ Regardless of PCV 7 or PPSV 23	○ Single dose of PCV13
Adults: Above 19 years		○ One dose of PCV13 followed by one dose of PPSV23 at 8 weeks later

**Hemophilus influenzae* vaccine: Universal immunization program-recommends pentavalent vaccine for all children above 6 months of age and hence receive HIB vaccine universally.

Preoperative preparation: All patients need to have a betadine shampoo head bath two times a couple of days prior to surgery. If they want to shave the whole head, they can do that, or else required amount of shaving can be done on the table under anesthesia. Patient is admitted on the previous day of surgery, undergoes preanesthetic check-up and is kept nil orally for at least 6 hours prior to surgery time.

Anesthesia: Anesthesia is induced by volatile anesthetics using oxygen, nitrous oxide, sevoflurane of 1 minimum alveolar concentration (MAC). Intubation is done after paralyzing the patient with atracurium as a muscle relaxant in appropriate doses. Maintenance of anesthesia is done using anesthetic gases and 0.5 MAC of sevoflurane. IV Infusion of fentanyl is given in the dose of 2–3 micrograms/kg/hour is continued throughout the procedure.

Adult patients are induced using IV propofol in the dose of 2 mg/kg instead of volatile anesthetics. Maintenance of anesthesia is same as stated above. No muscle relaxants are given 45 minute to 1 hour before testing the stapedius reflex. Low concentration of volatile anesthetics are added to prevent awareness. Dose of fentanyl is increased as and when required during the procedure.

Candidacy for CI has also expanded to include very young children and those with multiple handicaps and syndromic associations. In this context, CI surgeons face a multitude of challenges while performing surgery for such individuals. A meticulous assessment of the candidates' temporal bone anatomy and their general condition for fitness for anesthesia during surgery becomes paramount in performing the implant procedure without any untoward incidents.

Peroperative preparation and surgical technique: After thorough preparation of the pinna and postaural region with Betadine, the ear canal is washed with saline and a Betadine wick is kept in the ear canal. This is just to warn the surgeon with Betadine trickling into the field if he/she accidentally opens the ear canal, called 'Betadine sign'. A mini postaural incision with superior lazy 'S' extension is marked. The position of the BTE processor and receiver stimulator is marked with the help of templates (Fig. 14.3).

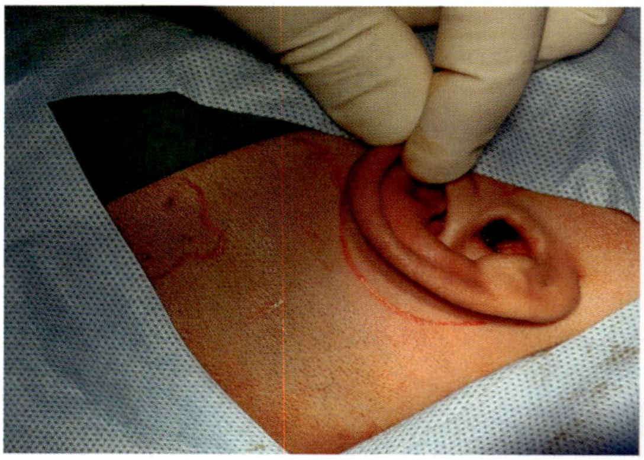

Fig. 14.3: Postaural incision and position of the receiver stimulator marked

Ivoban is draped onto the operating field after injecting xylocaine 2% with 1: 2,00,000 adrenaline into the incision site. The postaural incision is taken and skin flaps are elevated both anteriorly and posteriorly (Fig. 14.4).

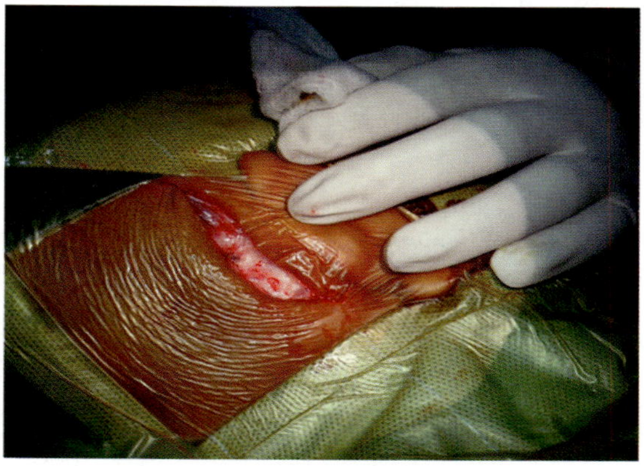

Fig. 14.4: Incision and elevation of skin flaps

The superiorly based periosteal flap is elevated (Fig. 14.5). We have noticed that superiorly based flap is better in complete coverage of the receiver stimulator at the end of the surgery rather than a Palva's flap.

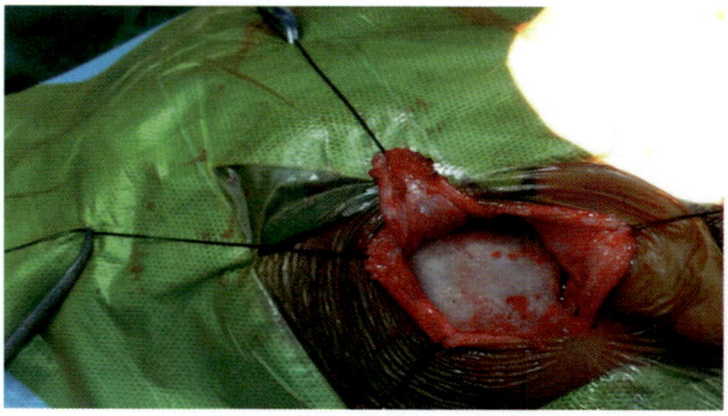

Fig. 14.5: Skin flaps are elevated and superiorly based periosteal flap

Small pieces of periosteal tissues are taken and kept in saline to use for sealing the cochleostomy or the round window after insertion of the electrode. Mastoid retractors are placed and cortical mastoidectomy is done with overhanging cortical margins to prevent the loop of the electrode array slipping out of the mastoid cavity later. Body of the incus is exposed in the aditus, lateral semicircular canal bulge and digastric ridge are identified. Posterior canal is thinned out and posterior tympanotomy is performed by drilling through the facial recess triangle between incus bridge, facial canal and chorda tympani. If one finds air cells in this area, it will be easy to enter middle ear, otherwise thick bone will make posterior tympanotomy little challenging (Fig. 14.6).

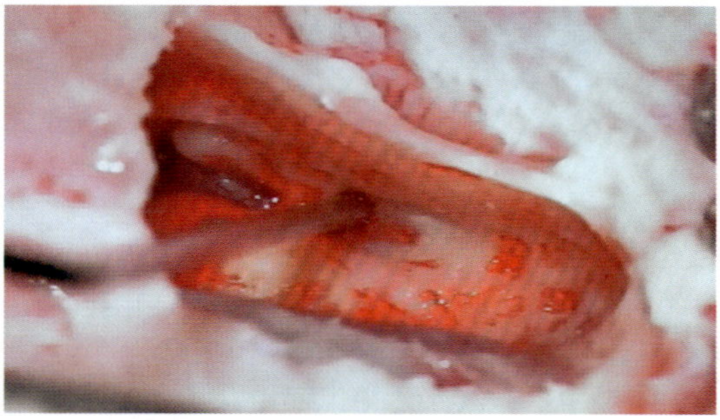

Fig. 14.6: Cortical mastoidectomy showing posterior tympanotomy site

One should drill carefully while doing posterior tympanotomy by using 3 mm, 2 mm, 1.4 mm cutting burrs initially and later with 2 mm, 1.4 mm and 1 mm diamond burrs. Always drill **horizontal to the facial nerve** and never vertical to it, to avoid facial nerve injury in case one accidentally exposes the nerve. Use of facial nerve monitor will warn the surgeon whenever he/she is very close to facial nerve and avoid injury. Posterior tympanotomy should be wide enough to expose the incudostapedial joint, stapedius, promontory and round window niche (Fig. 14.7).

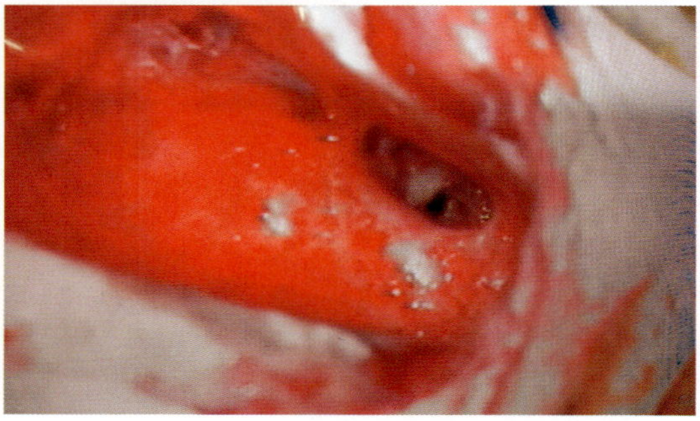

Fig. 14.7: Posterior tympanotomy

If the superior lip of the round window, called 'operculum' is obscuring the visibility of round window membrane, one needs do drill it away gently with the help of 1 mm Skeeter diamond drill. In majority of normal cochleae, it will be possible to expose the whole round window membrane clearly. In these cases, one can do round window insertion of electrode to have least intracochlear damage. If one can visualize only a portion of the round window, either because of forward facial nerve or rotated cochlea, extended round window cochleostomy or regular cochleostomy can be performed for electrode array insertion (Fig. 14.8).

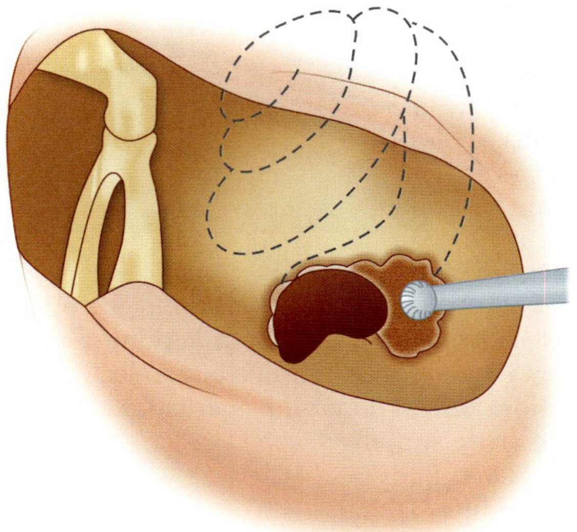

Fig. 14.8: Extended round window cochleostomy

Once the round window is exposed it is recommended to keep gelfoam soaked in dexamethasone on the membrane and keep some pieces of gelfoam soaked in adrenaline in the middle ear and aditus area. Dexamethasone will diffuse through the round window membrane and help to preserve residual hearing. Adrenaline will help to achieve hemostasis. Now it is time to make bed for the receiver stimulator. The site and the size of the bed is marked with the help of template. The drilling of the bed is done initially with cutting burrs and later with diamond burrs. The size of the bed should be perfect and the margins should be vertical. In children one can leave an island of thin bone in the center and expose the dura all-round to allow the thickness of the template to sink so that the receiver stimulator sits flush with outer cortical bone (Fig. 14.9).

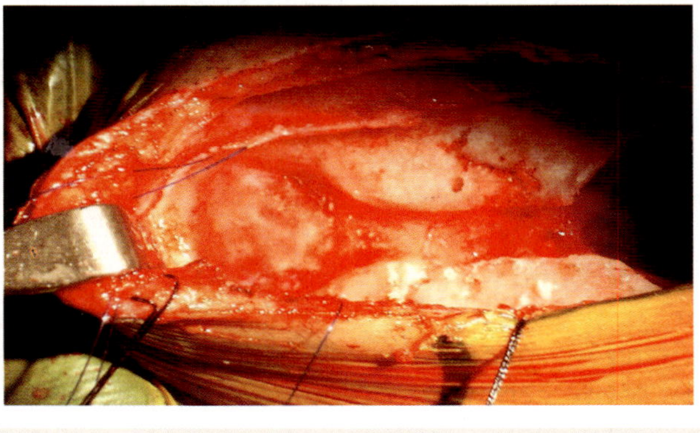

Fig. 14.9: Implant bed with tunnel for electrode array

Once the bed is made, it is connected to the mastoid cavity by drilling a tunnel for the electrode array with a small hook at the junction of tunnel with the mastoid cavity. A thorough normal saline wash is given around the bed and hemostasis is achieved. All the gelfoam from the middle ear and mastoid is taken away and saline wash is given. Now we are ready for implantation.

At this point, the surgeon and the staff nurse change their gloves and cover the operating area with a fresh sterile hole towel and switch off the monopolar cautery. Sterile implant is taken out of the box and kept on a fresh sterile towel spread on the table. In case of round window insertion, one should make a horizontal incision in the lower part of the membrane with a no. 23 hypodermic needle and you will observe perilymph oozing out. In case of extended round window insertion, one has to drill the bone adjacent to the inferior lip of round window to have a proper entry into the scala tympani. If one is planning regular cochleostomy, drill anteroinferior to the round window membrane with 1 mm skeeter drill at low speed till one exposes the endosteum of the cochlea. Now the endosteum is opened with the help of 0.2 mm right angle pick and a drop of injection Healon (sodium hyaluronate) is injected into the cochlea. Further drilling is done with 0.7 mm diamond drill to enlarge cochleostomy to the required size. The size of the cochleostomy can be assessed by the help of cochleostomy gauge. Sodium hyaluronate prevents bone dust and blood entering the cochlea. This is called 'soft surgical technique' and causes least intra-cochlear damage. Now the implant receiver stimulator package is anchored in the bed (Fig. 14.10). The active electrode array is taken out of the sheath and held proximal to the active electrodes with jeweller's forceps or AOS (advance off stylet) forceps.

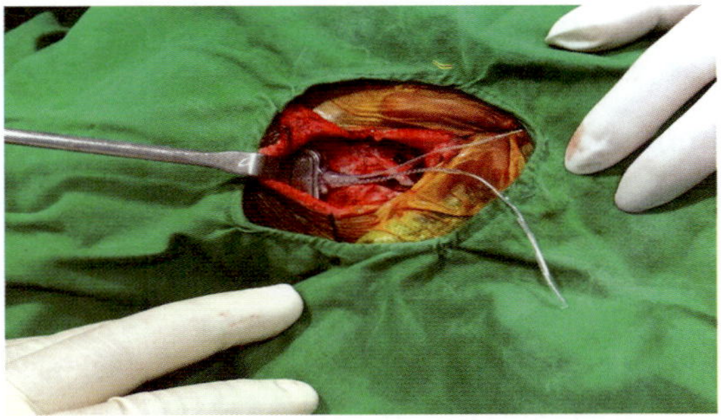

Fig. 14.10: Implant housed in subperiosteal pocket

The electrode is inserted very gently into the cochlea either through the round window or cochleostomy in an atraumatic way. One should take time to insert the electrode array very slowly and gently to avoid damage to the electrodes and to reduce intracochlear trauma (Fig. 14.11). Once complete insertion is accomplished, the round window or the cochleostomy is sealed with periosteum taken at the beginning of surgery (Fig. 14.12).

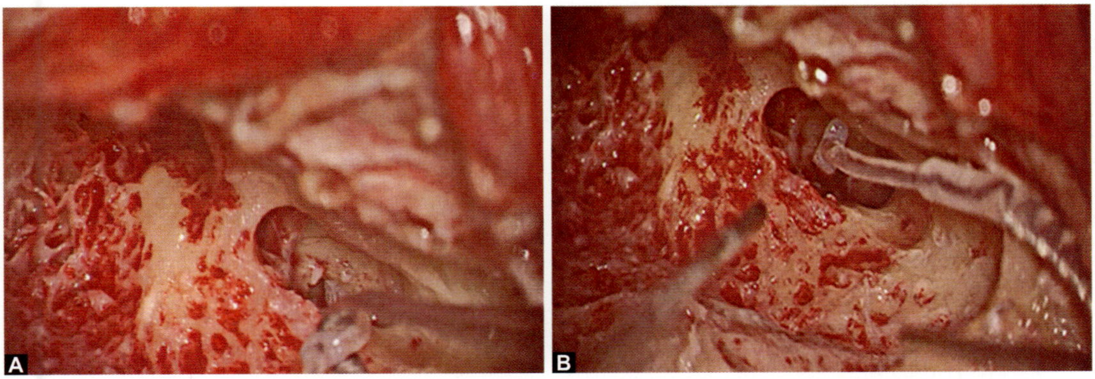

Fig. 14.11: (A) Electrode insertion through round window; **(B)** Implant electrodes *in situ*

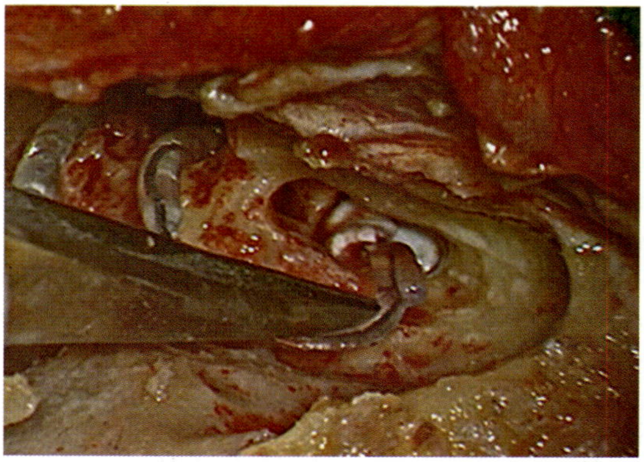

Fig. 14.12: Round window sealed with connective tissue

This will prevent chances of meningitis in case of child developing middle ear infection in the postoperative period. The remaining portion of the electrode array is folded in to the mastoid and ground electrode is tucked underneath temporalis muscle. Now the implant is ready for intraoperative testing. The receiver stimulator is connected to the laptop with coil, coil cable and processor with all aseptic precautions.

Intraoperative monitoring: The purpose of intraoperative assessment is two-fold. The first is to ensure that the device is properly placed in the cochlea and the second is that it is responding to stimulation and is functioning.

Prior to insertion of the implant, it is good practice to measure the electrode impedance when the implant is in a sealed cover. At this point the electrode impedances are typically high and indicate open electrodes. If a short circuit electrode is seen, the implant is discarded and the backup implant is selected (extremely rare). This test also indicates that implant is communicating with the processor. Verification of the placement is done in two ways: (i) Recording of electrical stapedius reflex (ESR) and (ii) recording of electrically evoked compound action potentials (ECAP). Recording of ESR can be done with all the implants currently available in the market. The presence of the ESR indicates proper placement and functioning of the reflex arc. ECAPs are now recorded by software that automatically set the appropriate parameters. Presence of ECAPs indicates synchronous firing of electrically stimulated auditory nerve fibres. In most cases this may suffice, but in cases of thin nerve, common cavity, and cases where ECAPs are not obtained advanced manual settings may be necessary.

Then the wound is closed in layers and mastoid dressing is given. The position of the electrode array can be checked either by C arm or a digital mastoid X-ray (modified Stenver's view in unilateral cases and transorbital view in cases of bilateral implantation) (Fig. 14.13).

Complications of Cochlear Implantation

I. **Intraoperative complications**
1. CSF gusher from cochleostomy
2. Dural injury—CSF leak
3. Misplacement of electrodes
4. Tip roll over
5. External auditory canal breakdown

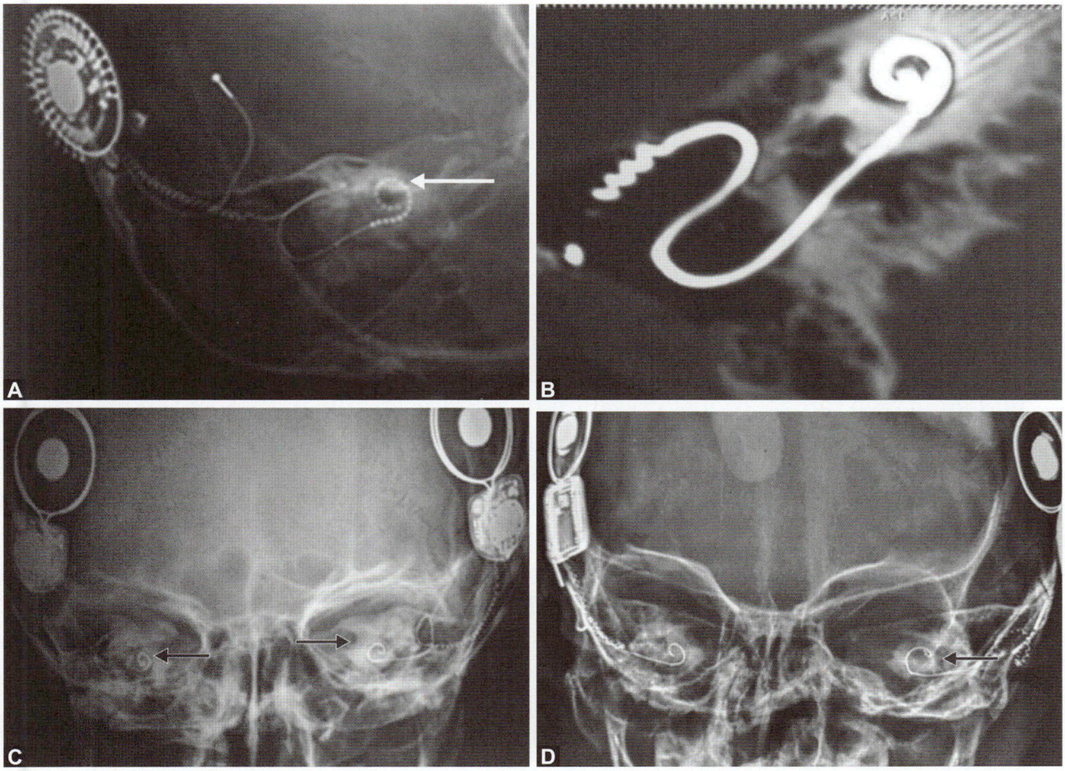

Fig. 14.13: (A) Modified stenver's view–unilateral implant, **(B)** CT scan showing electrode array, **(C)** Transorbital view (bilateral CI), **(D)** bilateral CI with tip fold over in left implant (shown by arrow)

6. Facial nerve injury
7. Emissary vein bleeding

II. **Postoperative complications**
1. Hematoma formation
2. Flap infection and wound breakdown
3. Displacement of receiver stimulator
4. Cholesteatoma formation
5. Meningitis
6. Device failure:
   - Hard failure
   - Soft failure
7. Facial nerve stimulation
8. Electrode migration

Switch-on and Mapping

Generally, after 2 weeks to 1 month postsurgery, the switch-on is done to give enough time for wound healing. The family/caregiver/recipient need to be aware and would have been preoperatively and postoperatively counselled regarding the responses to be expected at switch on. Information regarding the usage of processor, accessories, care and maintenance of processor and its accessories, Bluetooth accessories, apps if any is to be provided. The magnet strength of the external processor coil needs to be optimally set. If not set appropriately it may cause redness at magnet site and breakdown of skin. Care about using appropriate magnet strength is stressed.

Also, the mapping process needs to be explained. Even after initial counselling parents might feel that child is going to start responding and talking immediately post switch on. During switch on they are again explained about what to expect and about post-implant (re) habilitation process.

The first check during switch on is the impedance check. Impedance measurement is done to check the electrodes inserted. This will give information about the open or short electrode(s), atypical impedances. Neural responses (ECAPs) are conducted and can be used to approximately decide the level of stimulation to be provided to the recipient. The responses at switch on in children vary from crying, startle, smiling, eye movements, eye widening, eye blinks, or just cessation of activity. Adults with post-lingual hearing impairment may feel that the sounds are different from what they were used too. They may feel that it sounds garbled, cartoon-like or robotic.

Mapping is the process to provide appropriate input through the processor into the implant system. The threshold and comfort levels are recorded. The threshold (T level) is the least amount of electrical stimulus required for the recipient to perceive sound. The Comfort/Most comfortable level (C or M level) is the amount of electrical stimulus required for a loud but comfortable/most comfortable perception of sound. At switch on the maps that are provided to the recipient are progressive maps with variable dynamic ranges wherein the recipient initially hears sounds through a map with a reduced range. Later the MAPs that provide a wider dynamic range make more sounds audible are used. As per a multicentre study (Vaerenberg, Smits, De Ceulaer, et al., 2014) most centres (76%) send the CI user home with incremental MAPs after the switch-on session. These MAPs contain progressively higher maximum levels allowing the CI user to accommodate to each MAP before switching to the next one.

It needs to be explained to families/recipients that the mapping process in isolation does not show good listening skills and speech and language development, but that their consistent effort in therapy will show the results. As (re)habilitation starts, mapping is done regularly at intervals to adjust these levels further. Thresholds and most comfortable levels can be accurately measured in adults. In children, these are done by observing behavior or with a conditioned response to the stimulus along with objective inputs such as ECAP and ESR thresholds. Parameters like coding strategy, pulse width, the rate of stimulation are modified if required. The mapping is frequent initially and at a lesser frequency later and is scheduled in consultation with the therapist and the audiologist after reviewing progress with earlier maps.

(Re) Habilitation

The CI recipient must undergo (re)habilitation process to develop listening, speech and language and communication skills in cases of children and in case of adults they need to give meaning to the new sounds and develop communication repair strategies. A naturalistic approach rather than a structured approach is used in children with cochlear implants. Children who are implanted later in age may have to use a combination of the two approaches.

The type of (re)habilitation depends on factors like listening skills, the age at implantation, duration of implant use, cochlear anatomy, cognition, and associated issues. Primarily in children, especially who are implanted early the auditory-verbal approach for habilitation is widely used. The child will attend therapy sessions wherein the caregiver / parents observe and follow-up on the activity at home. Evaluations are carried out at regular intervals to see if the child is progressing as expected or if any modifications need to be done in the therapy process. Ongoing assessment helps to evaluate the listening, speech and language skills that will provide information for appropriate planning.

Therapy goals are made depending on the child's present level of functioning which will be changed or modified according to the progress the child makes. Usually, the areas that are focused on are audition, speech, language, cognition, literacy skills, pragmatics, and communication development. Parent guidance is crucial because the generalisation for the goals will happen if the child gets enough repetitions at home. These must be done creatively, naturally, so that the child understands the concept in every context. Families need to be explained in detail about the selection of a language for communication. Families often get confused between the medium of instruction of language in school system vs primary language spoken at home.

The educational thrust and direction of early identification and cochlear implantation is obviously mainstreaming. There are numerous options concerning the communication mode, language choice, and the number of sessions of therapy, choice in education, which need to be deliberated on. Children with CI will have to make their way through an educational and social environment that is not primarily geared to their needs. Counselling and support are going to be needed within the school as well as at home. These services could be provided in a meeting with school staff. Information can be passed on in the form of written material regarding the acoustic environment required, seating arrangement of the child, the language content and usage.

The outcomes after cochlear implantation depend on many factors like age at implantation, duration of deafness, appropriate selection of candidates, cochlear anatomy, insertion of electrodes during surgery, duration of use of implant, quality of intervention, psychological status, cognitive skills, other associated issues and parental/ family involvement.

REFERENCES

1. American Speech-Language-Hearing Association (2008). Guidelines for audiologists providing informational and adjustment counselling to families of infants and young children with hearing loss birth to 5 years of age [Guidelines]
2. Basavaraj, V (1981). Test for assessing syntax in Kannada, doctoral thesis, University of Mysore
3. Cochlear implants and vaccination recommendations (2017), https://www.cdc.gov/vaccines/vpd/mening/public/dis-cochlear-faq-gen.html
4. Dutt, S.N., Kumar, A (2019). The methodology and electro-physiological classification of pre-operative trans-tympanic electrically-evoked auditory brainstem response (TT-EABR). *Indian J Otolaryngology Head Neck Surgery* 71, 1–4 . https://doi.org/10.1007/s12070–019-01585–2.
5. Karanth P. Communication DEALL Developmental Checklists. Bangalore: Com DEALL Trust, 2007.
6. Lakkanna S, Venkatesh K, and Bhat JS (2008). A Development. Bakersfield, CA; Omni Therapy Services.
7. Luterman D (2003). Counselling parents about cochlear implants, ASHA leader, leader. FTR2.08102003.6

8. Moog JS, and Geers A (1975). Scales of early communication skills for hearing-impaired children. Published by CID—Central institute for the deaf, 825 South Taylor Ave., St. Louis, MO 63110; Web: http://cid.edu
9. Pearson, Nicole; Muñoz, Karen EdD; Landon, Trenton J. PhD; Corbin-Lewis, Kim PhD Counselling skills in audiology, The Hearing Journal: March 2019—Volume 72—Issue 3—p 50,51 doi: 10.1097/01.HJ.0000554354.53822.78.
10. Robins DL, Casagrande K, Barton M, Chen CA, Dumont-Mathieu T, and Fein D (2014). Validation of the modified checklist for autism in toddlers, Revised with follow-up (M-CHAT- R/F) Pediatrics; 133(1): 37–45. doi: 10.1542/peds.2013–1813
11. Sennarogulu L and Bajin D (2017). Classification current management of inner ear malformations. Baalkan Med Journal; 34:35–409.
12. Teagle HF, Roush PA, Woodard JS, Hatch DR, Zdanski CJ, Buss E, Buchman CA (2010) Cochlear implantation in children with auditory neuropathy spectrum disorder ear and hearing.Vol 31(3):325–35. doi: 10.1097/AUD.0b013e3181ce693b.
13. Vaerenberg B, Smits, C, De Ceulaer, G, *et al* (2014). "Cochlear implant programming: A global survey on the state of the art," The Scientific World Journal, Vol., Article ID 501738, 12 pages,. https://doi.org/10.1155/2014/501738.

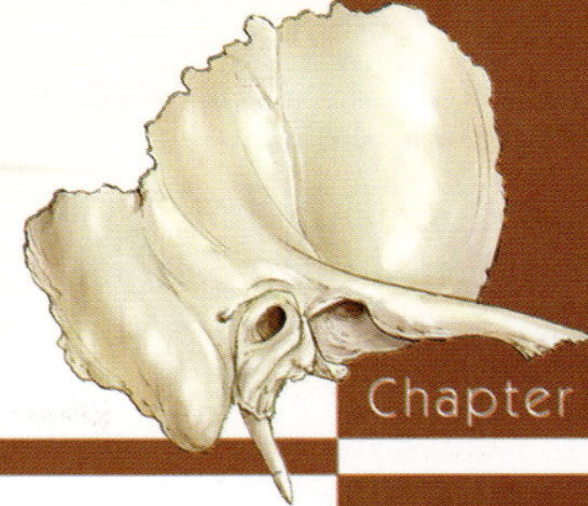

Chapter 15

Translabyrinthine Approach to the Internal Auditory Canal

Produl Hazarika • Dipak Ranjan Nayak • Ajay Bhandarkar • Kabikanta Samantaray

Introduction

The translabyrinthine approach is a surgical approach to the cerebellopontine angle, or CPA. It is used in the surgical extirpation of lesions of the cerebellopontine angle, including acoustic neuroma. The surgery for vestibular schwannoma has been evolved considerably in the last century. Following the mortality up to 80% associated with traditional neurosurgical approaches till the development of translabyrinthine approach. This approach is a unique and intricate approach to the lateral skull base that has been refined and perfected over the past several decades (John et al., 1999).

Historical Perspective

The first surgical attempt to remove acoustic neuroma was made in 1891 by McBurney, with a mallet and chisel. Charles Ballance described the first successful complete removal of an accoustic neuroma (House and House, 1964, House and Charles, 1979). The translabyrinthine approach was initially described by Panse in 1904 and first used to resect a cerebellopontine angle tumor by Quix in 1912. This approach was not considerd as a standard approach until William House published a microsurgical approach of 47 resections with no mortalities in 1964. Before William House's era, there was no cooperation between otologists and neurosurgeons in posterior fossa surgery. This concept was changed after neurosurgeon William Hitselberger joined William House as a team (McRacan and Brackmann, 2015). Thus the House and his team truly popularized this approach (Doig, 1970). Morrison and King (1973) have described a modification of this approach in combination with a transtentorial component for the resection of vestibular schwannomas and other lesions of the cerebellopontine angle and related structures.

Anatomy

The internal auditory canal is a cylindrical neurovascular channel providing a tunnel for the facial, cochlear and vestibular nerves, the nervus intermedius, the internal auditory artery and vein from the posterior cranial fossa into the petrous bone. The average meatus is about 8 mm long and 4 mm wide. But variations in size and degree of pneumatization of the encasing petrous bone have an impact upon the size, shape and orientation of the IAC. The vertical diameter may lie between 2 and 7 mm. But difference of 1 to 2 mm would usually be considered abnormal.

The IAC has 3 distinguishable regions (Fig. 15.1):

1. The porus (meatus) or inlet located on the posterior surface of the temporal bone.
2. The canal proper
3. The fundus, abutting upon the medial aspect of the labyrinth

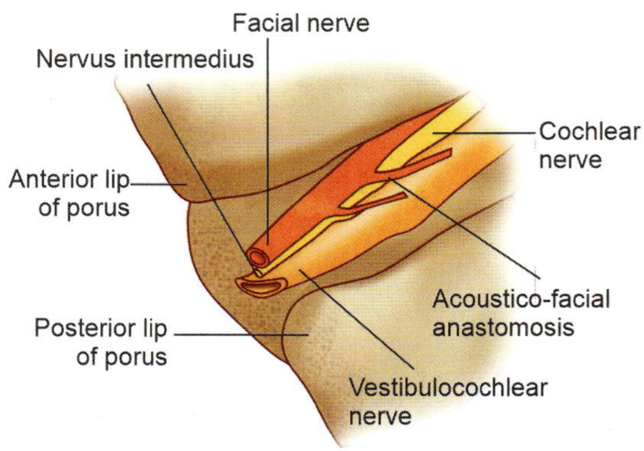

Fig. 15.1: Structure at the porus of the internal auditory canal

The position of the roof of the meatus can be determined by orientation of the posterior semicircular canal. The canals ampulla at its anterior end is in the axis of the IAM at its lateral end and the line of that meatal axis makes an angle 60° with the direction of the superior canal behind it.

The lateral end of the meatus lies consistently at a depth of 28 mm medially to the inner surface of the squamous temporal bone, above the bony external meatus. The lateral or posterior lip of the porus is sharply defined and concave, while the medial or anterior lip is represented by the appearance of a gutter extending from the canal along the petrous face. The posterior lip of the porus lies about 1 cm in front of the bony scala overlying the fovea in which the saccus endolymphaticus is lodged.

The term 'semilunar lip' is used clinically to denote the combined inferior, superior and posterior margins of the porus. Neoplasm arising within the IAC often erode this lip. Thus widening the porus and canal as well as shortening the length of the floor, roof and posterior wall. The walls of the meatus are smooth and featureless. The space ends laterally at the fundus where a bony plate separates its lumen from the vestibule and the lateral end of the canal. In places it is very thin, and is perforated at the macule cribroase for the transmission of nerve fibres from one space to the other.

The fundus is divided into an upper and lower region by the transverse horizontal crest. Above the crest two depressions are separated by a vertical bar of bone. The anterior leads the facial nerve into its canal, while the posterior, the superior vestibular area, corresponds to the elliptical recess of the vestibule and transmits the superior vestibular nerve (Fig. 15.2).

The vertical bony bar subdividing this upper area of the fundus is an important surgical guide to the position of the facial nerve during operations within the meatus. Below the transverse crest, a large anterior area is perforated by a spiral band of openings, the

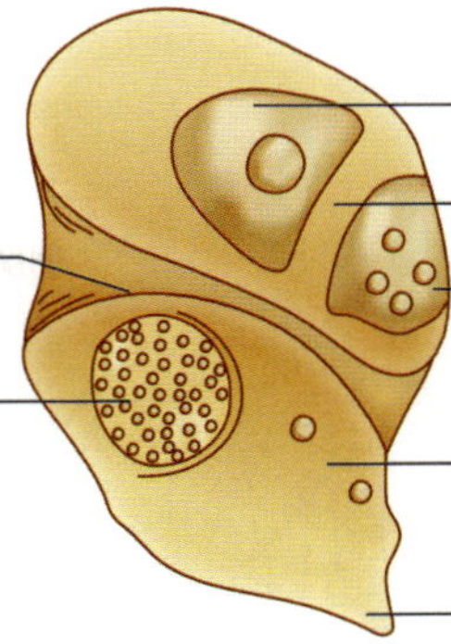

Fig. 15.2: Cross-section of internal auditory meatus

tractus spiralis foraminosa, which follows the curve of the cochlea, and transmits cochlear nerve fibres. The inferior vestibular area occupies the smaller posterior region below the horizontal crest. Here inferior vestibular fibres from the saccule are joined by fibres from the posterior semicircular canal ampulla to form the inferior vestibular nerve. These latter fibres, constituting the posterior ampullary nerve enter the meatus through a small hole, the foramen singulare Morgagni, on the posterior wall just medial to the inferior vestibular area. They are surgically accessible there, from the middle ear, just below the round window. The dura mater at the porus fuses with the periosteal lining of the meatus. Within the meatus the structures are invested with a thin coating of piamater, and floating in cerebrospinal fluid extending from the cisterna magna.

Translabyrinthine Approach to the IAM Indications (Fig. 15.3)

1. Small intracanalicular tumors like acoustic neuromas and medium-sized lesions up to 3.5 cm in diameter in the cerebellopontine angle can be completely removed by this route alone.
2. Large neuromas, 4 cm in diameter or more, can be removed either by a combined translabyrinthine transtentorial operation or by a combined translabyrinthine sub-occipital approach.
3. Other lesions of the IAM and angle such as developmental cholesteatoma, meningioma, angioma or neuromas arising for V, VII, IX, X or XI may also be removed by these approaches provided VIII nerve function is permanently lost.
4. Useful in patients who have persistent symptoms from idiopathic endolymphatic hydrops and who have irreversible loss of auditory function on the affected side.
5. This procedure is sometimes required, after stapedectomy failure or following sudden spontaneous loss, provided there is no useful function and when distracting tinnitus cannot be relieved by antidepressive or other therapy.
6. The translabyrinthine operation of chronic suppurative petrositis and labyrinthine with recurrent meningitis and posterior fossa arachnoiditis.

Limitations

1. The sacrifice of any residual hearing in the operated ear
2. In the past it has been said the approach is limited to smaller tumors. There is no tumor too large to be approached by translabyrinthine operation, this approach puts one

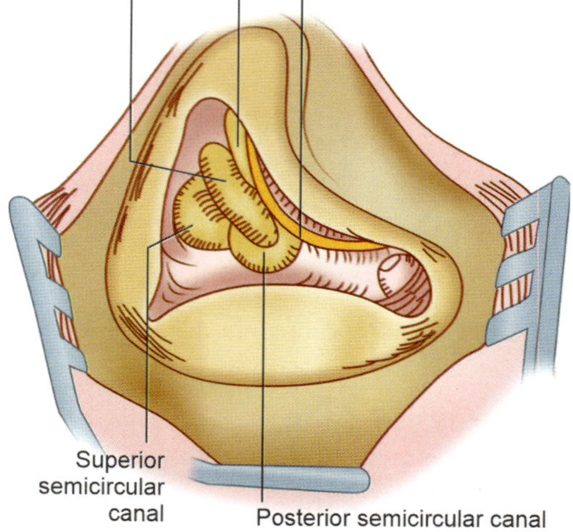

Fig. 15.3: Exposure of the facial and the semicircular canals

directly into the center of the tumor at its origin. Intracapsular removal of the tumor allows the capsule to be displaced toward the opening by surrounding brain structures. (Otolaryngologic Clinic of North America, Vol. 25 no. 2 April 1992 by Derald and Donglas Green.)

Technique

1. **Position of patient and skin flap:** A postauricular incision is made approximately 2 cm behind the postauricular crease. Posterior curve of the incision allows access to the area behind the sigmoid sinus.
2. **Cortical mastoidectomy:** An extensive cortical mastoidectomy is performed.

Labyrinthine Dissection

Bone is removed in the sinodural angle along the superior petrosal sinus. The opening along the superior petrosal sinus gradually deepened and widened until the labyrinthine bone is encountered. The lateral and posterior semicircular canals are then progressively removed and the facial nerve, which lies anteriorly, is carefully approached. The lateral semicircular canal is opened, and the common crus of the superior and posterior semicircular canals is identified deep in three dissection. The removal of bone with rotator movement in a wide plane rather than making a narrow grove allows safe identification of the blue line of the semicircular canal (2.3, 3.1, 4.0 mm diamond burrs, angled handpiece, suction irrigation). The superior semicircular canal is followed to its ampulla. The ampulla of the superior semicircular canal is preserved as a landmark to find the end of the superior semicircular canal is preserved as a landmark to find the end of the superior vestibular nerve, Bill's bar and the facial canal. The vestibule is then opened and the facial nerve is skeletonized from the genu inferiorly to near the stylomastoid foramen. The facial nerve is skeletonized from a posterior direction, where it occurs is needed to approach the cerebellopontine angle

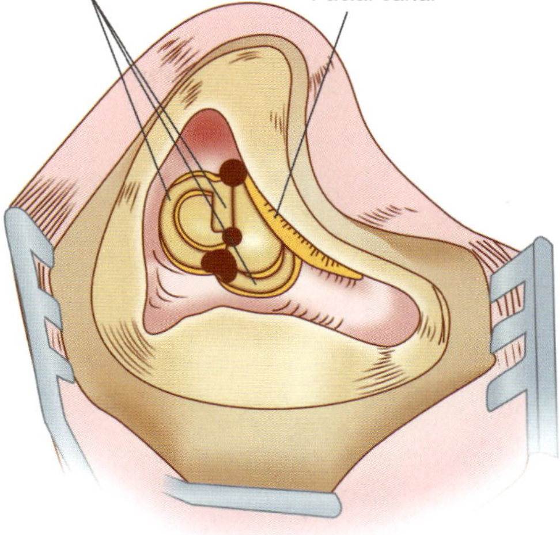

Fig. 15.4: Three canals being opened

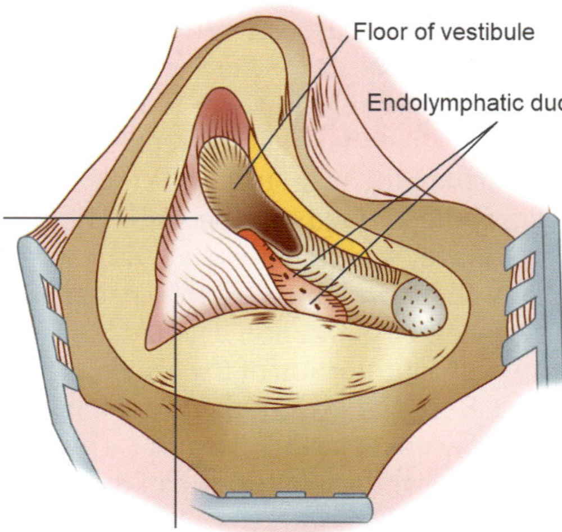

Fig. 15.5: The three canals have been drilled further and the vestibule is opened

(Figs 15.4 and 15.5). The final removal of bone along the facial nerve is accomplished with a diamond burr. As the facial nerve is skeletonized, the cribriform area of the superior vestibular nerve entering the vestibule is seen. It is important to skeletonize the facial nerve adequately so that the vestibule can be seen in this area.

Internal Auditory Canal Dissection (Fig. 15.6)

After the labyrinthine bone has been removed to the level of the vestibule, dissection of the bone surrounding the IAC is started. The bone to be removed for exposure of the IAC forms a wedge or triangle. One side is the roof of the IAC. The second side is the floor of

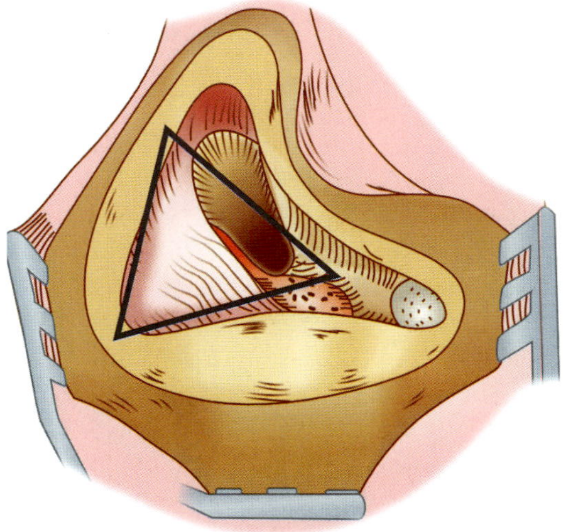

Landmark of IAC

Fig. 15.6: Landmark triangle of internal auditory canal consisting of floor of labyrinthectomy dissection anteriorly, posterior fossa dura posteriorly, superiorly roof of internal auditory canal

the labyrinthectomy dissection and the third side is the posterior fossa dura as it extends between the other two sides. The dissection is started along the superior petrosal sinus and then gradually enlarged in all directions towards the IAC. In approaching the IAC one must remember that the medial wall of the vestibule represents the lateral wall of the IAC fundus where the nerves enter the inner ear structures therefore minimal bone removal on the medial wall of the vestibule will expose the IAC. The IAC can be recognized by color change in the bone. In cadaver specimen or the living surgical specimen without a tumor, the color of the canal will be dark blue. In the specimen with a tumor, the color is usually red from the vascularity of the tumor. The IAC is skeletonized by removal of bone 180 degrees around the posterior portion of the canal extending from the area of the fundus to the canal extending from the area of the facial canal and petrous apex to the superior midpoint of the Porous acousticus (3.1, 2.3 and 1.4 mm diameter diamond burrs, small suction—irrigator). Exposure at the superior lip of the Porous acousticus is limited. The posterior superior portion of the IAC can be well exposed. The inferior border of the IAC can be defined. If the dissection is carried, anteriorly a small white discoloration in the bone appears which represents the cochlear aqueduct which when entered release cerebrospinal fluid extension. Anterior to the cochlear aqueduct will involve the jugular bulbs and the 9th, 10th and 11th cranial nerves. A thin layer of bone is preserved over the superior portion of the IAC. This layer of bone has to be removed for wide exposure of the IAC and the posterior fossa dura. Wide exposure eliminates blind dissection through a small keyhole into the IAC and bleeder from the sectioned nerve can be dealt with ease. The thin plate of bone is removed.

Dural Incision (Fig. 15.7)

The exposed dura of the IAC is slit along the long axis of the canal at its inferior border with 1.0 mm right angled hook. This prevents injury to the facial nerve superiorly in the occasional cases of variation (sometimes a tumor may push the nerve posteriorly).

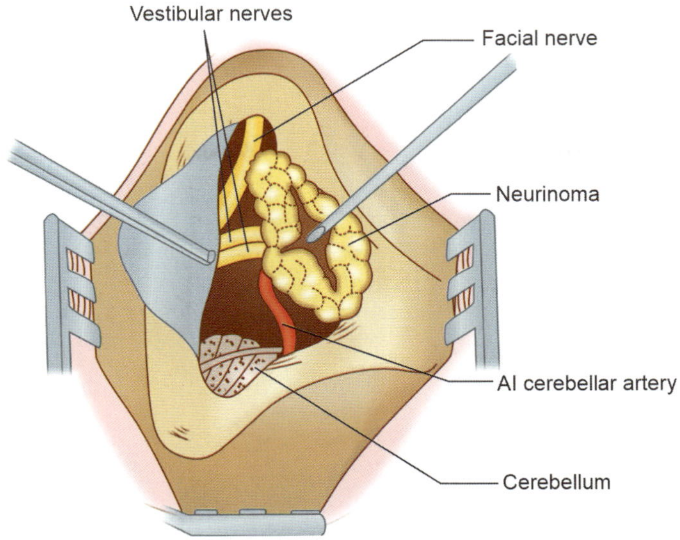

Fig. 15.7: Dural flap reflected to expose the CP angle

Identification of the Facial Nerve

The lateral of the IAC is dissected, and the plane of the facial nerve is established by uncovering the labyrinthine segment of the facial nerve. The facial nerve is located anterior to the superior vestibular nerve with the Bill's bar separately the 2 nerves. The ampulla of the superior vestibular nerve is preserved for easy identification of the superior vestibular nerve. A brush like termination of the superior vestibular nerve is encountered at its termination in the ampulla. A one millimeter hook is inserted deep to the vestibular nerve to palpate the Bill's bar (Nelson). Probing with a hook to identify Bill's bar is not advised by some because the type of the hook may go through the meatal foramen and induce a postoperative facial palsy. Superior vestibular nerve occupies a recess medially which can be safely probed. The superior vestibular nerve is cut with a neurectomy knife from its attachments in the ampulla area. When the superior vestibular nerve is lifted up the facial nerve is seen as it exits the fallopian canal into the IAC vestibulofacial anastomosis that occur here should be carefully sectioned with a neurectomy knife. Directly inferior the transverse crest is seen which divides the IAC into a superior and inferior portions. Inferior vestibular nerve lies laterally and auditory nerve lies medially. The inferior vestibular nerve is cut using a neurectomy knife. After the lateral end of the facial nerve is identified and separated from the tumor, all tumor remnants are removed along with the cochlear and vestibular nerve (Fig. 15.8).

Dura is sutured mastoidectomy cavity obliterated with temporo-parietal fascia or strips of abdominal fat. Aditus is obliterated with a small piece of muscle postaural incision closed in layers. The patient is kept on the operating table until responding well and then is transferred directly to the ICU.

Complications

1. **Facial paralysis** is a possible complication of the VIII nerve section or following removal of intracranial tumors, despite all precautions. It may present as late as the

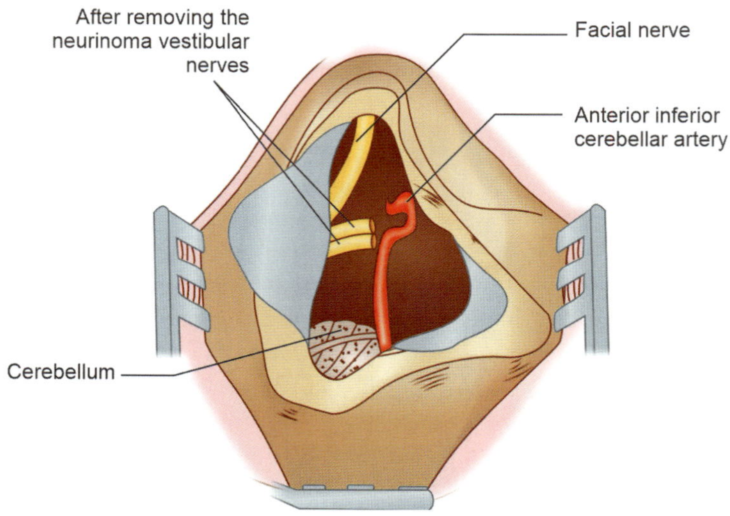

Fig. 15.8: Post resection of acoustic tumor

fifth or sixth day. A partial or delayed palsy may progress to become complete. It is doubtful if steroids are of further value after 2 weeks. Recovery must be awaited and eye protected by artificial tears, moisture chambers and soft contact lens. A suitable shield or lateral tarsorrhaphy / lid loading with gold plate may be considered.

2. **Headache** is the immediate postoperative period.

REFERENCES

1. John P, *et al.* Translabyrinthine approach. Operative Techniques in Neurorsurgery,1999; 2(2):52–57
2. C. McBurney, M.A. StarrA contribution to cerebral surgery: diagnosis, localization and operation for removal of three tumors of the brain: with some comments upon the surgical treatment of brain tumors. Am J Med Sci, 1893; 55 : 361–87.
3. House HP, House WF. Historical review and problem of acoustic neuroma. Arch Otol, 1964; 80:601–04.
4. William F. House and Charles M. Acoustic tumors, volume II: Management. Edited by Luetje, 280 pp, illus, university park press, Baltimore, MD, 1979.
5. McRacan and Brackmann. Historical perspective on evolution in the management of lateral skull base surgery. Otolaryngol Clin North Am, 2015; 48.3:397–405.
6. Doig JA. Surgical treatment of acoustic neuroma. The translabyrinthine approach. Proceedings of the Royal Society of Medicine. 1970;63:775.
7. *Schuknecht* HF, *Gulya AJ*. Anatomy of the Temporal Bone with Surgical Implications-Published in 1986 by Lea and Febiger, Philadelphia.
8. Harold Ludman. Mawson's disease of the ear, Year Book Medical Publishers, 1988.
9. Brackmann DE and Green JD 'Acoustic Neuroma' Translabyrinthine Approach for Acoustic Tumor Removal-Otolaryngol Clin North Am. 1992 Apr;25(2):311–29.
10. Morrison AW. Translabyrinthine approach to the Internal Auditory Meatus –J R Soc Med. 1978 Apr;71(4):269–73.
11. Disease of the Nose, Throat, Ear, Head and Neck-Ballenger 14th edition.
12. Ralph Nelson. Temporal bone dissection Mannual. House Ear Institute, 1983.

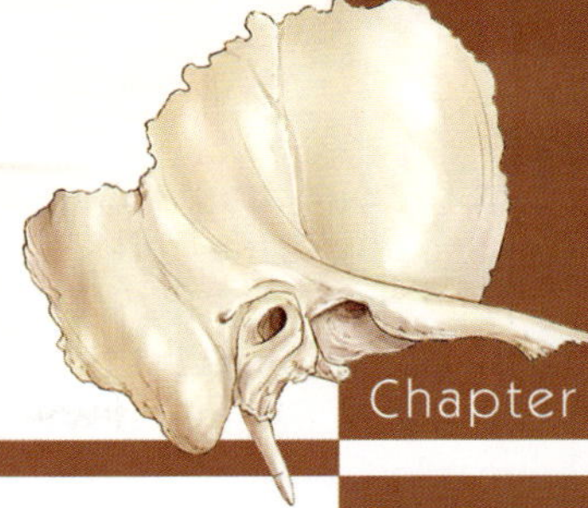

Chapter 16

Surgical Refinements to the Translabyrinthine Approach to the Cerebellopontine Angle

Sampath Chandra Prasad Rao • Mario Sanna

Introduction

The TLA is a lateral approach used for accessing various tumors of the cerebellopontine angle (CPA), most commonly vestibular schwannoma (VS). This was first described by Rudolf Panse in 1904 and was first performed for VS in 1911 by Franciscus Hubertus Quix from Utrecht University, Netherlands. But due to unsatisfactory results this approach was criticized by Harvey Cushing and Walter Dandy, two of the pioneers of neurosurgery of that time and thereafter this approach fell into disrepute.[1] After the advent of microscopes in otology, William House at the House Ear Institute in Los Angeles re-discovered the TLA (TLA) marking the beginning of the era of modern skull base surgery.[2–5] Subsequently, there was a developing opinion that while small tumors could be removed through the TLA, larger lesions were best approached suboccipitally as the TLA failed to provide a large surgical field.[6] To overcome this limitation of the TLA, the proponents of this approach enlarged it by additional bone removal over the middle and posterior fossae and by the addition of the transapical extensions (where bone is drilled out to various degrees around the IAC), thereby obtaining a wider surgical view and a better control over the tumor and surrounding structures. This facilitated removal of even very large tumors with anterior and medial extensions.[1,7–10] Furthermore, this approach could be combined with other skull base approaches like the transcochlear approaches described by William House[11] or transotic approaches described by Ugo Fisch[12,13] for additional exposure.

Over the years, we have introduced some technical modifications to the TLA that allowed us to reduce the mortality rate to <1%with minimal morbidity.[14] Identifying FN by using the ampullary nerve as a landmark rather than the Bill bar, lowering the high jugular bulb, and extending bone removal around and anterior to the IAC (transapical extension) were the major refinements added to the original technique.

The Enlarged Translabyrinthine Approach (ETLA)

Rationale

The limited view provided by the classic translabyrinthine approach, prevented considering this valuable approach for the removal of large acoustic tumors, more so in the presence of limiting anatomical obstacles such as a high jugular bulb, an anteriorly placed sigmoid sinus, a low dura, and a small mastoid cavity.[15]

The purpose of the ETLA approach is the same as with the conventional TLA; that is to obtain lateral access to the internal auditory canal (IAC) and the CPA, thereby allowing removal of CPA lesions without cerebellar retraction. In the conventional TLA, a thin shelf of bone is left over the middle cranial fossa dura, the sigmoid sinus and the jugular bulb. In the ETLA, bone is drilled out over these structures to completely expose the middle cranial fossa dura, the posterior fossa dura, sigmoid sinus, retrosigmoid dura and the jugular bulb along with the contents of the IAC. This allows retraction of structures during surgery and thereby enabling exposure and hence removal of even very large VS. The advantage in exposure obtained by the enlarged approach when compared to the conventional TLA is shown in Fig. 16.1. Another difference between the two approaches is that in the enlarged approach, the bone around the IAC is drilled by 270 degrees compared to 180 degrees in the conventional approach providing the surgeon with additional anteromedial exposure (Fig. 16.2). In our center, we have abandoned the conventional TLA in favor of the enlarged approach.

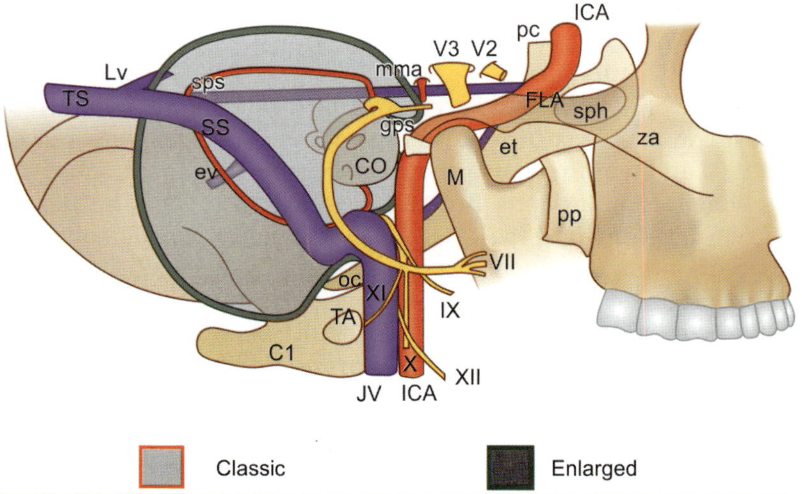

Fig. 16.1: Exposure of the CPA and the surrounding areas obtained by the ETLA is much larger than the classic TLA. TS: Transverse sinus, LV: Longitudinal venous sinus, SS: Sigmoid sinus, SPS: Superior petrosal sinus, ev: emissary veiw, OC: Occipital condyl, TA: Transverse process of attas, JV: Jugular vein. Cranial nerves–V2, V3, VII, IX, X, XI, XII

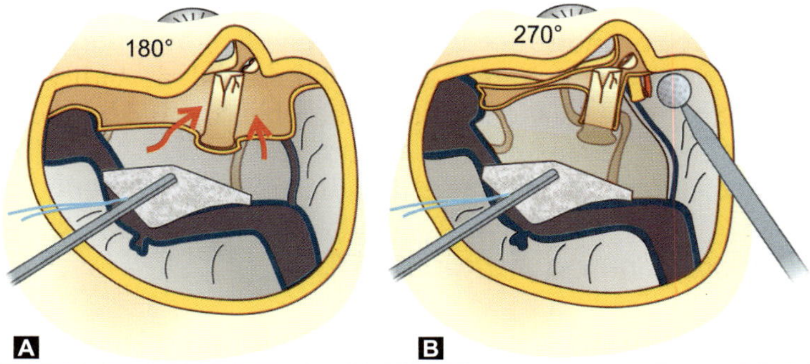

Fig. 16.2: Illustrations showing the difference between the **(A)** conventional 180 degrees exposure, and **(B)** the 270 degrees exposure of the internal auditory canal

Indications

- *Tumors of any size with poor preoperative hearing*: This approach is indicated for tumors wherein hearing preservation is not essential due to poor preoperative hearing (grade 3 or worse according to the modified Sanna classification). With the wide exposure that this approach provides, the surgeon can focus on total eradication of tumor.
- *Large tumors irrespective of preoperative hearing*: This is indicated in VS greater than 1.5 cm in diameter in the extra-canalicular portion, regardless of the preoperative hearing. Very large tumors, even those larger than 4 cm in diameter (grade 5) can be safely removed by the ETLA.
- *Neurofibromatosis type 2 (NF 2) with large tumors*: NF 2 commonly presents with bilateral VSs and this makes hearing preservation or rehabilitation very important. While hearing can be preserved in small tumors by opting for hearing preservation surgeries like the retrosigmoid or the middle cranial fossa approaches, it is difficult to ensure this in larger tumors.[16] In such a scenario, the ETLA is the preferred approach in NF 2, wherein large tumors can be removed and preserving the cochlear nerve can be attempted for a simultaneous cochlear implant (CI). Likewise, when it is not possible to preserve the cochlear nerve, an auditory brainstem implant (ABI) can be placed in the same sitting, by this approach.[17]

Contraindications

- *Only hearing ear*: This procedure is contraindicated in the only hearing ear. However, this has become a relative contraindication currently due to the option of simultaneous ipsilateral CI or ABI as mentioned above or a contralateral CI.[18]
- *Ipsilateral chronic otitis media*: This procedure is contraindicated in the presence of active infection. However, the approach can be used in cases of simple tympanic membrane perforation with no active infection, while the external auditory canal is closed as a cul-de-sac. If there is an active infection, a subtotal petrosectomy is performed, with eradication of the infection, obliteration of the cavity with abdominal fat, and closure of the external auditory canal as a cul-de-sac. The ETLA is then performed as a second stage surgery.

Surgical Technique

Mastoidectomy (Left Ear)

A C-shaped postauricular skin incision is placed starting from 2–3 cm superior to the attachment of auricle, at the level of the dome of the helix, continuing 4–5 cm posterior to the retroauricular sulcus, and ending just below the mastoid tip (Fig. 16.3). The skin flap is reflected anteriorly and maintained in position with two hooks. The musculoperiosteal layer is incised in a T-shaped fashion using a cutting diathermy (Fig. 16.4) and is elevated. Monopolar diathermy is applied to transect the muscles attached to the mastoid tip that helps to raise the flap. Bleeding from the mastoid emissary vein usually occurs at this step and it can be controlled by the use of bone wax. The posterior margins of the musculoperiosteal flaps are sutured to the skin which helps in achieving hemostasis from the skin incision and at the same time keeps the flaps retracted (Fig. 16.5). We do not recommend the use the conventional retractors which limit the access and exposure.

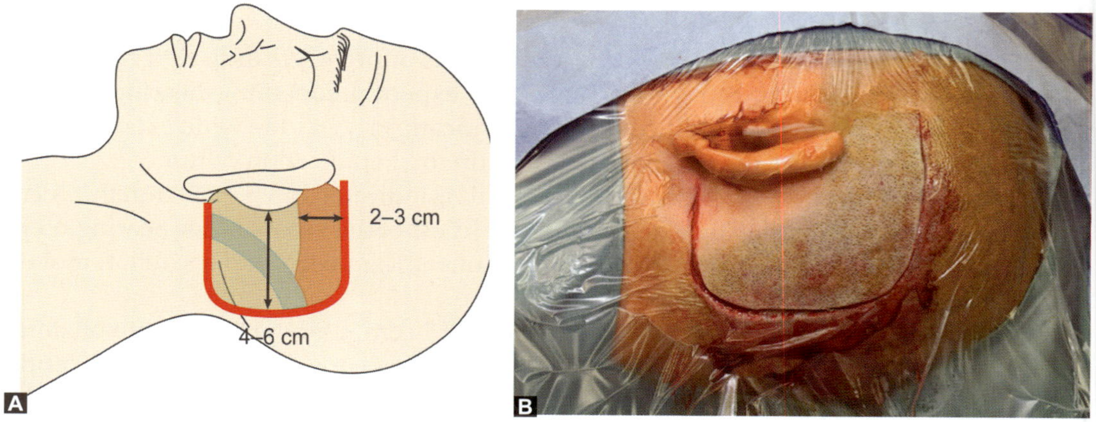

Fig. 16.3: Right postauricular skin incision for the ETLA

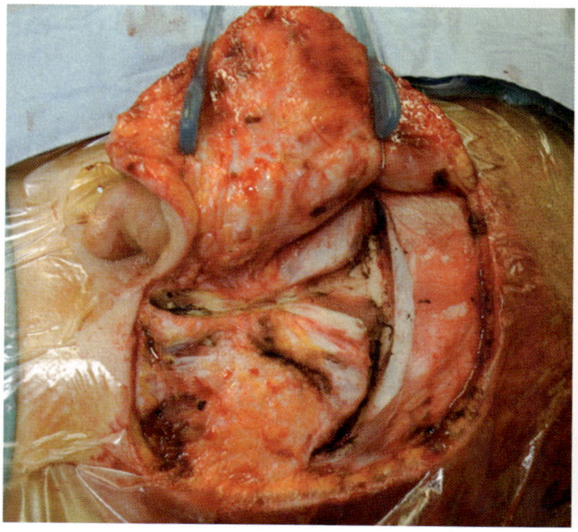

Fig. 16.4: The musculoperiosteal flap is incised using a monopolar diathermy in a 'T' fashion. The vertical incision extends up to the mastoid tip

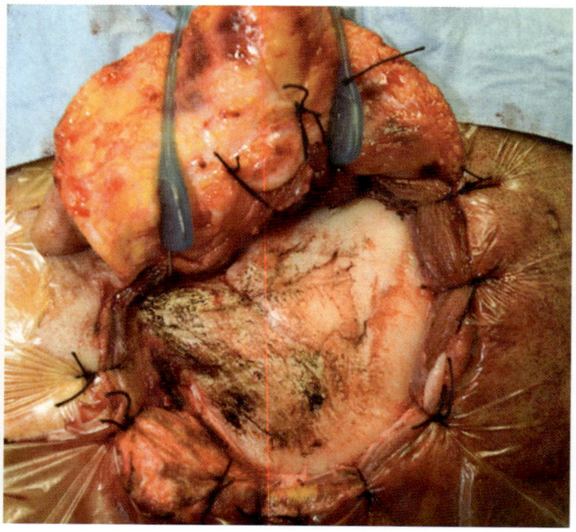

Fig. 16.5: The musculoperiosteal flaps are held by sutures

An extended mastoidectomy is then performed. The middle cranial fossa dura and the sigmoid sinus are identified, leaving a thin shell of bone overlying them. Bone 2–3 cm posterior to the sigmoid sinus is also drilled using a large cutting burr (Fig. 16.6). The mastoid air cells are exenterated, and the antrum is widely opened. The digastric ridge is identified, the facial nerve skeletonized and the retrofacial air cells drilled out. Using a large diamond burr, the remaining bone covering the middle cranial fossa and the sigmoid sinus as well as the posterior fossa dura posterior to the sinus are further drilled and removed. The sinodural angle must be clearly exposed to know the exact location of the superior petrosal sinus exiting the sigmoid sinus. The sigmoid sinus is followed down to the jugular bulb, and the three semicircular canals are delineated.

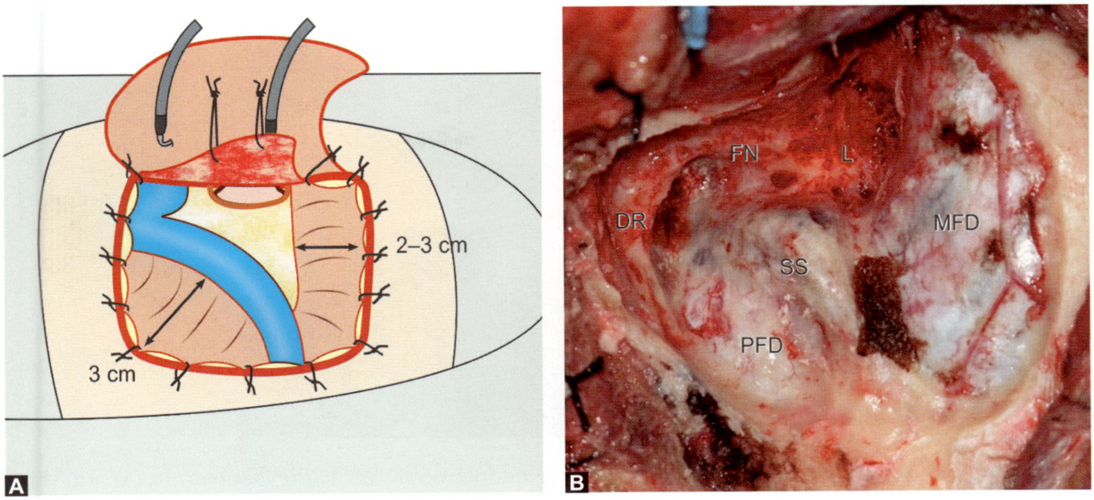

Fig. 16.6: (A) Extensive removal of bone over the middle cranial fossa as well as posterior to the sigmoid sinus (SS) is essential in the ETLA. **(B)** Mastoid air cells are well exenterated to demonstrate the labyrinth (L) and the mastoid segment of the facial nerve (FN). An adequate bone exposure will extend to about 3 cm posterior to the sigmoid sinus. DR: Digastric ridge, MFD: Middle fossa dura, PFD: Posterior fossa dura

Labyrinthectomy, Access to the IAC and the CPA

The labyrinthectomy starts by opening the lateral semicircular canal using a medium-sized cutting burr. The posterior semicircular canal is next opened, followed by opening the superior semicircular canal (Fig. 16.7). The anterior end of the lateral semicircular canal is left *in situ* to protect the facial nerve lying anteriorly. The last part of bone over the middle cranial fossa dura adjacent to the labyrinth is finally removed using a rongeur

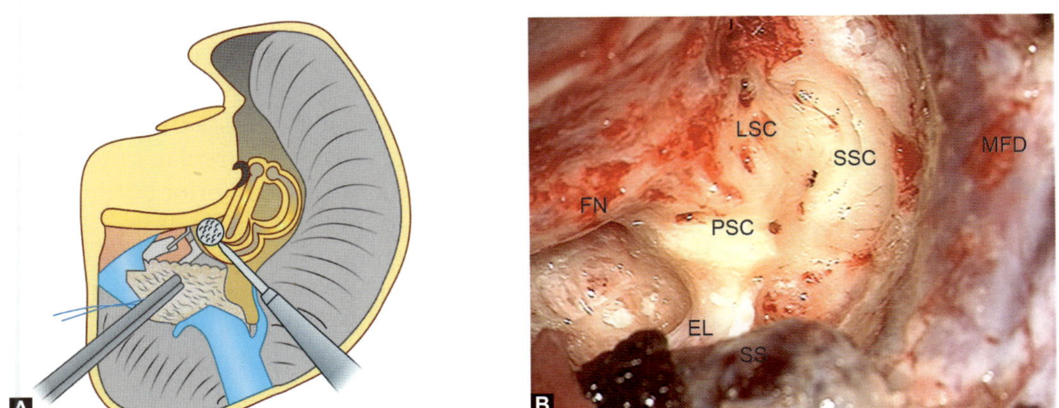

Fig. 16.7: (A) Note the suction-irrigator is pushing the sigmoid sinus away from the working burr. **(B)** The three semicircular canals have been opened. Note the endolymphatic duct (EL) extending from the medial surface of the posterior canal (PSC) to the posterior fossa dura (PFD). SS: Sigmoid sinus, FN: facial nerve, MFD: middle fossa dura, LSC: lateral semicircular canal, SSC: Superior semicircular canal

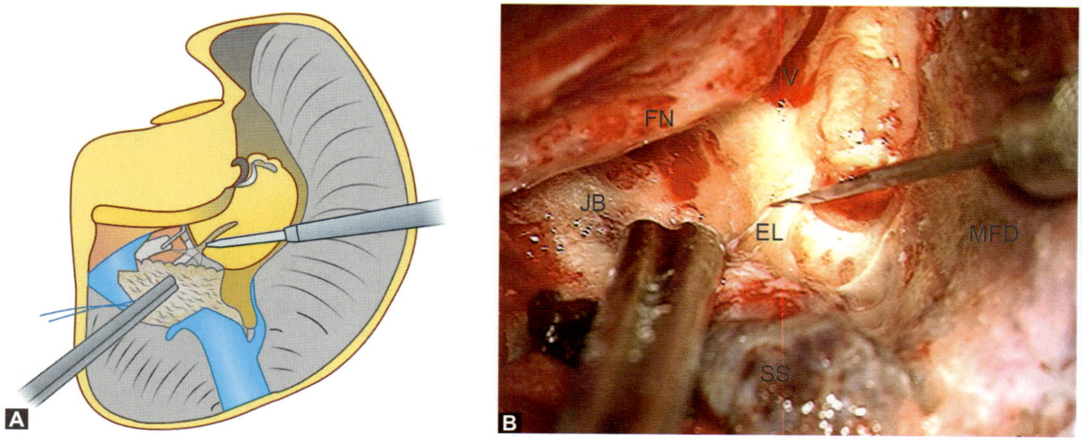

Fig. 16.8: A beaver knife is used to cut sharply the endolymphatic (EL) duct (shown in **(A)** and **(B)**) to allow dural retraction. The semicircular canal have been drilled out and the vestibule (Ve) can be seen. FN: Facial nerve, JB: Jugular bulb, MFD: Middle fossa dura, SS: Sigmoid sinus

after separating the bone from the dura by the use of a septal dissector. The ampullae of the lateral and superior semicircular canals are drilled. However, the anterior part of the ampullae of these two canals should be left to protect the labyrinthine segment of the facial nerve and to serve as a landmark for the superior vestibular nerve.

The vestibule is then opened widely. It is important to avoid drilling the floor of the vestibule in order to avoid inadvertent entry into the IAC. Similarly, drilling the roof of the vestibule may result in injury to the facial nerve, as the nerve runs immediately lateral to the vestibule. The endolymphatic duct is transacted by the use of beaver knife (Fig. 16.8). This step facilitates the complete drilling of bone overlying the posterior fossa dura and the subsequent dural retraction. The bone left over the posterior and middle fossa is successively drilled out. During this step the cochlear aqueduct can be identified. This is an important landmark for the glossopharyngeal nerve, which lies immediately inferior to it. In small or medium-sized VSs, opening the cochlear aqueduct allows the CSF to drain. This does not occur in large tumors, because the duct is occluded by the tumor. After a wide exposure of the dura is accomplished, following the posterior fossa dura allows the porus of the IAC to be identified. The ampulla of the superior semicircular canal serves as a landmark for the superior border of the IAC at the fundus. The inferior border of the canal is identified by drilling the retrofacial air cells up to the cochlear aqueduct. Further cautious drilling at the level of the fundus leads to the identification of the horizontal crest as well as the superior ampullary canal. Bone between the superior border of the IAC and the middle fossa dura and between the inferior border of the IAC and the jugular bulb can be further drilled, depending on the size of the tumor. We routinely drill the bone 270° around the IAC (Fig. 16.2).

Identification of the Facial Nerve at the Fundus

The original technique described by House for identifying the facial nerve at the fundus depends on the identification of the vertical crest (Bill's bar). However, we have modified this technique. By drilling inferiorly at the fundus the inferior vestibular nerve is exposed while in a more superior plane the horizontal crest is identified, which separates the inferior vestibular nerve from the superior vestibular nerve. The superior vestibular nerve is followed laterally where it leaves the fundus of the IAC. The nerve then lies in a tiny canal that enters the ampulla of the superior semicircular canal as the superior ampullary nerve (Fig. 16.9). The superior ampullary nerve is dissected from its canal using a 90° hook with the tip facing inferiorly (Fig. 16.10A). The superior ampullary nerve is separated from the facial nerve by a vertical crest of bone, called the Bill's bar which protects the facial nerve while this step is being carried out. The hook is moved medially toward the fundus, with subsequent separation and establishment of a good plane of cleavage between the superior vestibular nerve and the anteriorly lying facial nerve. Once the superior ampullary nerve is detached and reflected medially and posteriorly,

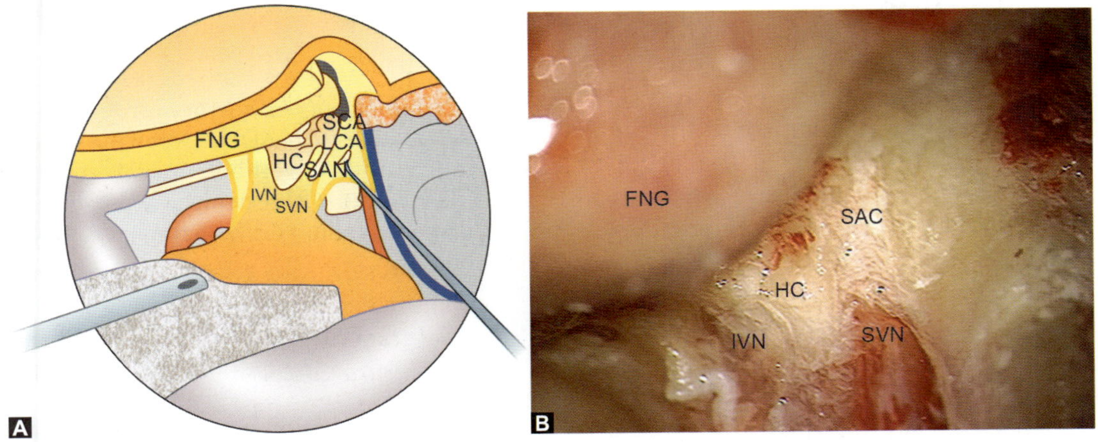

Fig. 16.9: The superior vestibular nerve (SVN) has been followed laterally into the superior ampullary nerve canal (SAC) where the superior ampullary nerve enters the lateral canal ampulla. FNG: Facial nerve genu, HC: Horizontal crest, I: Incus, IVN: Inferior vestibular nerve, LCA: Ampulla of the lateral semicircular canal, SCA: Ampulla of the superior semicircular canal

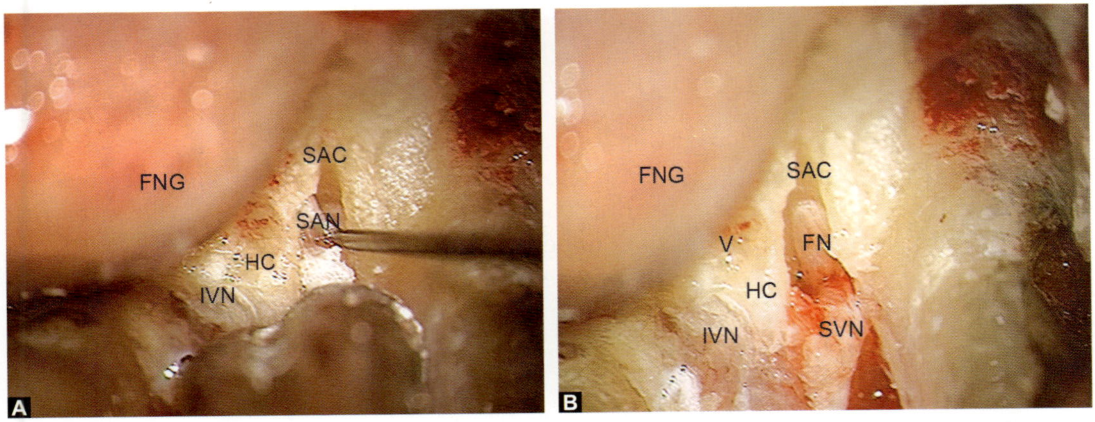

Fig. 16.10: (A) A small hook is used carefully to dislodge the superior ampullary nerve (SAN) from the superior ampullary canal (SAC), **(B)** After reflecting the superior vestibular nerve (SVN) medially, the facial nerve (FN) can be seen anteriorly. FNG: Facial nerve genu, I: Incus, HC: Horizontal crest, VC:Vertical crest (Bill's bar), SVN: Superior vestibular nerve, IVN: Inferior vestibular nerve, V: Vestibule

the facial nerve can be clearly observed (Fig. 16.10B). The relationship between the facial and cochlear nerves and the horizontal and vertical crests is well appreciated. Careful dissection of the superior vestibular nerve continues medially. Often here one may encounter adhesive bands between the superior vestibular nerve and the facial nerve (Fig. 16.11), which may bleed on manipulation, thus obscuring the plane of dissection. To control this, a piece of dry Gelfoam® is placed on the facial nerve which also helps to protect the nerve during further dissection. Our technique of identification of the facial nerve by identification of the superior ampullary nerve and the horizontal crest rather than the vertical crest ensures proper identification and hence greater protection to the facial nerve.

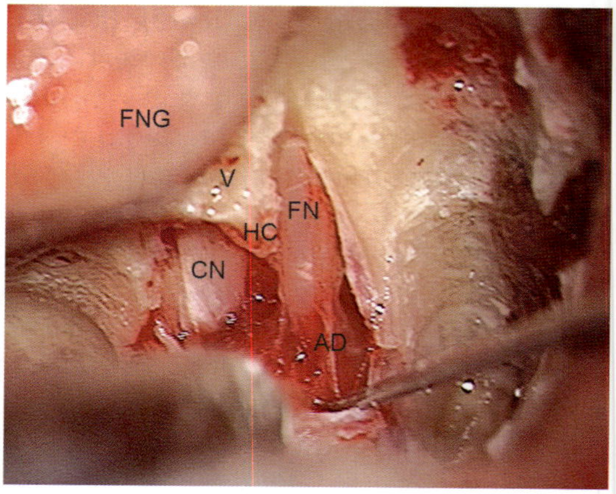

Fig. 16.11: While the dissection of the vestibular nerves is further progressed medially, adhesions (AD) between the facial nerve (FN) and the vestibular nerves start to be encountered. CN: Cochlear nerve, FNG: Facial nerve genu, HC: Horizontal crest, V: Vestibule

Opening the Dura

Before opening the dura of the posterior fossa, the lines of incision are coagulated with a bipolar cautery. Careful coagulation over the dural surface leads to its retraction, thus providing a wider access. The dotted red line represent the dural incision (Fig. 16.12). Using the neurosurgical scissors, a small snip is made just anterior to the sigmoid sinus and immediately inferior to its junction with the superior petrosal sinus and the dura is

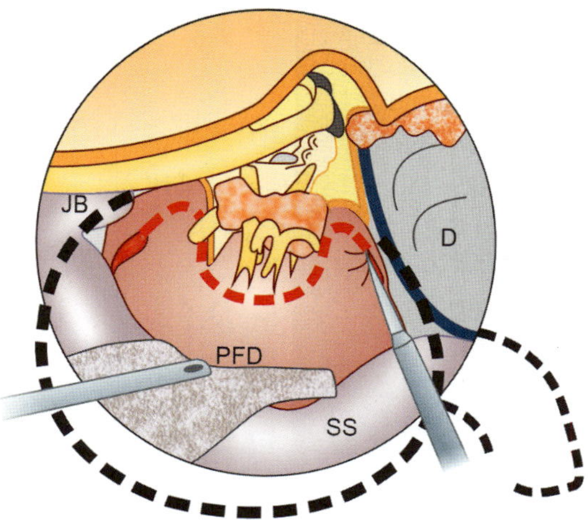

Fig. 16.12: Bipolar coagulation of the posterior fossa dura is done before incision of the dura. The dashed lines indicate the outlines of the dural incision. JB: Jugular bulb, PFD: Posterior fossa dura, SS: Sigmoid sinus, D: Dura

opened. Once sufficient opening of the dura has been achieved, Merocel® is inserted and slipped further into protect the underlying structures while the dural incision is being completed. The superior dural incision runs parallel and just inferior to the superior petrosal sinus up to the limit of bony drilling. The inferior incision starts just in front of the distal part of the sigmoid sinus, and follows the sinus and jugular bulb course to the porus, where it joins the superior incision.

Bloodless Techniques for Tumor Removal

After the dura has been opened, the tumor in the CPA can be visualized, and the arachnoid of the lateral cistern is identified and opened. This allows CSF to drain out, leading to a collapse of cerebellum which results in an increased working space. In a case of a large tumor, it is difficult to achieve this, due to compression of the cistern by the tumor (Fig. 16.13). In large tumors, they may be debulked at the centre to reduce their size. Intracapsular debulking is performed by using microscissors and bipolar coagulation. It is extremely important to find the plane of cleavage that lies between the arachnoid adherent to the tumor capsule and the arachnoid surrounding the other structures in the CPA. Once this plane of cleavage has been obtained, Gelfoam® is placed on this plane to prevent blood from entering the CPA (Fig. 16.14). The outer surface of the tumor is coagulated using a bipolar. Using this manoeuvre in all the directions, the tumor retracts and comes separated from the surrounding structures.

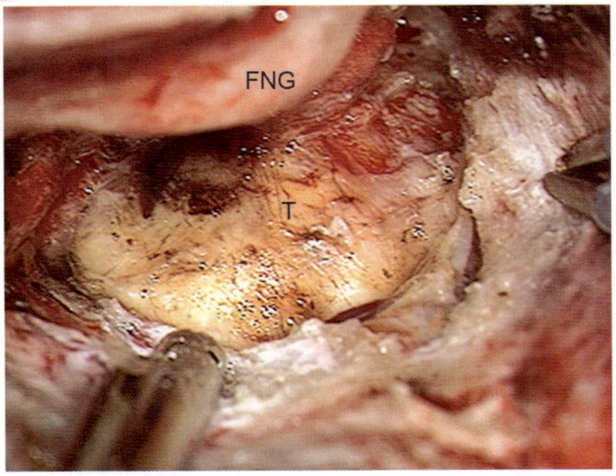

Fig. 16.13: After opening in the dura, the tumor (T) can be seen filling the cerebellopontine angle. FNG: Facial nerve genu

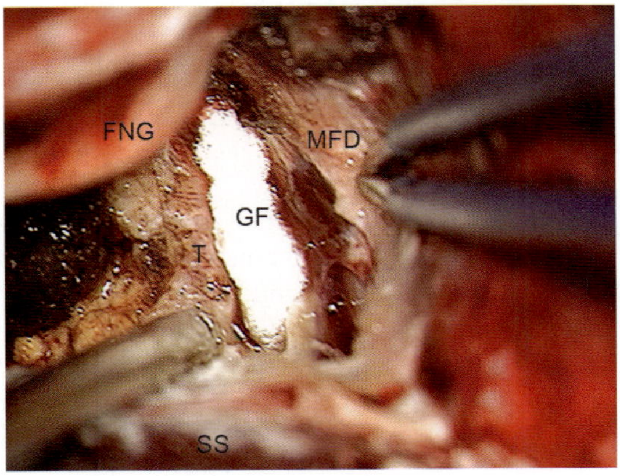

Fig. 16.14: After coagulating the arachnoid at the superior surface of the tumor (T), a plane of cleavage is looked for. A large piece of Gelfoam® (GF) is used to fill the gap around the tumor (T) to prevent blood from filling the CPA. FNG: Facial nerve genu, MFD: Middle fossa dura, SS: Sigmoid sinus

The superior surface of the tumor is dissected (Fig. 16.15). The trigeminal nerve is frequently found adherent to the tumor. The tumor surface is repeatedly coagulated and incised, thereby reducing the size of the tumor. The posterior aspect is further dissected and the interface between the tumor and the brainstem can be perceived. Tumor is then dissected from the facial nerve. Since the plane of cleavage between the tumor and the facial nerve has already been established at the fundus of the IAC, dissection proceeds in a lateral to medial direction. Localization of the facial nerve at the porus is achieved by following it from the

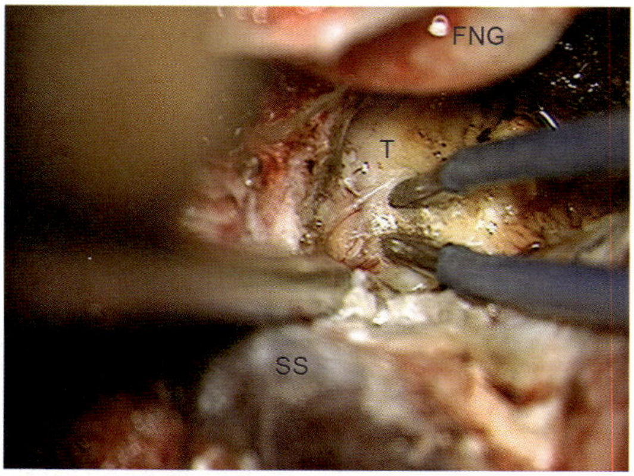

Fig. 16.15: The outer surface of the tumor is coagulated from all directions to achieve adequate tumor retraction from surrounding tissues. FNG: Facial nerve genu, SS: Sigmoid sinus, T: Tumor, Tent: Tentorium

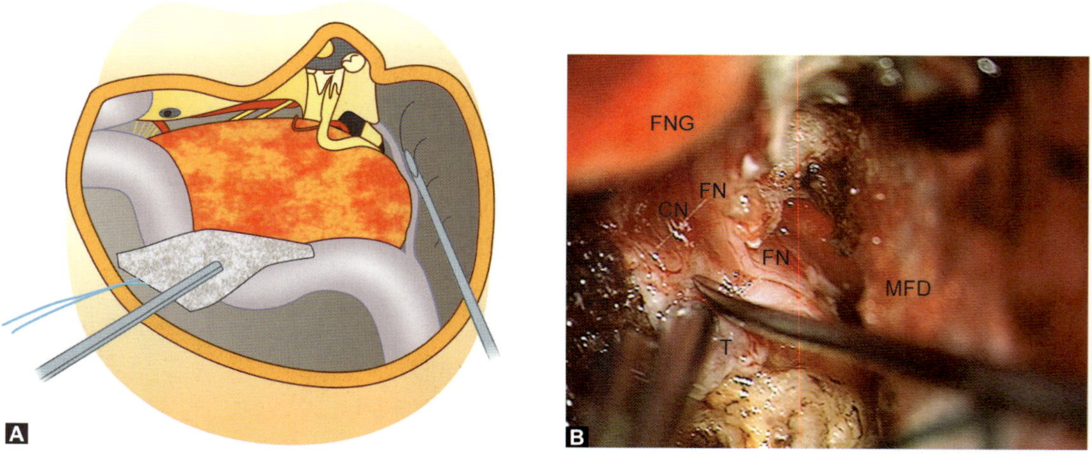

Fig. 16.16A and B: The facial nerve (FN) can be followed from within the internal auditory canal, and it can be seen angulating anteriorly over the porus and lying adherent to the anterior surface of the tumor (T). The identification in this dangerous area where the nerve is usually adherent to the surrounding structures can only be achieved with the help of the transapical extension. CN: Cochlear nerve, FNG: Facial nerve genu, MFD: Middle fossa dura, SS: Sigmoid sinus, V: Trigeminal nerve, VNs: Superior and inferior vestibular nerves

fundus (Fig. 16.16). Care should be taken not to force any traction on the facial nerve while carrying out the dissection. At the level of the porus, the facial nerve is usually adherent to the tumor and frequently becomes thin and splayed, thereby becoming vulnerable. Very gentle manipulation is necessary in this step (Fig. 16.17).

The facial nerve at the level of the brainstem is then identified and the last part of the tumor is carefully dissected from the facial nerve and the brainstem. It is important to neither coagulate nor apply traction to these important structures (Fig. 16.18). The integrity of the facial nerve is determined using the facial nerve stimulator. The anesthetist raises the blood pressure and Valsalva maneuver is performed to look for bleeding points. Hemostasis is achieved.

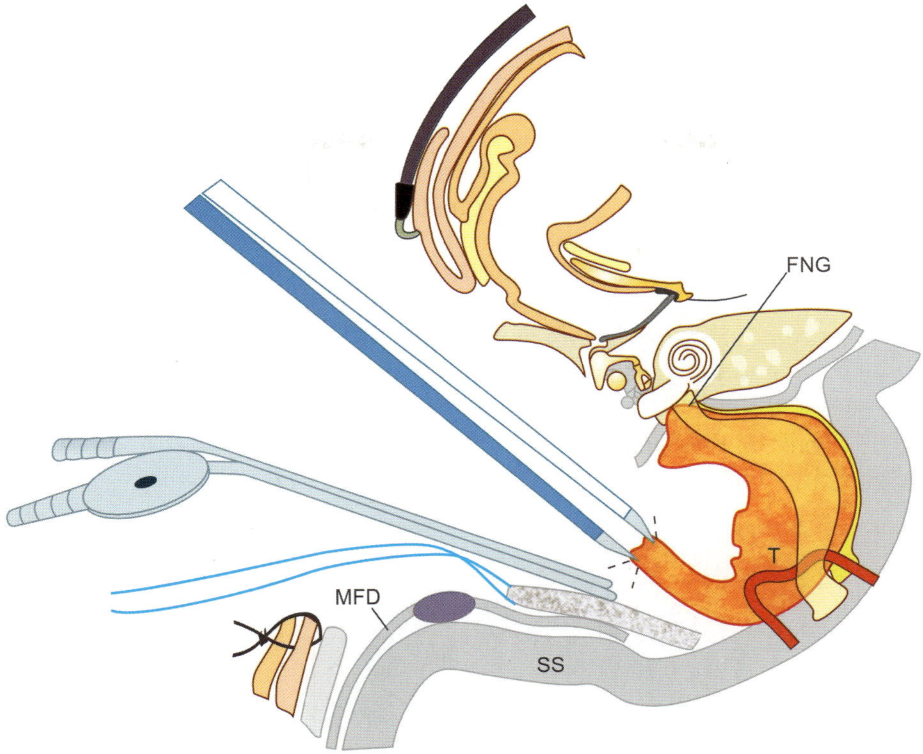

Fig. 16.17: After reducing the core and the walls of the tumor, dissection of the facial nerve is continued. Very delicate maneuvers are made in this area. FNG: Facial nerve genu, MFD: Middle fossa dura, SS: Sigmoid sinus, T: Tumor

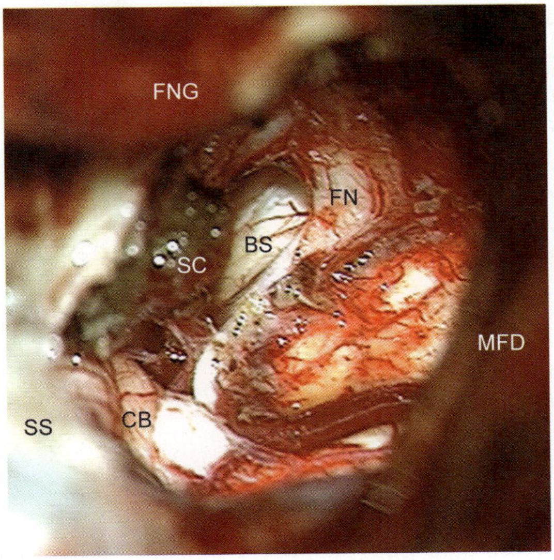

Fig. 16.18: CPA after total tumor removal. Note the integrity of the facial nerve (FN) together with its vasculature. BS: Brainstem, CB: Cerebellum, FNG: Facial nerve genu, MFD: Middle fossa dura, SC: Surgicel®, SS: Sigmoid sinus

Closure

All the air cells, especially the retrofacial cells, should be observed to see if they have the communication with the tympanic cavity. If so, these cells are obliterated with bone wax to avoid CSF leak postoperatively. After the incus is disarticulated and removed, the aditus is obliterated with periosteum. Abdominal fat which has been harvested is sliced into several long, thin strips, and these strips are placed inside the CPA. The musculoperiosteal layer is closed using 1–0 Vicryl® (Fig. 16.19). This is followed by closure of the subcutaneous tissue and skin. A pressure dressing is applied.

In our experience, with the ETLA, tumor of very large sizes in the CPA can be safely removed. Wide removal of bone from the middle fossa dura, as well as extensive drilling of bone between it and the internal auditory canal, provides excellent control of the upper pole of the tumor and the trigeminal nerve area. Uncovering the sigmoid sinus and bone 2–3 cm posterior to it, and extensive bone removal creating a deep trough inferior to the internal auditory canal, obviate the need for a suboccipital or transotic approach, and

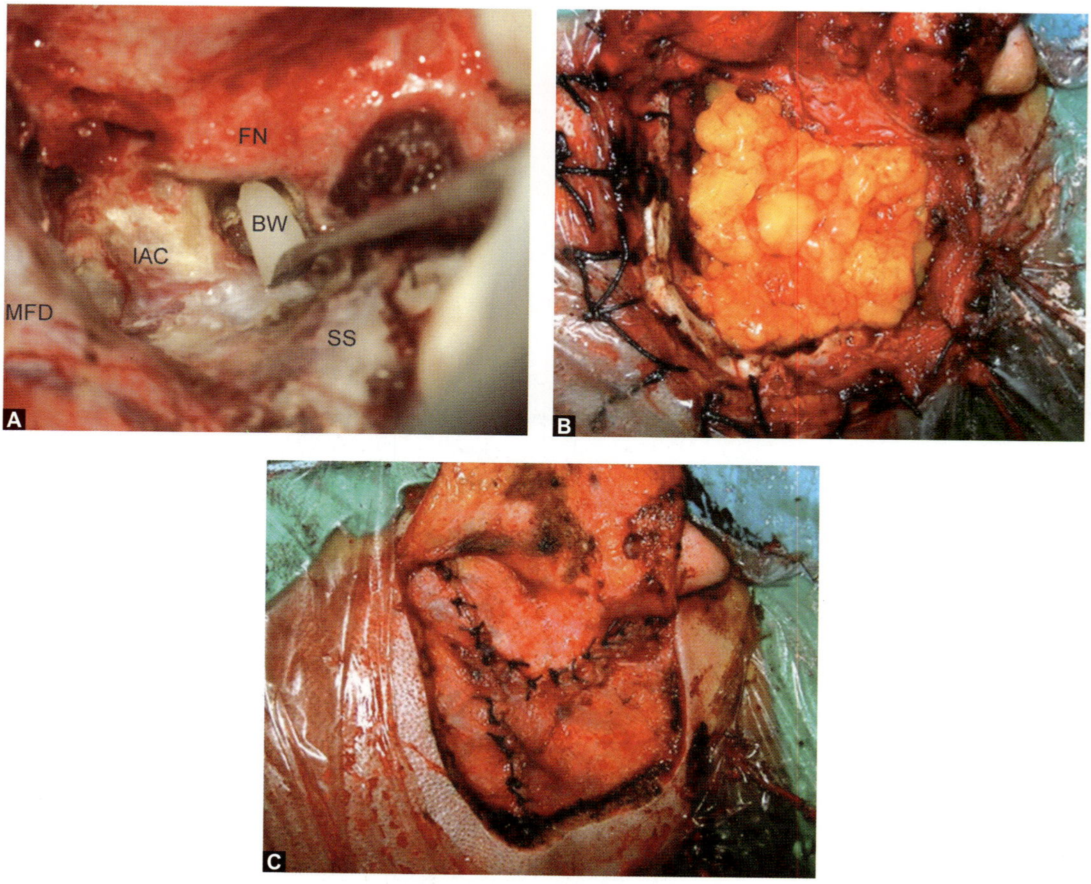

Fig. 16.19: **(A)** In a pneumatized temporal bone, cells superiorly and inferiorly to the internal auditory canal are obliterated with bone wax. IAC: Internal auditory canal, SS: Sigmoid sinus, FN: Facial nerve, JB: Jugular bulb, BW: Bone wax. **(B)** Abdominal fat is used to close the CPA and the bony defect. **(C)** The musculoperiosteal layer is approximated using 1–0 Vicryl®. After the musculoperiosteal layer is closed tightly, the skin flap is replaced and sutured

provide perfect control of the anterior pole of the tumor up to the lateral aspect of the prepontine cistern. In addition, extensive removal of bone between the internal auditory canal and the jugular bulb allows good visualization of the lower tumor pole. Tumors up to 6 cm in extrameatal diameter have been safely removed at the Gruppo Otologico, Italy, using this approach (Fig. 16.20).

- Completely uncovering the middle fossa dura, posterior fossa dura, sigmoid sinus and the retrosigmoid area is the most important aspect in the ETLA. Uncovering the above mentioned structures allows retraction and hence better visualization of all aspects of the tumor.

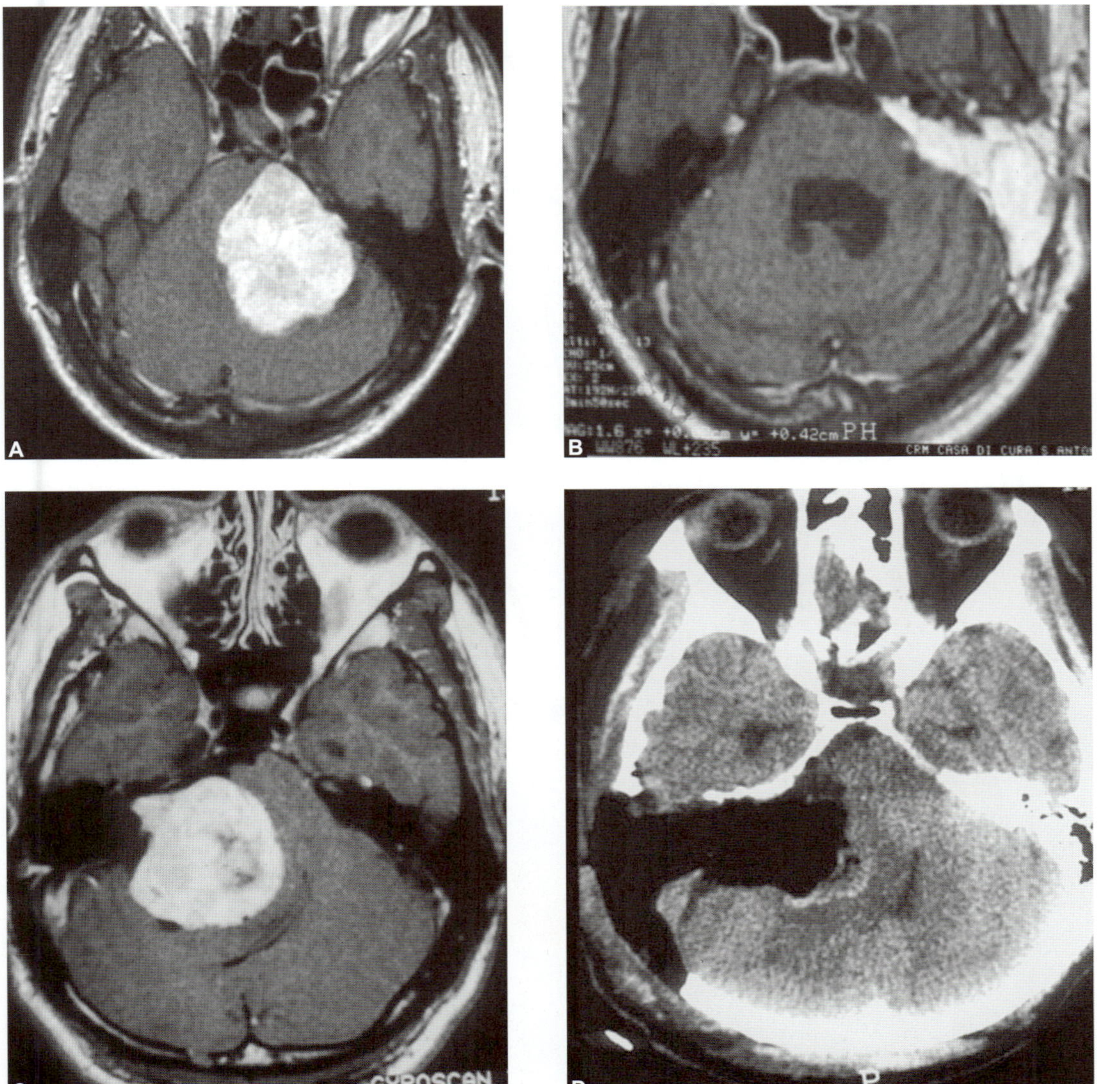

Fig. 16.20: Preoperative **(A)** and one week postoperative **(B)** MRI scan of a large grade 5 tumors which was removed totally with the ETLA. Preoperative **(C)** and one year postoperative **(D)** scans of another patient with a similar grade 5 tumor excised using a similar approach. Note that fat is inserted up to the petrous apex

- The facial nerve lies immediately lateral to the vestibule. The utmost care should be taken not to injure the nerve during drilling to open the vestibule.
- The IAC should be uncovered over 270° up to 310° in the ETLA creating 2 troughs, inferior and superior to the IAC. Sufficient removal of bone superior to the IAC is essential in order to control the area of the trigeminal nerve. Failure to do so leads to incomplete control of the superior pole of the tumor and of Dandy's vein.
- The fundus of the IAC is approached by first identifying the inferior vestibular nerve and the horizontal crest instead of the vertical crest (Bill's bar) as in the conventional TLA (Fig. 16.21). Then the superior vestibular nerve is identified and the drilling is

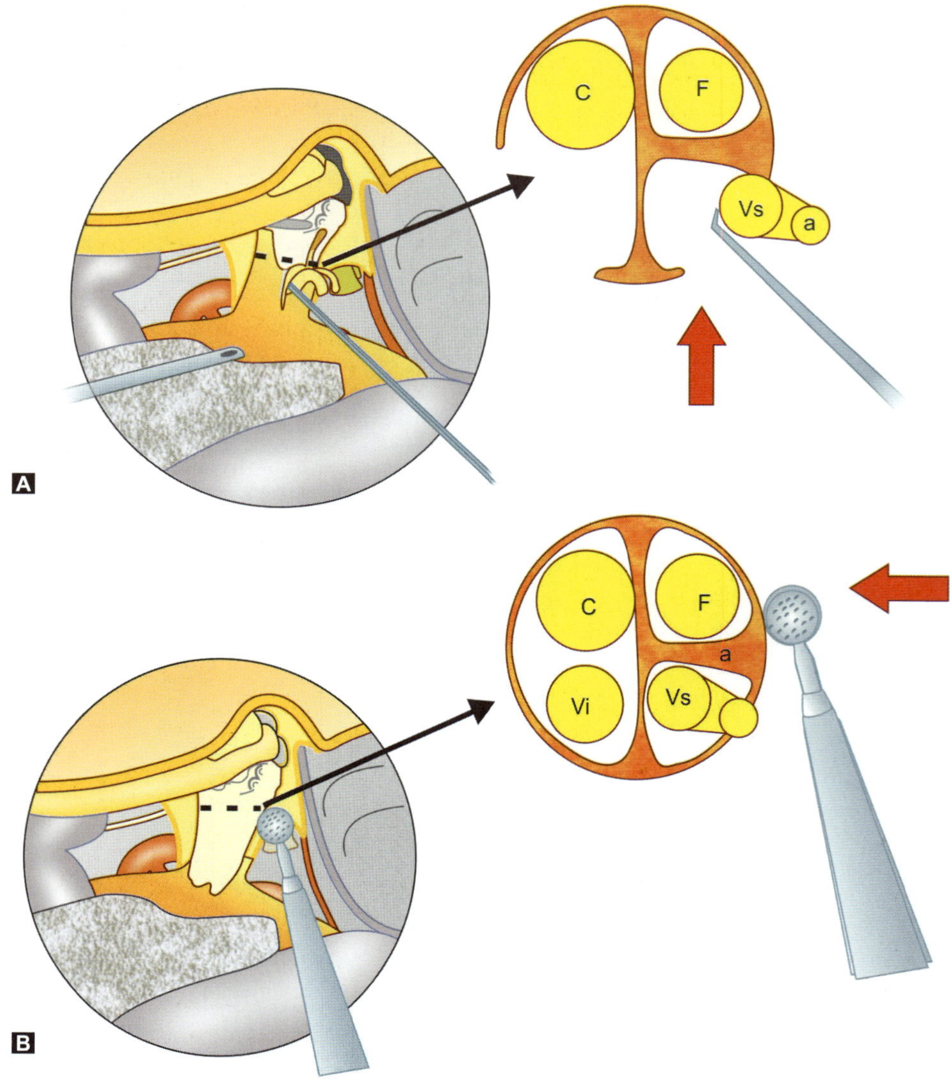

Fig. 16.21: (A) In our technique, we first identify the superior ampullary nerve (a) and then look for the facial nerve (F) after dissecting out this nerve along with the superior vestibular nerve (Vs). **(B)** In the conventional technique described by House the vertical crest (Bill's bar) is identified by drilling behind the superior vestibular nerve (Vs). Also seen are cochlear nerve (C), inferior vestibular nerve (Vi)

continued laterally until the ampullary nerve identified. Once the ampullary nerve is identified at the level of the fundus, it is dissected out and the vertical crest (Bill's bar) is identified medial to it. The facial nerve is then be identified medial to the Bill's bar.

- Facial nerve monitoring is helpful during tumor dissection. A train response given by the monitor indicates possible trauma to the facial nerve.
- It is important to maintain a bloodless surgical field in order to see clearly all the vital anatomy at all the time. This is ensured by dissecting the plane of cleavage between the tumor surface and the arachnoid and by bipolar coagulation of the veins and small arteries on the tumor surface. Once a plane is identified, Merocel® is inserted between the tumor and the arachnoid. Dissection proceeds with bipolar dissection of the tumor.
- During closure, long strips of abdominal fat are used to obliterate the CPA along with the bony defect. This is more effective in preventing CSF leakage than using the fat to obliterate the bone defect alone.
- Tumors up to 6 cm in extrameatal diameter can be safely removed using this approach.

Pitfalls

- The use self-retaining retractors for the skin and subcutaneous tissue is not recommended. Retractors impede surgical access leading to narrow working angle and deeper surgical field.
- Central debulking is important in dealing with a big tumor. Care should be taken while debulking soft or cystic tumors, so as not to penetrate the anterior or medial walls of the tumor and injure the adjacent structures, particularly the facial nerve and the brainstem.
- In small tumors, the AICA can be found looping around the tumor. It can also traverse between the facial nerve and the vestibulocochlear nerves.
- Towards the end of surgery, care should be taken while removing the incus to avoid fracturing the footplate, since this can create a communication between the CPA and the middle ear, with subsequent postoperative CSF leakage. We prefer periosteum to fat for the closure of the attic because it is easier to manipulate and provides a better seal.

Enlarged TLA with Transapical Extension (ETLA+TAE)

Rationale

This approach is an anteromedial extension of the ETLA, in which the IAC is drilled up to 320° (type I) or 360° (type II) of its circumference of the IAC (Fig. 16.22). This extension helps expose the anterior, superior and medial aspects of large tumors of the CPA.

Indications

This approach is indicated for large CPA tumors or tumors with marked anterior extensions, wherein hearing preservation is not intended. This includes large (or giant) VSs with anterior extension into the prepontine cistern and large meningioma of the posterior surface of the temporal bone centered on the IAC with significant anterior extension. It is also indicated in smaller tumors but with marked anterior extensions.

Limitations

Though this approach provides access to the prepontine cistern, it is difficult to remove tumors involving the petroclival region, like meningiomas, wherein the modified trans-cochlear approach is more suitable.

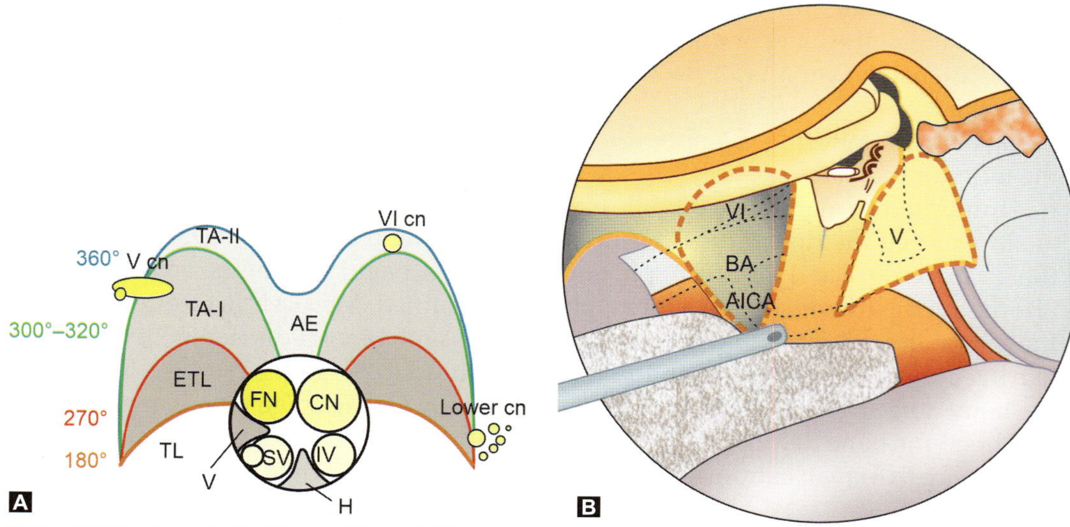

Fig. 16.22: (A) Amount of bone removal around the internal auditory canal in the different variations of the TLA. **(B)** The dashed line demonstrates the working area for extended bone removal. Note the fifth and sixth cranial nerves can be exposed and managed effectively. AICA: Anterior inferior cerebellar artery, BA: Basilar artery, V: Trigeminal nerve, VI: Abducens nerve, TL: Translabyrinthine, ETL: Extended translabyrinthine, TA-I: Transapical type I, TA-II: Transapical type II

Surgical Technique

The ETLA is performed as previously described. The IAC is identified and uncovered and bone is drilled out for 270° around the canal as previously described. Further drilling is carried superior and inferior to the IAC towards the petrous apex as required (Fig. 16.23A). In type I approach, up to 320° exposure around the IAC is achieved (Fig. 16.23B) leaving behind a thin segment of bone anteriorly. In type II approach, 360° of the IAC circumference is exposed (Fig. 16.23C). The contents of the IAC are pushed inferiorly to allow for drilling of the anterior wall of the canal (Fig. 16.24). Care should be taken to avoid injury to the superior petrosal sinus. The dura is opened as previously described.

Pearls

- In the case of tumors extending far anteromedially, the facial nerve is markedly displaced anteriorly. The transapical extension provides much better visualization of the nerve.
- In the case of giant tumors causing high intracranial pressure, the dura usually bulges, hindering access. In such cases, the tumor is first debulked from inside and after this the dura is opened to allow drainage of the CSF, which leads to drop in pressure and retraction of intracranial contents.
- After introducing this approach, we have abandoned the transotic approach for removal of anteriorly located tumors limiting its use only in the case of tumors with cochlear invasion, vertical internal carotid artery involvement or in case with very high jugular bulb and/or very advanced sigmoid sinus.

Pitfalls

- The facial nerve is at risk while performing the transapical drilling. Hence a diamond burr must be used and extreme care must be taken to avoid injuring the nerve.

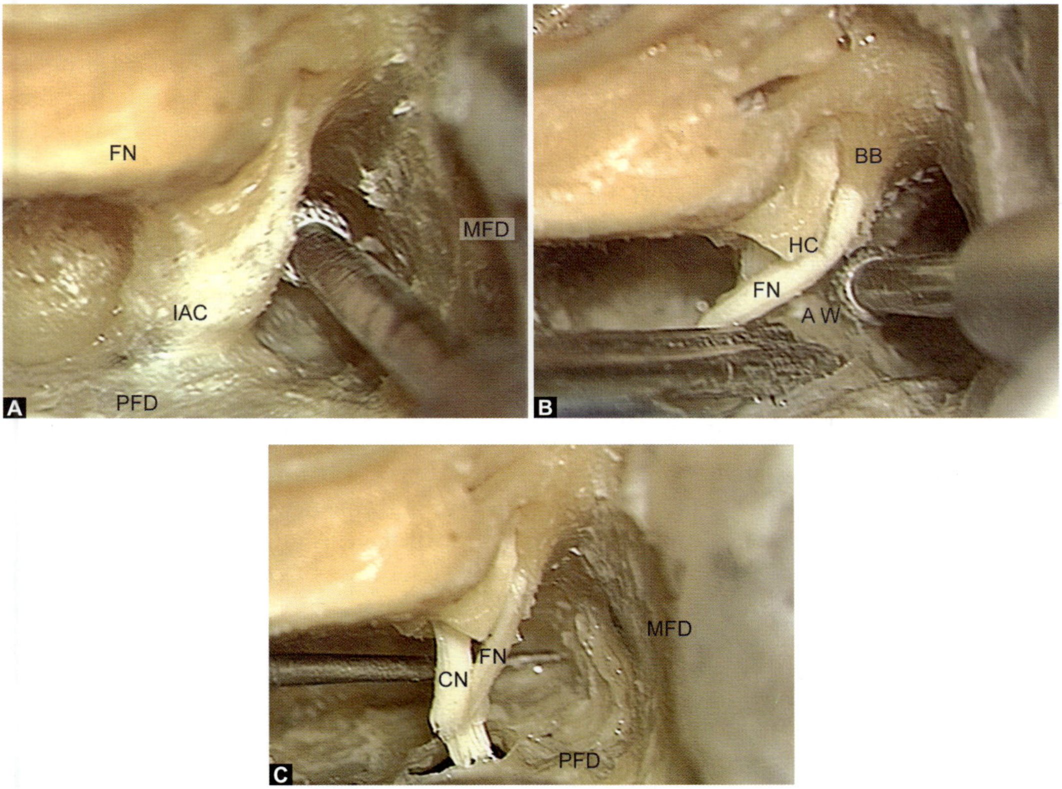

Fig. 16.23: (A) Extended TLA, **(B)** with TAE Type I and **(C)** Type II. CN: Cochlear nerve, FN: Facial nerve, IAC: Internal auditory canal, MFD: Middle fossa dura, PFD: Posterior fossa dura, HC: Horizontal crest, BB: Bill's bar, AW: Anterior wall

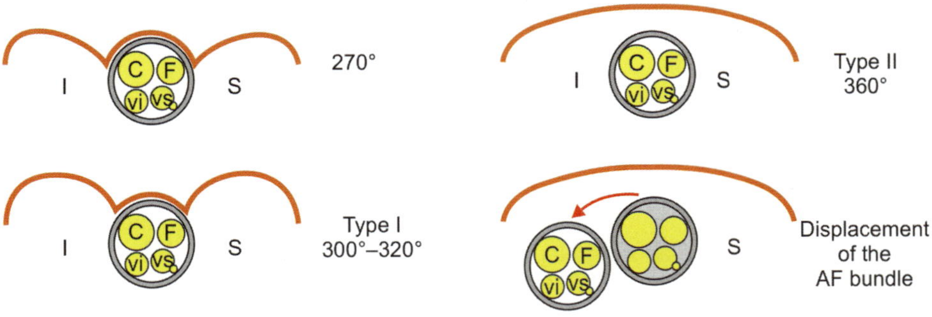

Fig. 16.24: Cross-sectional images of the internal auditory canal as seen in the ETLA exposure (270°), type I (300–320°), and type II TAE (360°). The contents of the internal auditory canal can be moved inferiorly. S: Superiorly, I: Inferiorly

A useful trick is to place the suction-irrigator between the drill and the nerve to afford protection.

- Care must be taken to avoid injuring the superior petrosal sinus while drilling the petrous apex superior to the IAC.

Pearls

- Completely uncovering the middle fossa dura, posterior fossa dura, sigmoid sinus and the retrosigmoid area is the most important aspect in the ETLA. Uncovering the above mentioned structures allows retraction and hence better visualization of all aspects of the tumor.
- The facial nerve lies immediately lateral to the vestibule. The utmost care should be taken not to injure the nerve during drilling to open the vestibule.
- The IAC should be uncovered over 270° up to 310° in the ETLA creating 2 troughs, inferior and superior to the IAC. Sufficient removal of bone superior to the IAC is essential in order to control the area of the trigeminal nerve. Failure to do so leads to incomplete control of the superior pole of the tumor and of Dandy's vein.

Conclusion

The ETLA is a safe approach that provides an excellent exposure for even very large tumors. The distinct advantages provided by the ETLAs are: The absence of cerebellar retraction, excellent exposure of the IAC and the CPA, extradural drilling and reduced incidence of postoperative CSF leaks. The ETLA and the ETLA+TAE have further increased the indications of the approach and helped tackled large, giant and anteromedially located tumors more effectively. Difficult anatomical and tumor-related situations can also be managed effectively with the ETLA. For similar tumor sizes, postoperative facial nerve function is better with ETLAs when compared to other approaches.

REFERENCES

1. Ben Ammar M, Piccirillo E, Topsakal V, Taibah A, Sanna M. Surgical results and technical refinements in translabyrinthine excision of vestibular schwannomas: the Gruppo Otologico experience. Neurosurgery 2012; 70:1481–1491; discussion 1491.
2. House WF, Hitselberger WE. Transtemporal Bone Microsurgical Removal of Acoustic Neuromas. Morbidity and Mortality of Acoustic Neuromas. Arch Otolaryngol 1964; 80:752–54.
3. House WF, Belal A, Jr. Translabyrinthine surgery: anatomy and pathology. The American journal of otology 1980; 1:189–98.
4. WF H. Translabyrinthine approach. In: House WF LC, ed. *Acoustic Tumors*. Baltimore: University Parke-Davis, 1979.
5. Hitselberger WE, House WF. Transtemporal Bone Microsurgical Removal of Acoustic Neuromas. Tumors of the Cerebellopontine Angle. Arch Otolaryngol 1964; 80:720–31.
6. Hardy DG, Macfarlane R, Baguley D, Moffat DA. Surgery for acoustic neurinoma. An analysis of 100 translabyrinthine operations. J Neurosurg 1989; 71:799–804.
7. Angeli RD, Piccirillo E, Di Trapani G, Sequino G, Taibah A, Sanna M. Enlarged translabyrinthine approach with transapical extension in the management of giant vestibular schwannomas: personal experience and review of literature. Otology and neurotology : official publication of the American Otological Society, American Neurotology Society [and] European Academy of Otology and Neurotology 2011; 32:125–31.
8. Sanna M, Russo A, Taibah A, Falcioni M, Agarwal M. Enlarged translabyrinthine approach for the management of large and giant acoustic neuromas: a report of 175 consecutive cases. The Annals of otology, rhinology, and laryngology 2004; 113:319–28.
9. Falcioni M, Russo A, Mancini F et al., Enlarged translabyrinthine approach in large acoustic neurinomas. Acta otorhinolaryngologica Italica : organo ufficiale della Societa italiana di otorinolaringologia chirurgia cervico-facciale 2001; 21:226–36.

10. Naguib MB, Saleh E, Cokkeser Y et al. The enlarged translabyrinthine approach for removal of large vestibular schwannomas. The Journal of laryngology and otology 1994; 108:545–50.
11. House WF, Hitselberger WE. The transcochlear approach to the skull base. Arch Otolaryngol 1976; 102:334–42.
12. Chen JM, Fisch U. The transotic approach in acoustic neuroma surgery. The Journal of otolaryngology 1993; 22:331–36.
13. Browne JD, Fisch U. Transotic approach to the cerebellopontine angle. Otolaryngologic clinics of North America 1992; 25:331–46.
14. Sanna M MF, Russo A, Taibah A, Falcioni M, Di Trapani G. Atlas of Acoustic Neurinoma Microsurgery. Stuttgart: Georg Thieme Verlag, 2008.
15. Gantz BJ, Fisch U. Modified transotic approach to the cerebellopontile angle. Arch Otolaryngol 1983; 109:252–56.
16. Rabelo de Freitas M, Russo A, Sequino G, Piccirillo E, Sanna M. Analysis of hearing preservation and facial nerve function for patients undergoing vestibular schwannoma surgery: the middle cranial fossa approach versus the retrosigmoid approach--personal experience and literature review. Audiology and neuro-otology 2012; 17:71–81.
17. Sanna M, Di Lella F, Guida M, Merkus P. Auditory brainstem implants in NF2 patients: results and review of the literature. Otology and neurotology : official publication of the American Otological Society, American Neurotology Society [and] European Academy of Otology and Neurotology 2012; 33:154–64.
18. Di Lella F, Merkus P, Di Trapani G, Taibah A, Guida M, Sanna M. Vestibular schwannoma in the only hearing ear: role of cochlear implants. The Annals of otology, rhinology, and laryngology 2013; 122:91–99.

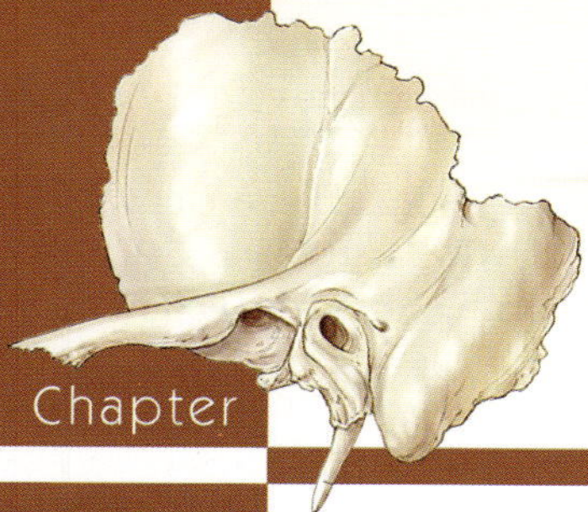

Chapter

17

Principle of Skull Base Surgery and Approaches to Lateral Skull Base Surgery

HN Udaybhanu • Dipak Ranjan Nayak • Produl Hazarika • Ajay Bhandarkar

Introduction

Skull base is that portion of the cranium lying and anteriorly to the neuro-axis, through which passes the 12 cranial nerves, major arterial and venous channels supplying the central nervous system. The skull base is composed of frontal and ethmoid bone anteriorly, occipital bone posteriorly, sphenoid and paired temporal bones in between. The following are the common discrete areas in the skull base of pathological importance.

1. Cerebellopontine angle
2. Jugular foramen
3. Area of petrous apex
4. Superior orbital fissure
5. Inferior surface of temporal bone
6. Other selected regions
   - Cavernous sinus
   - Pituitary

The various pathological conditions commonly encountered are:

1. Infection
2. Benign space occupying lesion (glomus, neuroma)
3. Primary and metastatic malignant neoplasm
4. Vascular abnormalities
5. Congenital defects
6. Traumatic lesions.

Historical Perspective: Although there were significant advancements in the related specialties in the past 25 years to tackle the conditions involving the skull base effectively, most of the conditions involving lateral skull base were considered inaccessible until recently, because of their close relations to the great vessels and major cranial nerves passing in this part of the skull base. Approaches to cerebellopontine angle for acoustic neuroma have already been described in Chapter 15. This chapter will discuss on the development of infratemporal fossa approach to the lateral skull base especially trans-temporal approaches. In 1961, Fairbanks-Barbosa was the first to report an infratemporal

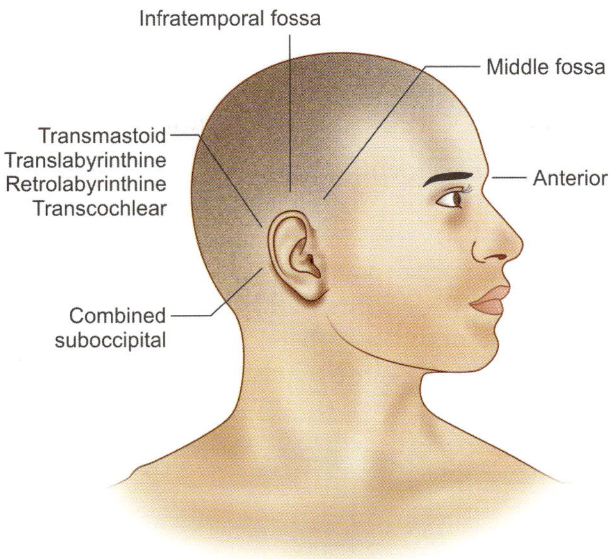

Fig. 17.1: Various skull base approaches.

fossa (ITF) approach, indicated for advanced tumors of the maxillary sinus. The surgical approach to infratemporal fossa through transtemporal route was described by Ugo Fisch (1977, 1979, 1984). There was a major breakthrough in the subsequent development of surgical expertise and microsurgical techniques for adequate management of these lesions. The pioneers who brought the revolution in the surgical techniques of skull base are: William House (1961); Glasscock (1978), Fisch (1977, 1978, 1982); Biller et al (1981) and Sekhar et al (1987). Hazarika et al (1990, 1992, and 1993) popularized the skull based surgery in India. In the modern era, Prasad (2014, 2017) popularized advanced infratemporal fossa approaches.

The lesions involving lateral skull base is more difficult to approach for their close relation to the neurovascular bundle consisting of great vessels and various cranial nerves, which necessitates thorough anatomical knowledge and expertise to tackle these tumors. Since lateral skull base lesions are more frequently encountered by the otolaryngology—head and neck surgeons, the present chapter will discuss about the principles of lateral skull base approaches (Fisch approach).

Principles of Lateral Skull Base Approaches

Lateral skull base approach can be further divided into:

1. Extended lateral approach (pre-auricular by Sekhar)
2. Infratemporal fossa approach (Fisch approach)

Infratemporal Fossa Approach (Fisch's Approach)

Infratemporal approach may be extended into three types depending on the extent of the disease.

- **Type A approach:** Access to the temporal bone in its infralabyrinthine and apical compartments mostly employed for glomus tumors.

- **Type B approach:** Access to the clivus
- **Type C approach:** Access to parasellar region and nasopharynx.

Steps for Surgery for Type A Approach

1. 'S/C' shape skin incision as shown in Fig. 17.2, involves wide undermining of the anterior skin edge
2. Elevation of periosteal flap, based on the posterior aspect of the membranous canal wall.
3. Transaction of external auditory canal at the bony cartilaginous junction and blind sac closure and sealing with periosteal flap in the inner aspect (Fig. 17.3).
4. Identification of the facial nerve trunk distal to stylomastoid foramen along the axis formed by the bisection of a line drawn between the pointer of tragal cartilage and mastoid tip.

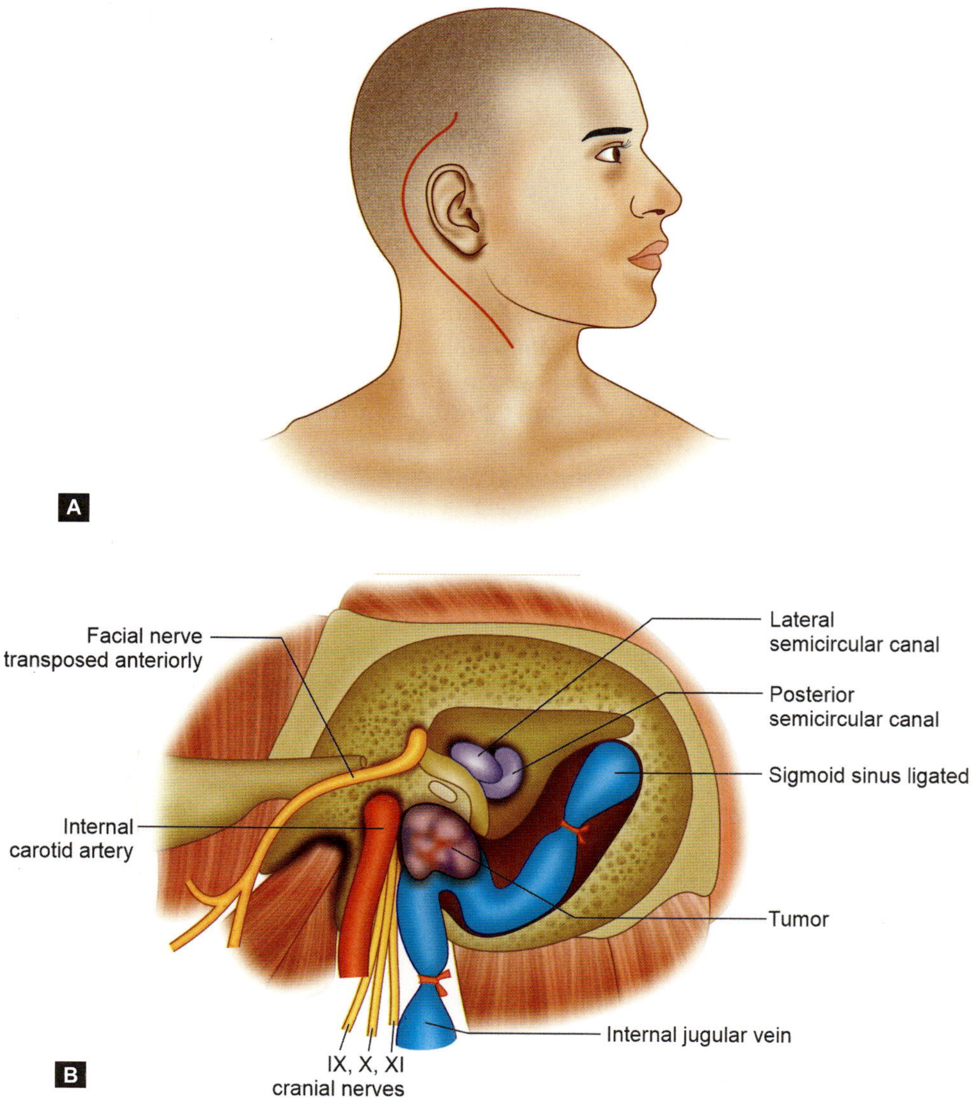

Fig. 17.2: Fisch approach type A, **(A)** Showing incision, **(B)** Final exposure before tumor removal

5. Identification of IX–XII cranial nerves, carotid and its branches and internal jugular vein (IJV) in the neck is followed by ligation of tumor feeding arteries like ascending pharyngeal, occipital and external carotid artery and IJV (Fig. 17.4).
6. Removal of the remaining skin of the bony external auditory canal tympanic membrane.

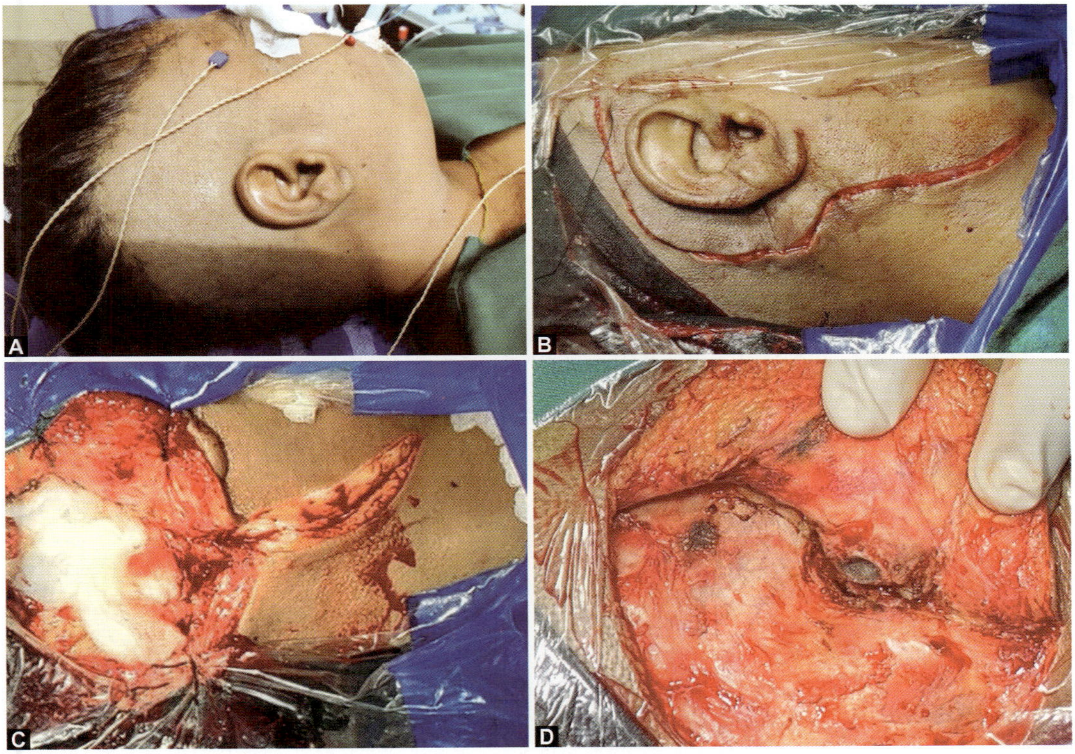

Fig. 17.3A and D: Surgical steps for Fisch approach type A (nerve monitor in place, incision, elevation of flap, transection of cartilaginous external auditory canal at bony cartilaginous junction)

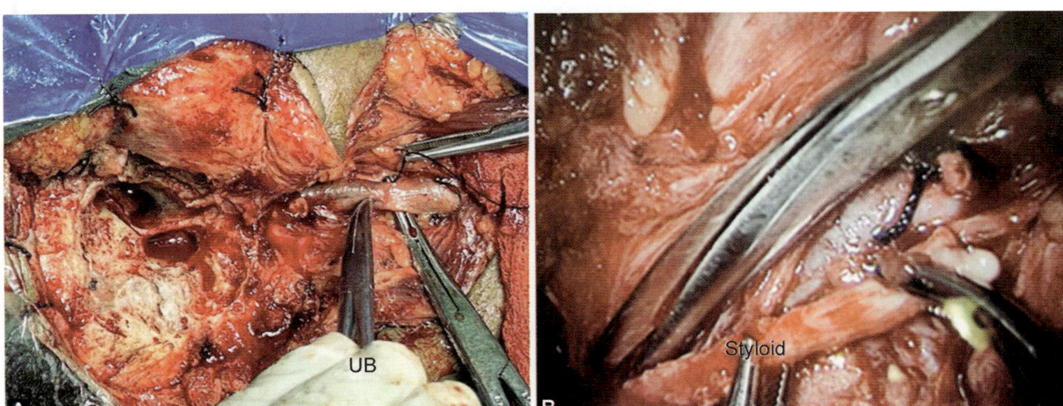

Fig. 17.4A and B: Mastoidectomy, skeletonization of facial nerve, tumor, identification of great vessels and nerves, ligation of IJV in the neck and division of styloid process

7. Subtotal petrosectomy by performing an extended radical mastoidectomy along with complete exenteration of petrous air cell system and contained mucosa.
8. Permanent anterior transposition of the facial nerve in the newly performed fallopian canal in the anterior attic wall (Fig. 17.5).
9. Permanent obliteration of eustachian tube.
10. Double ligation of sigmoid sinus after skeletonizing it completely in the glenoid fossa.
11. Insertion of infratemporal fossa retractor and further exposure of internal carotid artery by removal of styloid process and tympanic bone covering carotid foramen.
12. Mobilization of tumor poles anteriorly from carotid artery, superiorly from otic capsule, posteriorly from sigmoid sinus.
13. Separation of cranial nerves IX, X, XI from tumor surface if not filtrated. Nerves are sacrificed if infiltrated (Fig. 17.6).

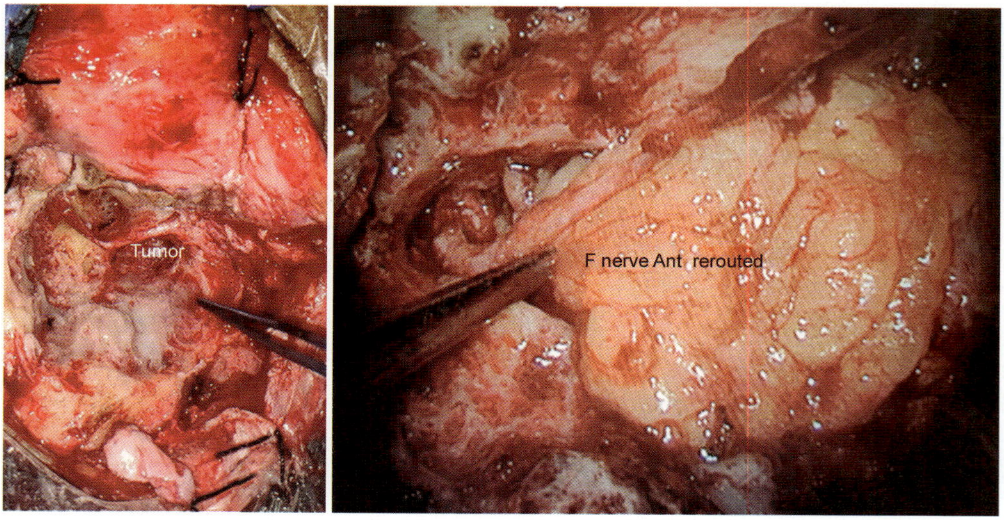

Fig. 17.5: Facial nerve before rerouting and after rerouting

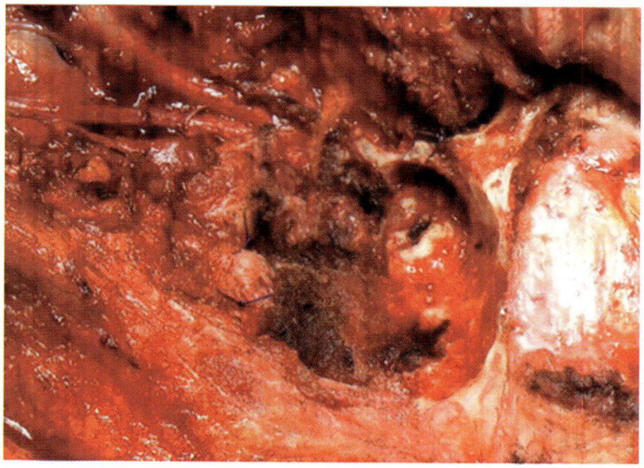

Fig. 17.6: Type A Fisch approach after complete glomus tumor removal on left ear. Control of bleeding done with inferior petrosal sinus

14. Intracranial intradural extension up to 2 cm can be removed.
15. Any extension larger than 2 cm is left *in situ* for later neurosurgical removal.

Type B Approach

Type B approach (Figs 17.7 and 17.8) provides access to the greater part of the clivus except for a small posterior area around the margin of the foramen magnum, which can be reached more easily by the type A approach. The surgical steps include:

1. C shaped skin incision in the postauricular region as shown in Fig. 17.7.
2. Elevation of the skin flap and blind sac closure of the external auditory canal.
3. Identification of the facial nerve in the retromandibular fossa and dissection peripherally up to second division.
4. Division of the zygomatic arch and mobilization with the attached masseter muscle and the temporalis muscle freed from their bony origin.
5. Subtotal petrosectomy as in type A.
6. Drilling of the glenoid fossa and disarticulation of TM joint.
7. Retraction of mandibular condyle and drilling of the tympanic bone lateral and anterior to the internal carotid artery.
8. Detachment of cartilaginous portion of the eustachian tube from the intratemporal horizontal portion and exposure of the foramen lacerum.
9. Division of mandibular nerve and middle meningeal artery after coagulation.
10. Drilling of the eroded bone until firm bone or dura is reached.
11. Mobilization of internal carotid artery from the carotid foramen to the horizontal portion.
12. Separation of the tumor mass from the adventia of internal carotid artery under direct vision and removal of tumor.
13. Closure of the wound after wiring of the zygomatic arch.

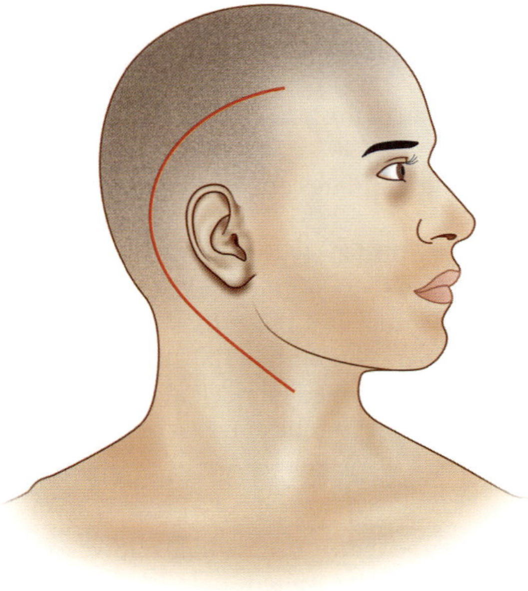

Fig. 17.7: Incision mark for Fisch Type B approach

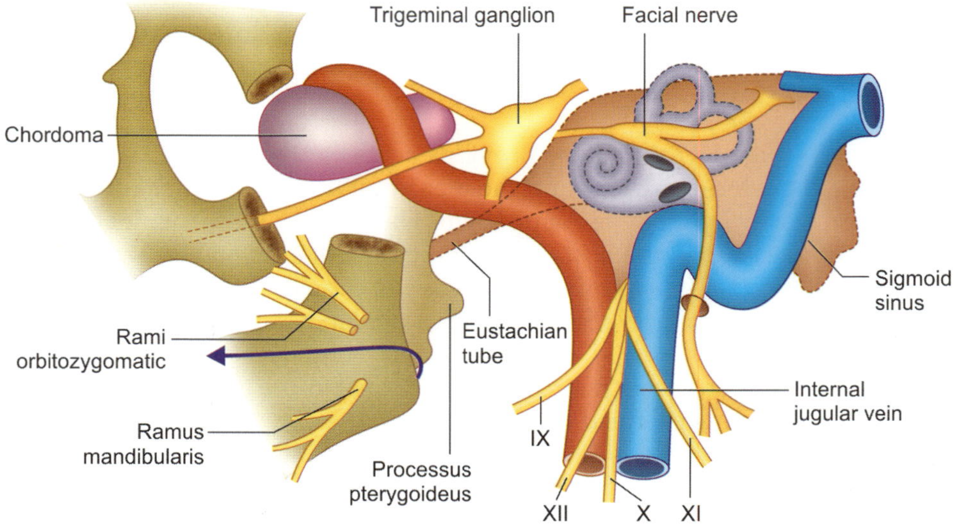

Fig. 17.8: Exposure of strucures in Fisch Type B approach

Type C Approach

An anterior extension of the Type B approach and permits access to the lesions of the nasopharynx, maxillary fossa, the eustachian tube, parasellar region, sphenoid sinus and the maxillary sinus.

Surgical Steps

1. Initial steps as in Type B.
2. Zygomatic arch is divided as far forward as possible and can include lateral orbital margin if necessary.
3. Detachment of the upper head of the lateral pterygoid muscle to expose lateral pterygoid plate
4. Removal of both the pterygoid plates and sectioning of maxillary division anterior to foramen rotandum
5. Following of the internal carotid artery as far as cavernous sinus
6. Entering of pterygomaxillary fossa and division of vidian nerve
7. Exposure of the maxillary sinus, nasopharynx and sphenoid sinus
8. Removal of tumor after separation of the vital structures
9. Malignant lesions should be removed enblock along with eustachian tube, the levator and tensor palate muscles, pharyngobasilar fascia and the pterygoid muscles.

Type D Approach

It is an anterior extension of Type C approach which allows to tackle the lesions involving anterior aspect of infratemporal fossa, sphenopalatine fossa, and lateral orbital wall that does not involve the carotid and middle ear. This approach is done with a preauricular incision, superiorly and anteriorly it is extended to orbit and inferiorly to the neck.

The steps include dissection of facial nerve into the stylomastoid foramen into the parotid gland.

Far-lateral approach: The far-lateral approach provides excellent exposure and access to the lesions anterior to foramen magnum resulting in complete excision of these lesions with reduced frequency of unwanted complications. This approach is used for lesions like meningioma, chordoma, chondroma, dermoid, etc. anterior to neuro axis around foramen magnum up to the vertebra-basilar junction. A modified park bench position is used for this approach, where the patient is placed in lateral position with side supports. A postauricular curvilinear incision starting 2–3 cm above and behind the pinna, which is continued posteriorly and inferiorly to the neck over the posterior border of the sternocleidomastoid muscle to the level of C3 or C4. The trapezius and sternocleidomastoid muscle, and the deeper splenius capitis, longissimus capitis, and semispinalis capitis are divided and reflected inferiorly as a single layer to expose the suboccipital triangle.

REFERENCES

1. Ugo Fisch. Infratemporal fossa approaches for extensive tumors of temporal bone and skull base. Neurological surgery of the ear,1977, Birmingham Alsculapius publication P. 34–53.
2. Fisch U, Pillsbury H. Infratemporal fossa approach to temporal bone and skull base. *Arch Otolaryngol,* 1979; 105:99–107.
3. Ugo Fisch: Otolaryngology clinics of North America (17) P. 513–51.
4. Ugo Fisch. Infratemporal fossa approach to temporal bone and skull base.JLaryngolOtol,1978; 92: P.:949–67.
5. Ugo Fisch. Infratemporal fossa approach of glomus tumor of temporal bone. Ann Otorhino laryng, 1982; 91:414–19.
6. Willium House. "surgical exposure of the internal auditory canal and its contents through the middle cranial fossa." Laryngoscope, 1961; 71:1363.
7. Biller, *et al*. Infratemporal fossa approach for lesion of skull base. Arch Otol, 1981; 107: 698–702.
8. Smith RR, *et al*. Surgical treatment of the cancer of the frontal sinus and adjacent areas. Cancer, 1954; 7: 991–94.
9. Sekhar, *et al*. Approach to large lateral and posterior cranial base tumors J Neurosurg 67:488–499, 1987.
10. Hazarika P, Nayak DR, Dinasingh A, *et al*. Anterior skull base-our experience. IJLO, 1997; *49*(4), 353–358.
11. Hazarika P(1), Nayak DR, Sahota J. Osteogenic sarcoma of sphenoid.IJLO. J Laryngol Otol. 1995 Nov;109(11):1101–4.
12. Hazarika P. Sahota J, Nayak DR, *et al*. Congenital internal carotid aneurysm. Int. J Paed Otolaryngology. 1993. 28, 63–8.
13. Goeppert H. Surgery of Skull Base Tumor. Edited by Gary J. 1991 .Churchi livingstone P. 59
14. North American clinics of Otolaryngology. Nass, *et al*. (1991) (24) 1465–1996
15. Laryngoscope. Glasscock (1978) 88: 905–33.
16. Ballenger Diseases of ear, nose, throat, head and neck 1992 edition.
17. Hazarika, Nayak, *et al*. Osteogenic sarcoma of sphenoid bone: an extended lateral skull base approach, JLO,1995; 109,11:1101–04.
18. Prasad S. Advanced techniques in the management of complex head and neck paragangliomas. OJOLHNS, 2017; 5:1–3.
19. Pai BS, *et al*. Far-lateral Transcondylar Approach to Anterior Foramen Magnum Lesions-Our Experience. Asian J Neurosurg. 2018 Jul-Sep; 13(3): 651–55.

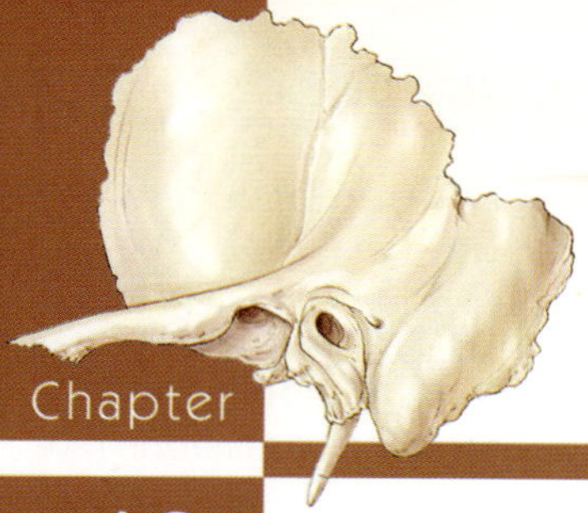

Chapter 18

An Introduction to Infratemporal Fossa Approaches

Sampath Chandra Prasad Rao • Ananth Chintapalli • Mario Sanna

"Skull base lesions are rare but serious conditions. It is important that their management be confined to specialized centers to avoid the problems encountered by the occasional surgeon and to allow experience to be consolidated in these centers".

—Ugo Fisch[1]

INTRODUCTION

The base of skull is an anatomical domain that separates the viscerocranium from the neurocranium. The unique aspect of the skull base pathology is its heterogenous nature that may arise from or involve this area and the fact that these lesions are in close proximity to the structures concerned with vital physiological functions of the human body, makes the reason that these lesions are often not dealt aggressively. The origins of the infratemporal fossa approaches can be traced to the description of glomus tumors by Rosenwasser in 1945.[2] Since then there has been a steady evolution and improvisation of the surgical management of the skull base lesions. FCW Capps in 1952 described vascular lesions in the middle ear and mentioned facial nerve rerouting in their surgical management.[3] Shambaugh in 1955 performed the endaural hypotympanic approach for limited glomus tumors which introduced the noesis of minimising hemorrhage and to preserve hearing.[4] It was the practice during the 1950s and 1960s that lesions with medial extension to the labyrinth and with carotid involvement were managed by radical mastoidectomy and irradiation.[5]

In 1964, MJ Shapiro and DK Neues described the skull base approach which included the ligation of the internal jugular vein and rerouting of the facial nerve in detail.[6] Farrior in 1966 extended the postauricular hypotympanotomy by removing the mastoid tip, mobilizing the facial nerve and thereby exposing the carotico-jugular region and the petrous apex and preserved the hearing.[7] WF House and ME Glasscock in 1968 described extended posterior tympanotomy approach preserving the posterior canal wall for glomus tympanicum.[8] Further development in the approaches of gaining access to the entire infratemporal fossa, control over the internal carotid, the peritubular region, the pterygopalatine fossa and as far up to the parasellar and clivus and even to the reaches of the nasopharynx were contributed by Gardner, Jackson, Glasscock between 1970s and 1980s. The most challenging is the management of the temporal bone and skull base neoplasms given the intimacy of the tumors with the ICA and the lower cranial nerves. This reflected in the technical limitations in complete surgical removal of the tumors earlier with the transcochlear and translabyrinthine approaches of the day, until Ugo Fisch in the early 1970s proposed the classification of glomus tumors and developed the infratemporal fossa approaches in which he employed the techniques of Shapiro and Neues. This approach crafted by Fisch was nurtured on the concept of permanent repositioning of the facial nerve anteriorly, resection of the mandibular condyle, the zygoma and a subtotal petrosectomy, which all gave an access to the entire petrous segment of the ICA, followed by a radical closure of the middle ear cleft.[9]

The subsequent years witnessed significant changes towards the approach of the skull base tumors particularly of those involving the jugular foramen in terms of planning, evaluation and classification of tympanojugular paragangliomas (TJP). Initially classified into types A,B,C and D by Fisch, further subclassification of type C and D TJPs by him into C1, C2, C3 and D1, D2 respectively gave a better understanding, much needed planning of the tumor resection and many more improvisations in the surgical techniques such as development of Fisch special infratemporal fossa retractor which facilitated anterior displacement of the mandible and thereby eliminating the need for condyle resection, usage of straight blunt suture needle for double ligation of the sigmoid sinus, successful anastomosis of CN XII–VII and V3–VII and staged approach of tumors with significant dural displacement increased the successful surgical outcomes of the ITF approaches and in turn the lateral skull base surgery. These advances in the surgical methods in handling these lesions and their persistent improvisation has succeeded in ramification of the cranial base surgery as a subspecialty and has seized to become an unsurpassable barrier to the otolaryngologists and neurosurgeons alike.

Evolving on the principle of finding adequate access by removing the bone from the skull base rather than retracting the brain, infratemporal fossa approaches developed into a system of approaches in itself comprising four types, each having their own indications and applications in skull base surgery. This article presents the system of infratemporal fossa approaches and their nuances.

INFRATEMPORAL FOSSA APPROACH TYPE A (ITFA-A)

Introduction

This is an extralabyrinthine approach passing from below the otic capsule mainly designed for extensive extradural lesions involving the jugular foramen area, infralabyrinthine and apical compartments of the petrous bone with anterior rerouting of the facial nerve as its key feature.

Principle

Primarily designed as a craniotemporocervical approach, gaining a wide access to the jugular bulb, jugular foramen, the petrous apex of the temporal bone along with the mandibular fossa and posterior portion of the infratemporal fossa is the prime objective of ITFA-A approach.

Indications

With its versatile access to the lateral cranial base, ITFA-A approach is the workhorse for addressing type C and type D tympanojugular paragangliomas and other jugulocarotid space lesions such as vagus and carotid body paragangliomas, carotid aneurysm, apart from cranial nerve neuromas of the IX, X, XI and XII nerves. Cholesteatoma with infralabyrinthine and apical extension, osteomyelitis of the temporal bone and rarer tumors of these compartments *viz* chondrosarcoma, cholesterol granuloma, meningioma, chordoma, myxoma, rhabdomyosarcoma, adenoid cystic carcinoma are other lesions which can be dealt with this approach.

Surgical Anatomy

The ITFA-A involves encountering a number of critical structures which more or less hamper its access to the intended areas. The structures hindering access to the lower lateral cranial base (Fig. 18.1): (1) Mastoid segment of the facial nerve, (2) tympanic bone, (3) posterior belly of the digastric muscle, (4) mastoid attachment of sternocleidomastoid muscle, 5. styloid process with its attached ligaments and muscles, 6. internal carotid artery, (7) internal jugular vein (8) lower cranial nerves—IX, X, XI, XII.

Enclosed within its lamellar bony canal, the mastoid segment of the facial nerve lies virtually lateral to the posterior half of the jugular bulb. The tympanic bone and its junctures with the mastoid, squamous and petrous portions corresponding the tympanomastoid, tympanosquamous sutures and petrotympanic fissure respectively, forms the anterior, inferior and a part of the posterior wall of the external auditory bony canal. With its vaginal process forming the sheath of the styloid process, the tympanic bone prevents an easy access to the deeper compartments of the lower lateral cranial base.

The sigmoid sinus progresses inferiorly as the jugular bulb within the jugular foramen. A tunnel shaped structure cradling the vital structures, this foramen is divided into an anteromedial compartment containing the glossopharyngeal nerve, the inferior petrosal

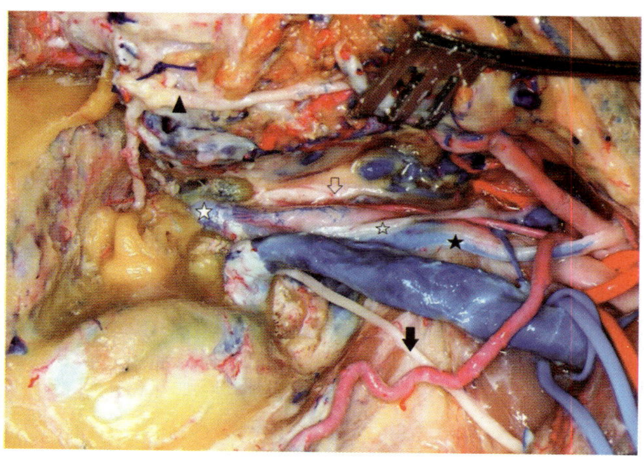

Fig. 18.1: After canal wall down mastoidectomy, removal of the tympanic bone and removal of the mastoid tip: Internal jugular vein (blue vessel loop), internal carotid artery (red coloured vessel loop), anteriorly transposed CN VII (solid black arrowhead), CN IX (hollow black down arrow), CN X (hollow black star), CN XI (solid black down arrow), CN XII (solid black star), vertical portion of petrous carotid (solid white star)

sinus and the meningeal branch of the ascending pharyngeal artery. The posterolateral compartment of the foramen harbours the jugular bulb, the vagus and the spinal accessory nerves.

The lower cranial nerves within the jugular foramen are oriented in a way where the glossopharyngeal nerve is the most lateral and the hypoglossal nerve is the most medial at their point of exit at the skull base. The IX cranial nerve exits along with the X and XI cranial nerves from the jugular foramen at a level superior to the hypoglossal nerve. The glossopharyngeal nerve crosses the internal carotid artery posteriorly lying lateral to it. After exiting the skull base from its canal, the hypoglossal nerve turns inferiorly to course along with the vagus for a brief distance in the upper neck and crosses the internal carotid artery in a posteroanterior direction whilst the vagus courses between the internal jugular vein and the internal carotid artery. The XI cranial nerve courses posteromedial to the IJV in about half of the cases and lies anterolateral to the transverse process of the C1 vertebra.

Surgical Technique

A wide postaural craniotemporocervical incision is applied that extends down to the neck. An anteriorly based subcutaneous flap is crafted followed by an inferiorly based musculo-periosteal flap (Fig. 18.2A and B). A posterior meatotomy is done and the external auditory meatal skin is transected. The meatal skin cuff is dissected and elevated from the surrounding tissue and delivered externally with the help of tissue hooks and sutured with an absorbable suture material. The conchal cartilage (within the pinna) and the tragal cartilage are released from their surrounding soft tissue and are sutured together creating a scaffold for blind sac closure to avoid iatrogenic fistula (Fig. 18.3A and B). The inferiorly based musculoperiosteal flap is elevated in continuum with the sternocleidomastoid muscle up to splenius capitis. The posterior belly of the digastric muscle is divided at its origin, the occipital artery encountered underneath the digastric is ligated (Fig. 18.4A to C). The glossopharyngeal nerve is identified traversing the ICA anteriorly. The vagus is identified

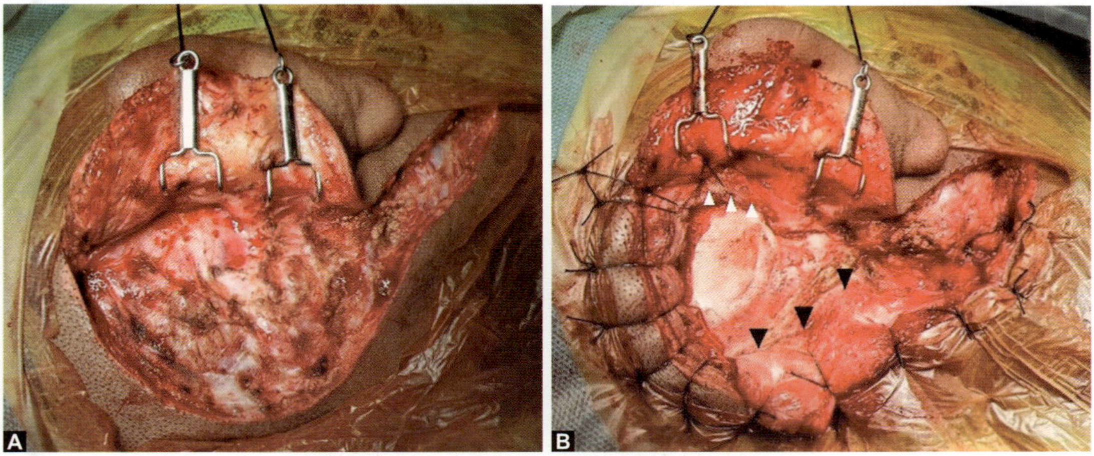

Fig. 18.2: (A) Elevation of a craniotemporocervical skin flap, **(B)** Raising of anterior based subcutaneous flap (white arrowheads) and an inferior based musculoperiosteal flap (black arrowheads)

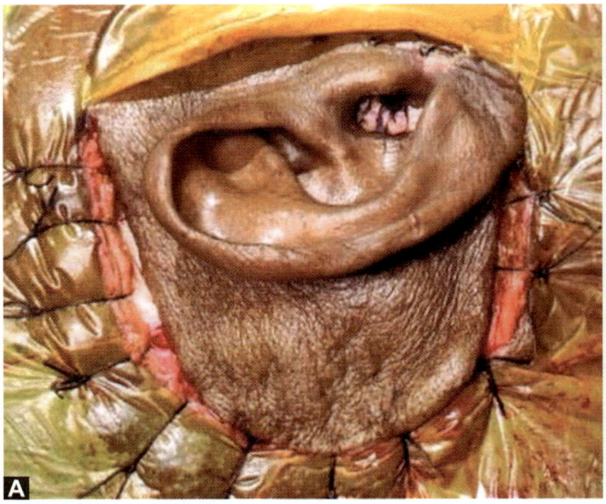

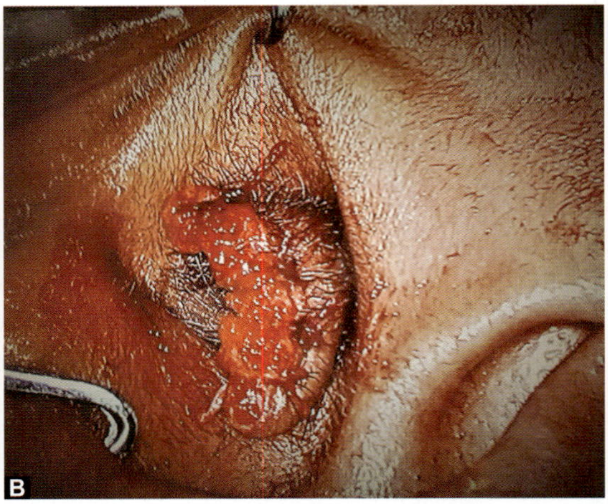

Fig. 18.3: **(A)** Blind sac closure of the external ear closed in two layers (outer everted canal skin and inner cartilage closure for scaffolding), **(B)** Showing the blind sac closure

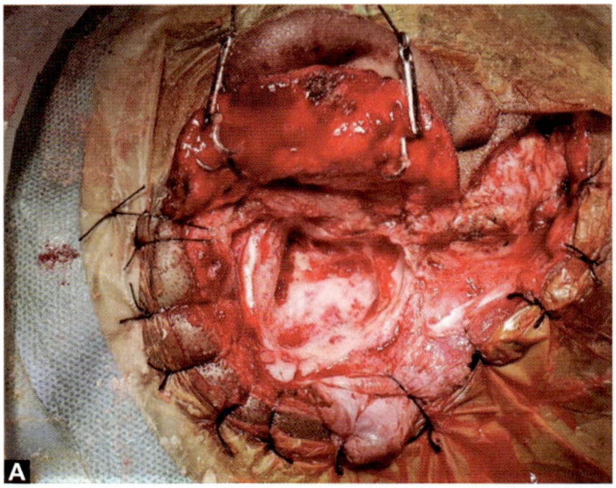

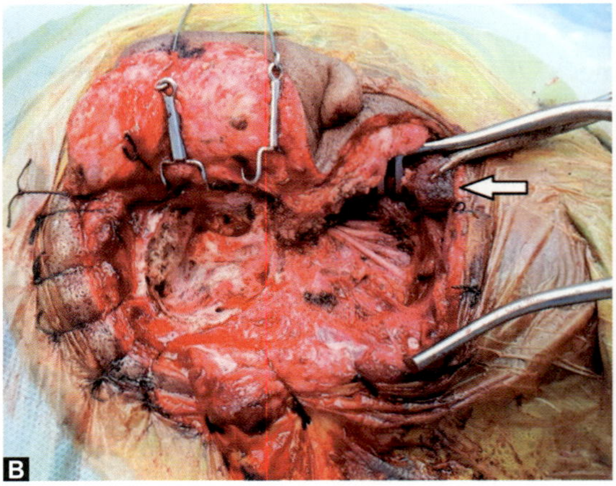

Fig. 18.4: **(A)** After cortical mastoidectomy and skeletonizing the dural plate and the sigmoid sinus plate, **(B)** Completion of canal wall down mastoidectomy and sectioning the posterior belly of the digastric muscle (white solid arrow) at its attachment to the mastoid tip and cervical exposure

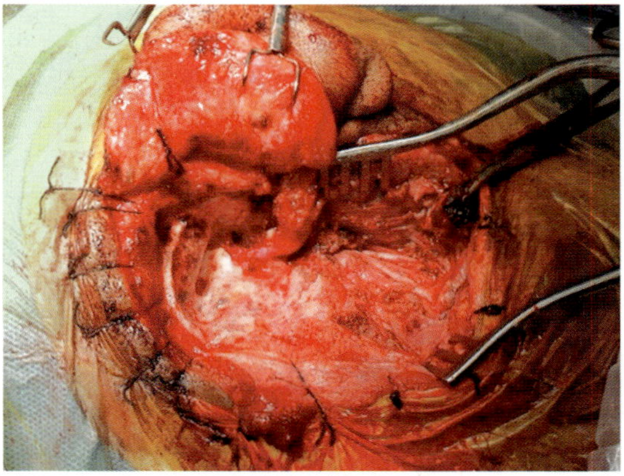

Fig. 18.4C: Facial nerve has been dislodged from its position in the fallopian canal after skeletonising it from the geniculate ganglion to the parotid segments

coursing between the IJV and the ICA and the hypoglossal is seen crossing the ICA anteriorly towards the tongue. The spinal accessory nerve is identified lateral to the IJV (in majority of cases) and passing anterolateral to the transverse process of C1 vertebra. The condylar emissary vein which lies in close proximity to the XI CN is cauterized when needed. The great vessels are marked with vessel loops. The dissection so far exposes the lateral surface of the temporal bone from the root of zygoma anteriorly to the occipitomastoid synchondrosis posteriorly along with its squamous and tympanic parts.

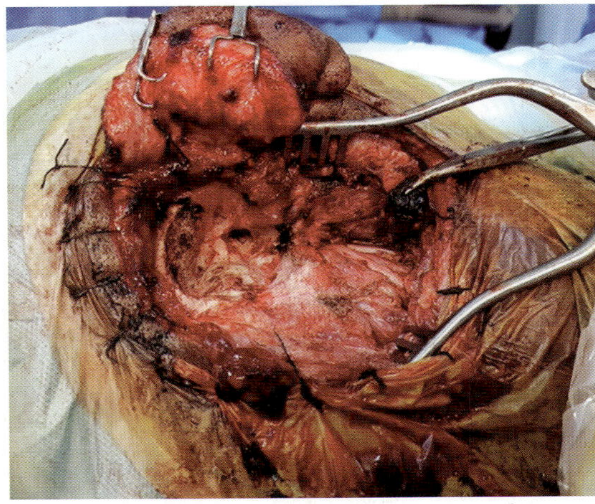

Fig. 18.4D: The jugular fossa is exposed after removal of the mastoid tip and drilling away of the entire tympanic bone

The canal wall down mastoidectomy is then performed, the tip of the mastoid is removed taking care to leave behind a cuff of soft tissue around the facial nerve at the stylomastoid foramen area. The tympanic bone is drilled and removed in toto (Fig. 18.4D). A neo bony canal is created at the root of the zygoma, the facial nerve is decompressed from the geniculate ganglion up to the stylomastoid foramen releasing the nerve from the fallopian canal. The dissection of the facial nerve (in its extratympanic segment) is carried within the parotid, thereby creating a soft tissue tunnel, which reduces the stretch injury of the nerve after its rerouting. The nerve is then positioned in the neo canal and secured with tissue glue. Now that the tympanic bone is excised and the facial nerve rerouted anteriorly, the jugular foramen is freely accessed after completion of subtotal petrosectomy. The tumor is exposed along its limits for a good control. The sigmoid sinus is skeletonized and decompressed leaving behind a ledge of bone at its superior aspect under which the surgical is packed, thereby compressing it extraluminally. Further compression is achieved by intraluminal packing of the sinus with Surgicel, completely ceasing the venous backflow from the transverse and the sigmoid sinuses.

After clipping the internal jugular vein in the neck with multiple ligaclips, the ligated portion of the IJV is then reflected superiorly. This expose and gives control over the inferior limit of the tumor. The upper limit of the tumor is then identified by drilling away the hypotympanic bone, the under surface of the cochlea and the petrous bone. The occipital bone posterior to the sigmoid sinus is drilled away to remove any tumor infiltration of this area. The final tumor resection is commenced only after all the tumor margins are exposed. The tumor resection over the jugular bulb is completed by meticulously resecting the lateral wall of the tumor with surface coagulation and addressing the venous bleed from the inferior petrosal sinus and the condylar emissary vein. The lower cranial nerves are preserved by sparing the medial wall of the bulb and the upper portion of the internal jugular vein (Fig. 18.5). Addressing the intradural extension of the tumors need a thorough preoperative evaluation and need to be done only after identifying and separating the AICA and PICA vessels.[10] The intradural component of the tumors are dealt either in continuum with the extradural tumor resection or executed in a staged manner.

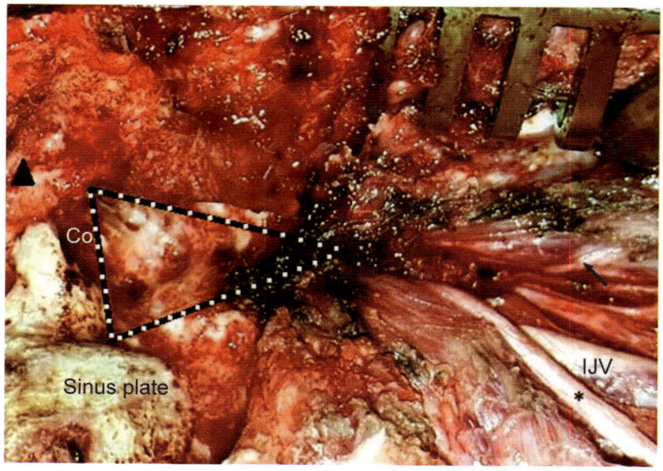

Fig. 18.5: Surgical exposure after canal wall down mastoidectomy, in toto removal of the tympanic bone and the mastoid tip: Internal jugular vein (IJV), cochlea (Co), transposed facial nerve (solid black arrowhead), XI cranial nerve (black asterix), X cranial nerve (black arrow). The jugular foramen (within the black and white dotted traiangle) from where the tumor has been removed

Management of the Internal Carotid

Management of the cervicopetrous internal carotid artery is the most crucial aspect in any ITFA. The management of the ICA begins primarily with a good preoperative assessment. A four-vessel angiogram gives the vascular architecture of the tumor and the site of surgery. A preoperative endovascular intervention of the cervicopetrous carotid is either an intravascular reinforcement with stenting or a permanent balloon occlusion. Advanced C3 and C4 tympanojugular paragangliomas, more than 180° encasement of the carotid by the tumor, preoperative evidence of stenosed segment within the carotid, extensive contribution of ICA branches to the tumor, revision surgery or a previous radiotherapy are some of the main indications which warrant a preoperative intervention of the ICA and allows a more aggressive tumor resection.[11]

The eustachian tube is obliterated with a muscle or periosteal plug, haemostasis secured with bipolar or Surgicel and the cavity obliterated with the abdominal fat harvest after treating it with an antibiotic preparation. The posterior belly of the digastric muscle is replaced and sutured. The musculoperiosteal flaps are repositioned and sutured to the temporalis muscle. And the wound closure is done in layers after placing a drain.

Complications

CSF leak is the most common postoperative complication encountered especially when the tumor involves the dura. Leaks with small dural deficits are effectively managed with tight compressive bandage. Moderate leaks collecting at the site of surgery can be aspirated percutaneously (in multiple sittings), till the CSF seizes to further collect. Significant leaks however require lumbar puncture and systemic diuretics (carbonic anhydrase inhibitors) to reduce CSF production.

Facial nerve paralysis is a known and accepted complication as a consequence of extensive manipulation, rerouting and also by tumor involvement in some cases.

Nevertheless, the recovery is expected generally within six months to one year, most of the cases settling with HB grade 2 and even grade 1 in few of them.

Lower cranial nerve involvement is a widely debated aspect of ITFA. In extensive and advanced lesions particularly in elderly age group, the LCNs are better spared. The fact that younger age group subjects show a better postoperative compliance prompts us to deal more aggressively in this group.[12,13]

INFRATEMPORAL FOSSA APPROACH TYPE B (ITFA-B) (Fig. 18.6)

Principle

A cochlear function preserving approach like ITFA-A, ITFA-B differs from the former with respect to the facial nerve that it is not transposed. Type B approach is primarily designed to be an extralabyrinthine approach, passing anterior to the otic capsule with the petrous apex and mid clivus portions as the target areas.

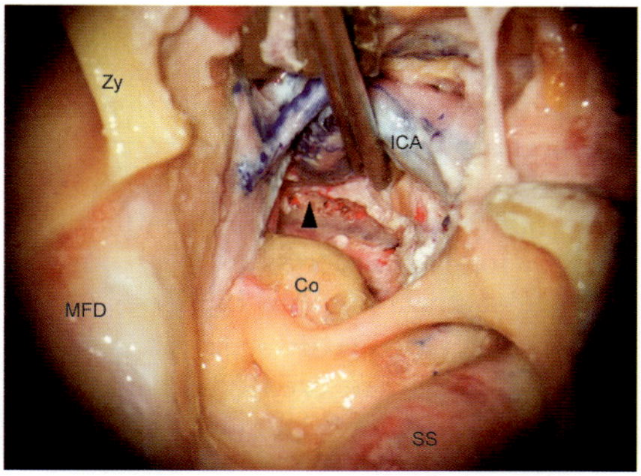

Fig. 18.6: ITFA-B exposure after a mini craniotomy involving only the root of zygoma and squamous portions of the temporal bone, removing the petrous bone anterior to the carotid artery and temporary transposing the vessel anteriorly gaining access to the petrous apex (solid black arrowhead); middle fossa dura (MFD); cochlea (Co); zygoma (Zy); sigmoid sinus (SS)

Indications

This approach is primarily designed for the lesions of the petrous apex such as apical and infralabyrinthine cholesteatoma and cholesterol granuloma of the petrous apex. Clival lesions such as chordoma, chondrosarcoma and extensive glomus tumors invading the clivus. Other rare tumors which are addressed in these anatomical domains are choristoma and melanoma of the eustachian tube and giant cell tumors of the petrous bone.

Surgical Anatomy

Given the wide exposure that is required for the type B approach, the dissection for creating the surgical corridor involves dealing with the anatomical structures impeding access to the infratemporal fossa such as: (1) The zygoma, (2) ramus of the mandible, (3) The temporomandibular joint, (4) parotid gland, (5) masseter muscle.

The understanding of the petrous apex in type B approach is such that its base is formed by the cochlea and the anterior surface of the internal auditory canal, roof by the middle fossa dura and the most anterior portions by the Gasserian ganglion, anterolaterally by the petro-occipital synchondrosis. Given the complex anatomy of the temporal bone and skull base and considering the fact that this already complex anatomy could further be distorted by the disease, a thorough orientation of the relationships of the surgical landmarks is all-important when performing these approaches. The main landmarks used in ITFA-B particularly during the manipulation of the petrous carotid are the cochleariform process, the basal turn of the cochlea, the eustachian tube, foramen spinosum, the foramen ovale, the middle meningeal artery, the mandibular nerve and the anterior foramen lacerum.[14] The other important landmark is the geniculate ganglion, that lies immediately above the cochleariform process and the greater superficial petrosal nerve which arises from the ganglion courses anteriorly, where it is joined by the deep petrosal nerve (from the plexus around the carotid) to form the vidian nerve at the anterior foramen lacerum and enters the pterygoid canal to distribute the parasympathetic innervation to the lacrimal gland, the nasal mucosa and the glands of the buccal mucosa.

Surgical Technique

A 'C' shaped incision (Fig. 18.7) commencing from the tip of the mastoid extending posteriorly around the ear pinna and moving anteriorly up to the orbital ridge is ideal for the desired bone dissection and for a mini craniotomy if required for gaining access to the intended target areas (Figs 18.8 and 18.9).

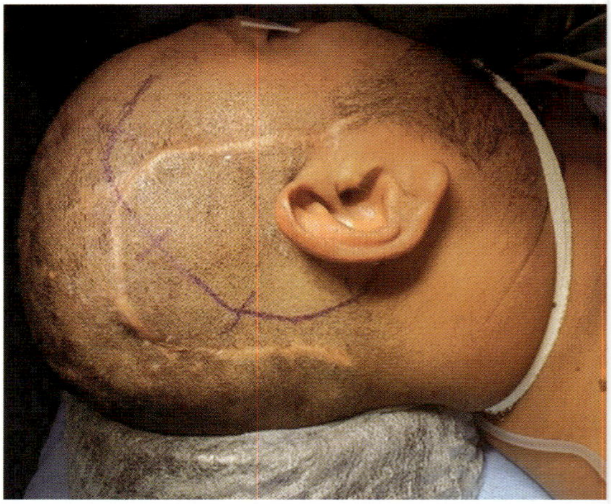

Fig. 18.7: Incision for ITFA-B in a patient with an extensive petrous apex cholesterol granuloma after a previous unsuccessful MCF approach elsewhere

The subcutaneous dissection is carried out and flaps are created in a way favourable for a mini craniotomy. Blind sac closure of the external auditory canal is performed as described in type A approach (Figs 18.10 to 18.12). The temporalis muscle is then exposed and cut as an inferior based pedicled musculoperiosteal flap. The subcutaneous plane is elevated in the plane superficial to the temporoparietal fascia, the temporal pad of fat is identified and entered deep to its plane to avoid injuring the frontal branch of the facial

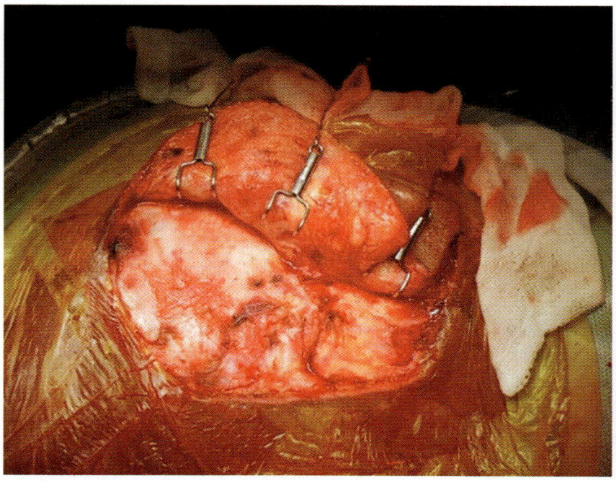

Fig. 18.8: Elevation of skin flap for type B approach

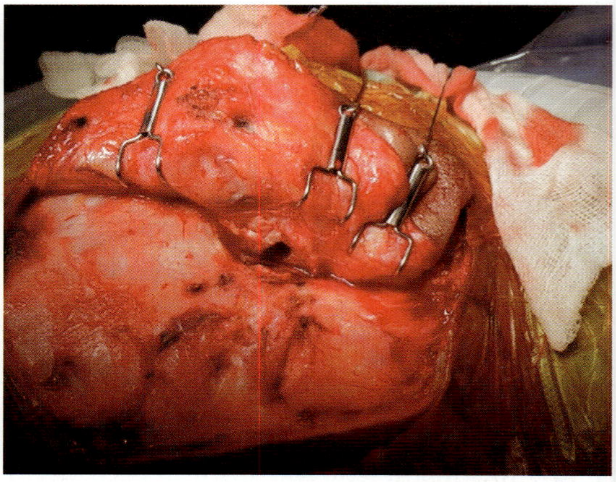

Fig. 18.9: Transection of the external auditory canal a couple of millimetres lateral to the bony cartilaginous junction

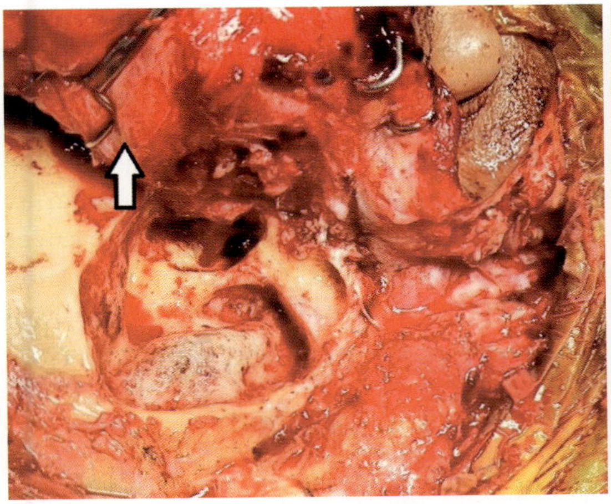

Fig. 18.10: Temporalis muscle flap reflected inferiorly (white solid arrow) and canal wall down mastoidectomy is performed

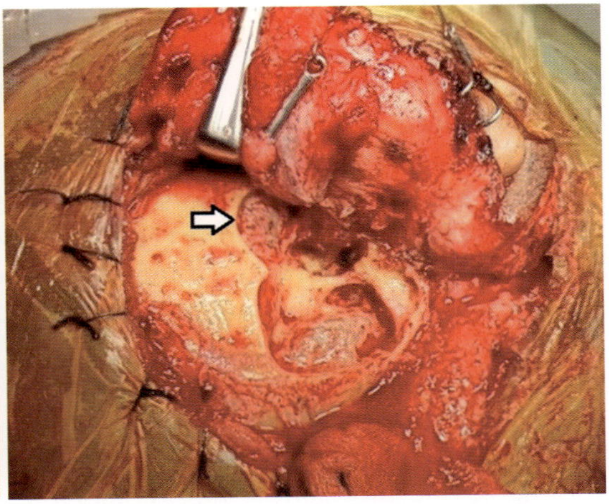

Fig. 18.11: A mini craniotomy (solid white arrow) involving the squamous and the zygoma root portions of the temporal bone

nerve. The dissection thus far exposes the complete lateral aspect of the temporal bone from the root of zygoma anteriorly, the tympanic bone, the squamous and mastoid portions up to the occipitomastoid synchondrosis.

A canal wall down mastoidectomy is then performed (Fig. 18.10). The tensor tympani muscle is identified at the cochleariform process, cut and reflected laterally taking care not to injure the greater superficial petrosal nerve lying immediately above the cochleariform process. A mini craniotomy involving the squamous portion of the temporal bone and the root of the zygoma and the middle fossa dura is exposed which creates a more anterior workspace and requires minimal brain retraction (Figs 18.11 and 18.12). Care is taken not to go too far anterior into the zygoma itself. The mini craniotomy hence created also involves separating the temporomandibular joint capsule from the under surface of the glenoid fossa and retracting it inferiorly along with the condyle of the mandible with the help of Fisch's special infratemporal fossa retractor and the temporalis muscle is reflected inferiorly away from the surgical field. The facial nerve is skeletonized but not decompressed and transposed as done in type A approach (Fig. 18.5). Here a retrofacial tymponotomy (Fig. 18.12) is performed when required for better instrumentation and surgical access to the hypotympanum. The entire tympanic bone is removed in toto from lateral to medial until the carotid canal is reached. The vertical segment and the genu

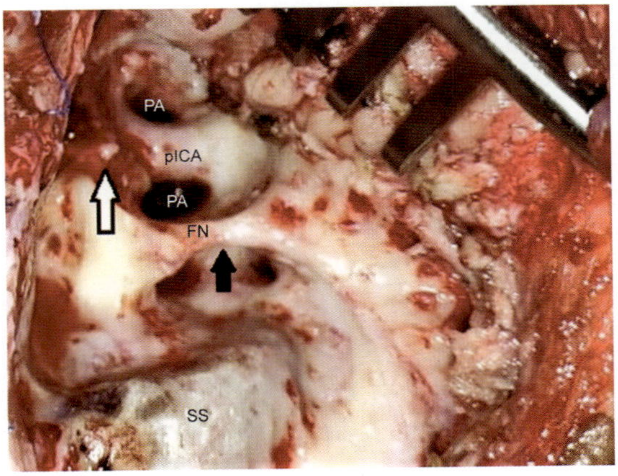

Fig. 18.12: In the same patient after skeletonizing the petrous carotid (pICA). Note the petrous apex (PA) accessed from both anterior and posterior to the petrous carotid and the cholesterol granuloma removed. Note the retrofacial tympanotomy (solid black arrow). The cochleariform process (solid white arrow) is shown for relationship with other landmarks. The sigmoid sinus (SS)

of the carotid is exposed by removing the hypotympanic bone and the portion of petrous bone between the basal turn of cochlea and the carotid canal. The horizontal portion of the carotid is decompressed by removing the bony eustachian tube. Drilling of the supratubal bone and the petrous bone anterior to the carotid canal is done, if necessary, to expose the laceral segment of the artery and the potential space thus created within the petrous pyramid enables to transpose the carotid artery anteriorly to access the petrous apex (Fig. 18.6). Removing the portion of bone posterior to the carotid canal exposes the lower clivus. Drilling the bone anteroinferior to the greater superficial petrosal nerve along the greater wing of the sphenoid uncovers the foramen spinosum and the middle meningeal artery within it. The vessel is ligated using ligaclips and is cut. Continuing the bone resection further medially along the greater wing of sphenoid leads to the foramen ovale and mandibular division of trigeminal nerve within it. Care is taken to cauterize the venous plexus around the foramen using bipolar forceps before the mandibular nerve is resected. The cartilaginous eustachian tube is sutured at the end of the procedure, the craniotomy bone flap is rewired, the temporalis muscle flap is reverted to its place and the abdominal fat harvest are used to obliterate the cavity (Fig. 18.13) and the wound is closed in layers after inserting the drain.

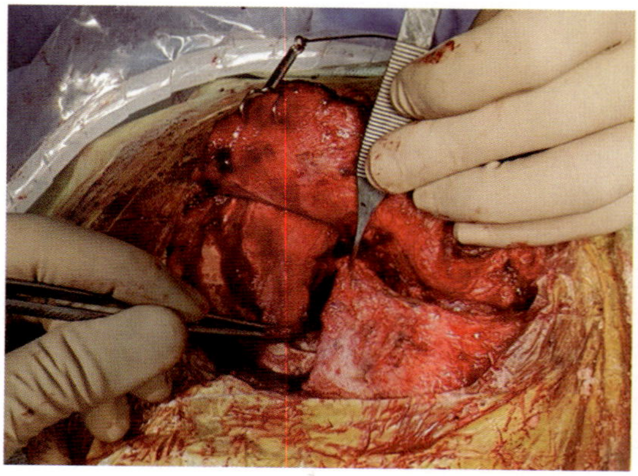

Fig. 18.13: Cavity obliteration with abdominal fat and flap repositioning followed by skin closure

Complications

As with type A, considering the morbidity, CSF leak is the most worrisome complication in ITFA-B as well. Need for craniotomy, manipulation of the tumor abutting the middle fossa dura and resection of intradural tumor, all increase the incidence and magnitude of CSF leak in type B approach as opposed to the type A.

Though not extensively manipulated and rerouted as done in type A, skeletonizing the facial nerve can still and may lead to certain degree of thermal and pressure injury causing postoperative paresis which in many cases is transient and shows a total recovery.

Another aspect of concern is the associated cosmetic defect due to manipulating the zygomatic complex and rotation of the temporalis muscle for obliteration of the wound. Mandibular dysfunction is transient as the condyle is preserved.

INFRATEMPORAL FOSSA APPROACH TYPE C (ITFA-C)

Introduction

The infratemporal fossa approach type C is one of the four subtypes described in the system of infratemporal fossa approaches. Its primary objective is to access as far as the petrous apex, clivus, pterygopalatine fossa, sphenoid sinus and cavernous sinus from the lateral aspect. Also, complex lesions like carcinoma of the nasopharynx with recurrence or persistence after irradiation can be managed with type C approach for a surgical solution.

Principle

The type C approach is crafted to be a cochlear function preserving procedure and to ingress the more medial and intricate anatomical territories like petrous apex, clivus, pterygopalatine fossa, sphenoid sinus, cavernous sinus and the nasopharynx of the skull base from its lateral aspect.

Indications

Based on its principle, the type C approach is indicated for lesions involving the infratemporal and pterygopalatine fossae, the petrous apex, the sphenoid sinus, cavernous sinus, the parasellar region, the nasopharynx and the peri tubal space. Adenoid cystic carcinoma, adenocarcinoma, melanoma, trigeminal neuroma of the infratemporal fossa, craniopharyngioma, pituitary adenocarcinoma amongst others of the parasellar region, nasopharyngeal carcinoma of the nasopharynx and the juvenile angiofibroma of the pterygopalatine fossa are some of the lesions that can be addressed with type C approach.

Surgical Anatomy

The salient concept of the ITF approaches is that the more medial the area of interest is, the wider the surgical field should become to accommodate the instrumentation and to gain the needed access. The surgical field of type C approach is anterior to the labyrinth and thus the surgical anatomy of ITFA-C is similar to that encountered for type B approach, but with a much wider and anterior dissection. The pterygoid process along with its laminae is the key anatomical structure in regard that the disease clearance is in reference to this structure. The orientation of the foramina and the neurovascular structures is important to avoid intraoperative complications. Foramen ovale and the sphenoid sinus lie posterior and superomedial respectively to the base of the pterygoid process. Hence the drilling of the greater wing of sphenoid bone leads to foramen rotundum and the maxillary nerve to access the pterygopalatine fossa. Further removing the vomer and medial pterygoid lamina which forms the lateral boundary of the choana, gives a wide workspace to the nasopharynx from the lateral aspect. The eustachian tube, mandibular nerve (foramen ovale) and middle meningeal artery (foramen spinosum) which lie lateral to the laceral segment of the internal carotid, have to be negotiated (Fig. 18.14). The pterygopalatine fossa is accessed after removing the pterygoid process. The vidian nerve and the maxillary nerve enter the pterygopalatine fossa from the vidian canal and foramen rotundum respectively

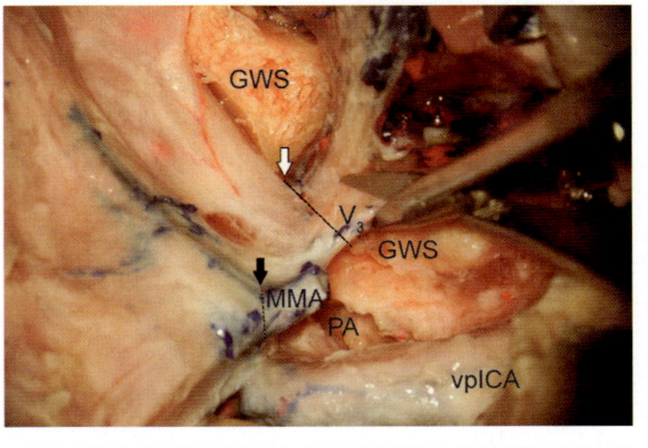

Fig. 18.14: The transected middle meningeal artery. V3 being cut. Foramen spinosum (black solid arrow); foramen ovale (white solid arrow); greater wing of sphenoid (GWS); petrous apex (PA); vertical segment of the petrous carotid artery (vpICA)

to form the sphenopalatine ganglion (Fig. 18.5). The maxillary nerve needs to be sacrificed to access the cavernous sinus. The abducens nerve lies in the lateral wall of the cavernous sinus while the ophthalmic division of the trigeminal, oculomotor and trochlear lie medial to its lateral wall.

Surgical Technique

A wide postauricular craniotemporal incision is given followed by the subcutaneous dissection, elevating the musculoperiosteal flaps and blind sac closure as described for type B approach. A canal wall down mastoidectomy is performed and the tympanic bone is removed in toto exposing the vertical portion of the internal carotid, hypotympanum and the capsule of the mandibular condyle. The intact capsule of the condyle is separated from the glenoid fossa as described in type B approach which can be retracted inferiorly with the infratemporal fossa retractor. An anterior craniotomy is carried out including the squamous portion of the temporal bone, the zygoma and the lateral rim of the orbital wall like in a fronto-temporo-orbito-zygomatic approach, which permits a wide exposure. Drilling is carried further superiorly, on the carotid canal after identifying its vertical segment exposing the genu of the artery, which lies in close proximity immediately anteromedial to the basal turn of the cochlea, taking care not to injure either of these vital structures. The horizontal segment of the carotid is exposed by removing the bony eustachian tube. Removing the supratubal bone allows exposure of the laceral segment.

The tensor tympani muscle is identified, cut and reflected anteriorly taking care not to injure the greater superficial petrosal nerve immediately above the cochleariform process. The bone anteroinferior to this nerve is drilled along the greater wing of the sphenoid till the middle meningeal artery within the foramen spinosum is identified. The artery is ligated with the ligaclips and resected. Drilling now continues more medially along the greater wing of sphenoid towards the foramen ovale and the mandibular division of the trigeminal nerve within it. The venous plexus in the foramen ovale is cauterized using bipolar forceps and the mandibular nerve resected. The dissection thus far exposes the periosteum over the greater wing of the sphenoid and the lateral lamina of the pterygoid process which is elevated along its attachment with the lateral pterygoid muscle. The drilling of the pterygoid process is according to the extent of the pathology and the area that needs to be accessed.

For the tumors involving the infratemporal and the peri tubal areas the bone of the skull base including the mandibular fossa, the bone around the foramen spinosum and ovale are removed leaving just a thin shell of bone over the middle fossa dura. The middle meningeal artery and the mandibular nerve are coagulated. The periosteum is elevated over the petrous apex and the clivus, the pterygoid process drilled away, the muscles are cut at their insertions and the lateral wall of the nasopharynx and nasal cavity are exposed. Tumor is excised en bloc leaving a safe margin of soft tissue.

For the exposure of the pterygopalatine and the sphenoid sinus, the pterygoid process and the base of the greater wing of the sphenoid bone is drilled out, the mandibular division of the trigeminal nerve and the middle meningeal artery are severed. The carotid is exposed up to its laceral segment after removing the bony eustachian tube. Further drilling of the bone exposes the inferior portion of the Gasserian ganglion through the middle fossa dura and thus exposing the foramen rotundum with the maxillary nerve and the sphenopalatine ganglion in the pterygopalatine fossa. The maxillary nerve is cut close to the Gasserian ganglion. The lateral and the medial pterygoid muscles are cut close

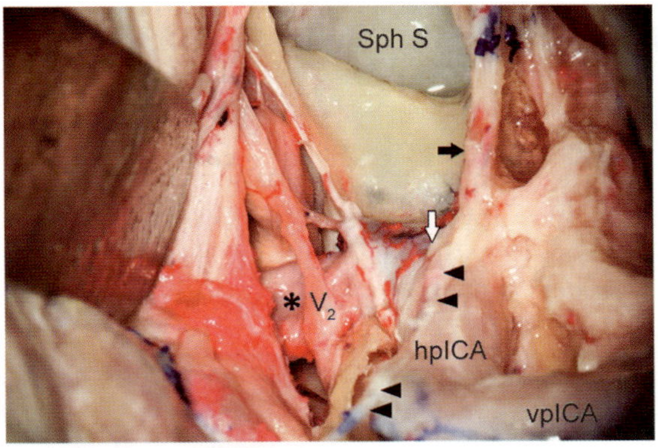

Fig. 18.15: Exposure achieved after the anterior craniotomy and drilling the bone anterior to the internal carotid and along the greater wing of sphenoid exposing the laceral segment of the vessel(solid white arrow); cavernous segment of the ICA (asterix); maxillary division of trigeminal (V2); the sphenoid sinus (Sph S); vertical (vpICA) and horizontal petrous internal carotid artery (hpICA). Note the greater superficial petrosal nerve over the ICA (black solid arrowheads) continuing further anteriorly beyond the foramen lacerum as the vidian nerve (solid black arrow)

to their attachments exposing the lateral wall of the nasopharynx. The sphenoid sinus is exposed laterally giving access to the sella region (Fig. 18.15).

For gaining access to the parasellar lesions, control over the cavernous sinus is achieved after sectioning the maxillary nerve on its inferolateral wall. The abducens is lateral to the carotid in the lateral wall of the cavernous sinus.

The wound closure is done by rotating the temporalis muscle flap into the defect after rewiring the zygoma arch. An additional defect, should there be any, is obliterated by an inferiorly based retroauriculo-occipital musculofascial flap or a sternocleidomastoid muscle flap.

Complications

Cosmetic defect of the wound site as a result of the zygoma complex manipulation, craniotomy and manipulation of the temporalis muscle is a known and accepted complication of this extensive procedure.

Infratemporal fossa hematoma postoperatively due to inadequate ligation of the middle meningeal artery is one of the complications encountered and has to be addressed immediately for it can cause pressure over the decompressed internal carotid.

Ascending infection from the nasopharynx may occur when the resected eustachian tube is not obliterated properly. Obliteration with a muscle flap reduces this complication. Injury to the frontal branch of the facial nerve may give raise to loss of function of the frontalis, orbicularis oculi leaving a cosmetic concern.

Difficulty in mastication secondary to retraction of the mandible, sectioning of the mandibular nerve, manipulation of the pterygoid muscles is an anticipated sequela. Reconstruction of the mandibular fossa with soft tissue reduces these problems to a considerable extent and the patients usually comply reasonably well over time. Anesthesia of the tongue due to loss of V3 is usually well tolerated.

INFRATEMPORAL FOSSA APPROACH TYPE D (ITFA-D)

Introduction

This approach is an even more anterior modification of type C and is considered along with the group of preauricular approaches to the skull base[15], where they share similar principles with some nuances. With the advent and improvisations in the anterior endoscopic approach, despite its limited access, type D approach has its own indications and place in the discipline.

Principle

Type D (Fig. 18.16) approach is performed in a similar way to type C but through a preauricular incision. The middle ear and the eustachian tube are left intact as a subtotal petrosectomy is not performed in contrast to type C approach. These particular approaches are reserved for addressing the tumors involving the anterior infratemporal fossa and the orbital apex but without involving the horizontal segment of intrapetrous internal carotid artery. Type D is carried out through either an extended preauricular skin incision (Type D1) or a hemicoronal incision (Type D2).[16]

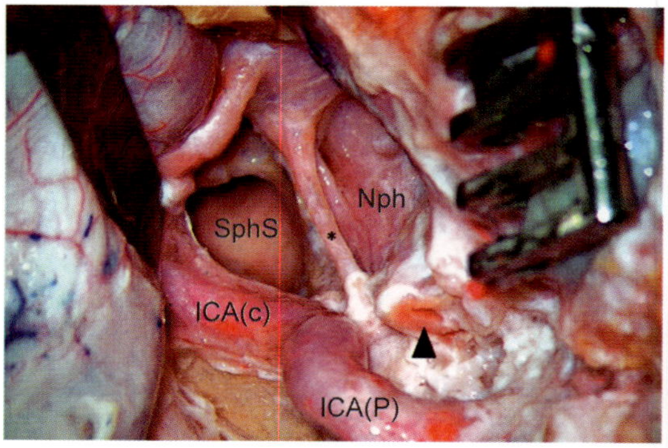

Fig. 18.16: The exposure achieved after a fronto-temporo-orbito-zygomatic craniotomy and retraction of the middle fossa dura: decompression of the petrous, ICA(P), laceral and cavernous, ICA(C) segments of the carotid; vidian nerve (black asterix); nasopharynx (Nph); cartilaginous portion of the eustachian tube (solid black arrowhead)

Indications

Type D approach is primarily for accessing benign and malignant neoplasms of the sphenoid and the clival areas, medial half of the petrous temporal bone, anterior portion of the infratemporal fossa, the nasopharynx, retropharyngeal and parapharyngeal spaces, ethmoid and the maxillary sinuses and intradural clivus-foramen magnum areas.[17]

Surgical Anatomy

The surgical anatomy in type D approach is similar to that encountered for type C approach. The dissection is anterior to the labyrinth, sparing the middle ear and the eustachian tube.

The structures encountered from lateral to medial are the superficial and the deep temporal fascia and subgaleal plane in between them, the parotid gland, the glenoid fossa and the temporomandibular joint, the infratemporal fossa, mandibular nerve from foramen ovale, middle meningeal artery from foramen spinosum. Further in the deeper fields are the pterygoid process and its laminae, the pterygopalatine fossa and its contents, optic canal, the superior orbital fissure and its contents, the anterior clinoid process and the Meckel's area.

The type D approach when combined with other preauricular group of approaches such as the transzygomatic and the frontotemporal orbitozygomatic approaches presents a wider access to the deeper fields with minimal brain retraction.

Surgical Technique

As this approach is an anterior modification of type C, a preauricular incision is used and the plane of dissection is maintained anterior to the middle ear, petrous internal carotid artery and the eustachian tube. In type D1 approach, it is an extended preauricular skin incision and in type D2 approach where a more anterior exposure of the pterygopalatine fossa and the lateral wall of the orbit is required, the incision used is hemicoronal skin incision.

The main trunk of the facial nerve and the frontal branch are dissected and preserved as done in type C. An extended zygomatic osteotomy is usually performed in type D1 approach where the zygomatic arch and a part of zygomatic bone are included in the osteotomy whereas in type D2 approach in more advanced lesions with tumor extending into the orbital apex through one of the orbital fissures, an orbitozygomatic osteotomy is required. The temporalis muscle is detached from the squama of the temporal bone, retracted inferiorly and the base of the middle cranial fossa drilled away. As mentioned earlier, subtotal petrosectomy is not done and the eustachian tube is preserved. The middle meningeal artery and the mandibular nerve can be sacrificed for a wider exposure. Further drilling of the pterygoid process gives access to the pterygopalatine fossa, sphenoid sinus, the nasopharynx, the orbit and the parapharyngeal space. A more superior exposure is achieved by drilling away the greater wing of sphenoid along the base of the middle cranial fossa.

Temporalis muscle flap is rotated inward in between the mandibular condyle and remnant of glenoid fossa to reconstruct the mandibular fossa and wound closure done in layers after placing drains.

Complications

Inadequate repositioning of the orbitozygomatic osteotomy would result in a cosmetic defect and seldom when the blood supply of the temporalis muscle flap is compromised resulting in a devitalized tissue. Injury to the intraorbital contents, hence every effort is made to preserve the periorbital fascia.

REFERENCES

1. Fisch U. Infratemporal fossa approach for lesions in the temporal bone and base of the skull. In Neuro-Otology and Skull Base Surgery 1984 (Vol. 34, pp. 254–266). Karger Publishers.
2. Rosenwasser H. Carotid body tumor of the middle ear and mastoid. Archives of Otolaryngology. 1945 Jan 1;41(1):64–7.
3. Capps FC. Glomus jugulare tumors of the middle ear. The Journal of Laryngology and Otology. 1952 Jul;66(7):302–14.
4. Shambaugh Jr GE. Surgical approach for so-called glomus jugulare tumors of the middle ear. The Laryngoscope. 1955 Apr;65(4):185–98.
5. Farrior JB. Infratemporal approach to skull base for glomus tumors: anatomic considerations. Annals of Otology, Rhinology and Laryngology. 1984 Nov;93(6):616–22.
6. Shapiro MJ, Neues DK. Technique for removal of glomus jugulare tumors. Archives of Otolaryngology. 1964 Mar 1;79(3):219–24.
7. Farrior JB. Glomus tumors: Postauricular hypotympanotomy and hypotympanoplasty. Archives of Otolaryngology. 1967 Oct 1;86(4):367–73.
8. House WF, Glasscock ME. Glomus tympanicum tumors. Archives of Otolaryngology. 1968 May 1;87(5):550–4.

9. Fisch U. Infratemporal fossa approach for glomus tumors of the temporal bone. Annals of Otology, Rhinology and Laryngology. 1982 Sep;91(5):474–9.
10. Fisch U, Mattox D. Microsurgery of the skull base. Thieme; 1988.
11. Bacciu A, Prasad SC, Sist N, Rossi G, Piazza P, Sanna M. Management of the cervico-petrous internal carotid artery in class C tympanojugular paragangliomas. Head and neck. 2016 Jun;38(6):899–905.
12. Bacciu A, Medina M, Mimoune HA, D'Orazio F, Pasanisi E, Peretti G, Sanna M. Lower cranial nerves function after surgical treatment of Fisch Class C and D tympanojugular paragangliomas. European Archives of Oto-Rhino-Laryngology. 2015 Feb 1;272(2):311–9.
13. Patel SJ, Sekhar LN, Cass SP, Hirsch BE. Combined approaches for resection of extensive glomus jugulare tumors: A review of 12 cases. Journal of neurosurgery. 1994 Jun 1;80(6):1026–38.
14. Aslan A, Balyan FR, Taibah A, Sanna M. Anatomic relationships between surgical landmarks in type b and type c infratemporal fossa approaches. European archives of otorhinolaryngology. 1998 May 1;255(5):259–64.
15. Sanna M. Atlas of microsurgery of the lateral skull base. Thieme; 2008.
16. Zhang M, Garvis W, Linder T, Fisch U. Update on the Infratemporal Fossa Approaches to Nasopharyngeal Angiofibroma. Rivista di Neuroradiologia. 2000 May;13(1_suppl):213–9.
17. Sekhar LN, Schramm VL, Jones NF. Subtemporal-preauricular infratemporal fossa approach to large lateral and posterior cranial base neoplasms. Journal of neurosurgery. 1987 Oct 1;67(4):488–99.

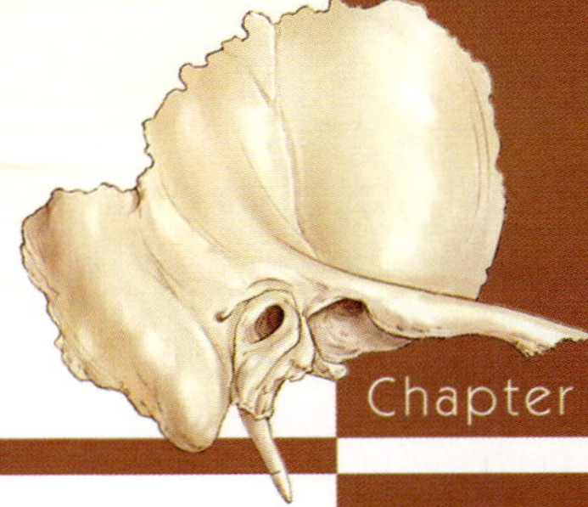

Chapter

19

Temporal Bone Resections for Malignancies of the Temporal Bone

Sampath Chandra Prasad Rao • Mario Sanna

Introduction

Temporal bone malignancies (TBMs) refer to a rare but distinct set of neoplasms originating within the confines of the temporal bone (TB) that account for approximately 0.2% of all head and neck malignancies. The annual incidence of such tumors is estimated to be between 1 and 6 per million population.[1,2] The incidence of TBMs at the Gruppo Otologico (Piacenza-Rome), which is a quarternary referral center for diseases of the skull base, is 130 (0.5%) cases for about 25,000 otological in-patient admissions over three decades. The rarity of these tumors can be adjudged by the fact that, in the last 15 years, there have been just about 20 series published dealing with squamous cell carcinomas (SCC) of the TB with a study population of over 20 patients, the largest series being that of Yin et al.,[3] with 95 subjects. Non squamous TBMs are even more rarely reported, most of them being limited to case reports. Because of the rarity of these tumors, it has been difficult for a single institution to analyze the data and formulate an optimal evaluation and treatment strategy.[4] Another impediment to the study of TBMs is the lack of a universally accepted staging system. There is no recognized American Joint Committee on Cancer (AJCC) or Union for International Cancer Control (UICC) staging system.[5] The T-staging that is currently available and still in the process of evolution, was adopted from a series of articles that were published by the Pittsburgh University[6–10] for SCC of the External Auditory Canal (EAC). A literature review indicates that unlike SCC of the EAC, there has been no serious attempt to classify and stage TBMs of other histologies and sites of origin other than the EAC.

However, over the years, morbidity and mortality in temporal bone resections have reduced significantly due to advances in neuroimaging, skull base surgery and neuroanesthesia. Moreover, the otologist/skull base surgeon of today is more compliant with the general oncological principles and practices than a few decades earlier. From very poor prognosis a few decades ago, using a combination of surgery and adjuvant radiotherapy (RT), up to 100% five year survival rates have been achieved by many authors for T1 and T2 tumors and up to 86% and 48% respectively in T3 and T4 tumors which indicates the progress made globally in the control of this disease.

Staging of TBMs

Staging of TBMs is important for determining prognosis and outcome after treatment. However, a standardized staging system has not yet been accepted internationally.[11] In 1980, Goodwin and Jesse,[12] divided SCC of the TB into three sites based on their origin (1) concha and cartilaginous meatus, (2) osseous meatus and (3) middle ear. This is valid as malignancies arising from each of these subsites have different tumor behavior and it would be unwise to compare them using the same parameters. For instance, tumors arising from the concha and the cartilaginous meatus tend to invade the soft tissues earlier than bone and behave more like cutaneous malignancies in other parts of the body. The tumors involving the osseous meatus tend to involve the bone anteriorly and posteriorly due to the thin skin. Similarly, tumors arising from the middle ear may involve the deeper parts of the TB sparing the EAC. The prognosis and management of tumors of each of these areas are different. Over the years many classifications have been proposed[6–10,13–15] but only the modified Pittsburgh classification for T staging for SCCs of the EAC has gained acceptance. There is still no consensus among authors for tumor staging in other parts of the TB.

Preoperative Management

Imaging is important in TBMs for accurate tumor and node staging since many patients have limited findings on physical examination. High-resolution computed tomography (HRCT) of the TB offers the most accurate method for evaluation of bone erosion due to malignancies. However, a reported limitation of CT is its inability to distinguish between tumor and fluid in the middle ear, soft tissue or mucosal thickening in the absence of bone erosion. Also, spread along fascial planes and neurovascular structures can be difficult to detect. Magnetic resonance imaging (MRI) can provide excellent differentiation between soft-tissue tumor margin, muscle and soft-tissue infiltration, and can help in distinguishing tumor from obstructive inflammatory changes. In addition, obstruction of the sigmoid sinus and encasement of the petrous internal carotid artery are better detected on MRI than CT, because of the vascular signal void seen on pre-contrast MRI and the flow enhancement of the sigmoid sinus seen on post-contrast MRI.[16] Tumor extension, especially cranial spread into the middle and posterior cranial fossa and caudal spread into the infratemporal fossa, is also better detected on MRI. Enhanced T1-weighted spin-echo images with fat-signal suppression are most suitable for this purpose. MRI has also made it possible to confidently diagnose perineural spread of malignancies.[17,18] Fat saturation Gadolinium-enhanced MR scans are often capable of detecting subtle tumor tracking along the Vth and VIIth cranial nerves, as well as other nerves that travel through the many foramina of the skull base, before the lesions have grown sufficiently large to affect the surrounding bone. Dental implants and densely calcified or ossified cartilages usually do not significantly degrade MR images as in CT.[19] Despite the advances in imaging it is still a challenge to exactly determine the size and extensions of TBMs. In their comparison of preoperative radiographic with intraoperative findings in 26 patients, Leonetti et al.[13] reported that anterior and inferior growth pattern were accurately assessed radiologically, while underestimations of tumor extent were seen with posterior, superior and medial tumor extensions. Another study showed statistical evidence that erosions of less than 2 mm on the anterior wall of the EAC are not recognized preoperatively by CT.[20] In our experience we have also often observed that peritumoral inflammatory changes show a much larger lesion on MRI than it actual actually is.

Surgical Techniques for TBMs

Surgery is the primary treatment of choice in TBMs. RT is used as an adjuvant treatment to surgery except in advanced tumors requiring palliation. The role of chemotherapy (CHT) is not established in TBMs. The surgical procedures employed for resection of TBMs are briefly described below.[21]

Lateral Temporal Bone Resection (LTBR)

This is the primary surgery of choice in T1 and T2 tumors. The approach entails a complete canal wall up mastoidectomy with an extended facial recess opening (Fig. 19.1). The incudostapedial joint is identified through the posterior tympanotomy and disarticulated (Fig. 19.2). The epitympanotomy is carried far anterior and the hypotympanotomy is carried far inferior and anterior through the hypotympanic portion of the tympanic bone (Fig. 19.3). Care must be taken not to damage the facial nerve and the dome of the jugular bulb. This step becomes challenging in case of a high jugular bulb. The epitympanotomy and hypotympanotomies are extended anteriorly along the anterior wall of the tympanic

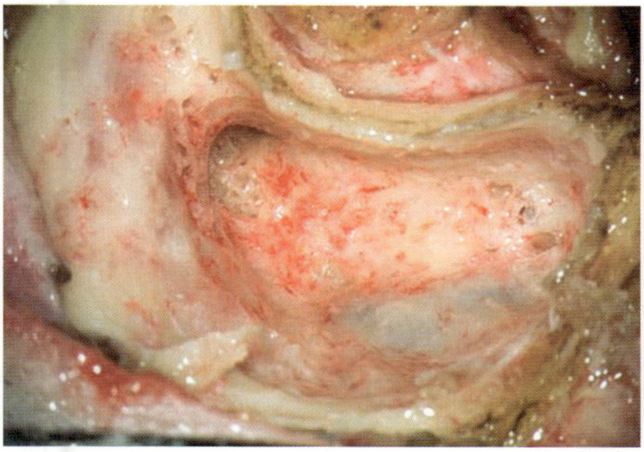

Fig. 19.1: The approach entails a complete canal wall up mastoidectomy with an extended facial recess opening

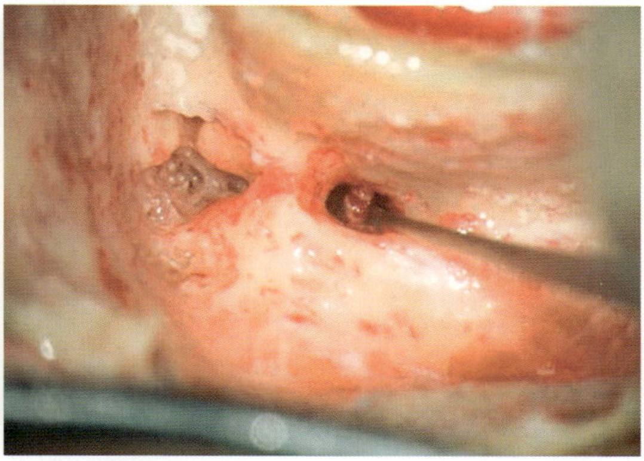

Fig. 19.2: The incudostapedial joint is identified through the posterior tympanotomy and disarticulated

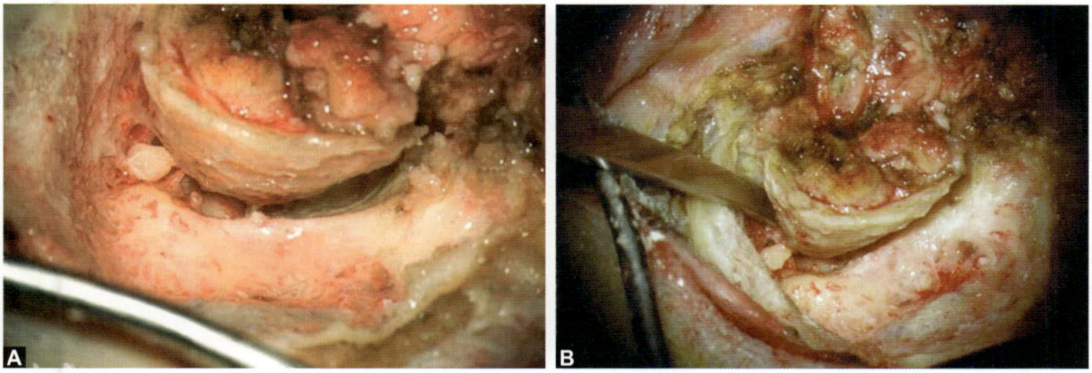

Fig. 19.3A and B: The epitympanotomy is carried far anterior and the hypotympanotomy is carried far inferior and anterior through the hypotympanic portion of the tympanic bone

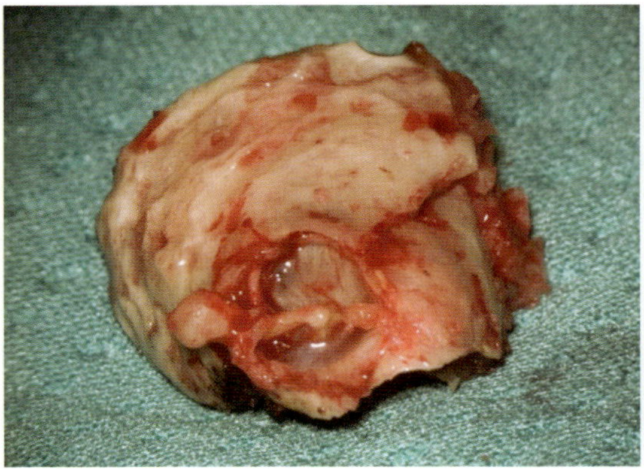

Fig. 19.4: The specimen resected en bloc includes the EAC, tympanic membrane and the malleus

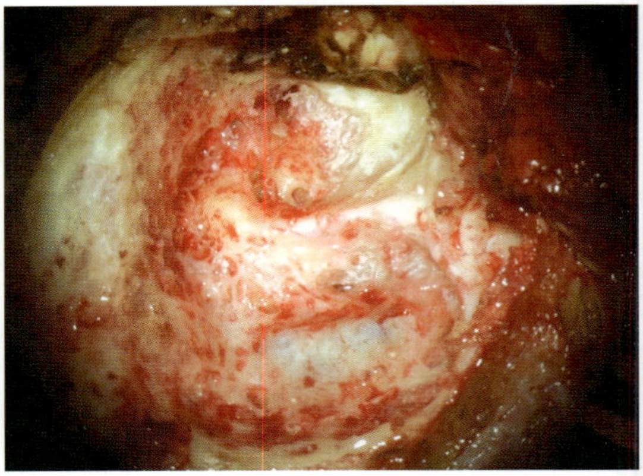

Fig. 19.5: The temporal bone cavity after LTBR

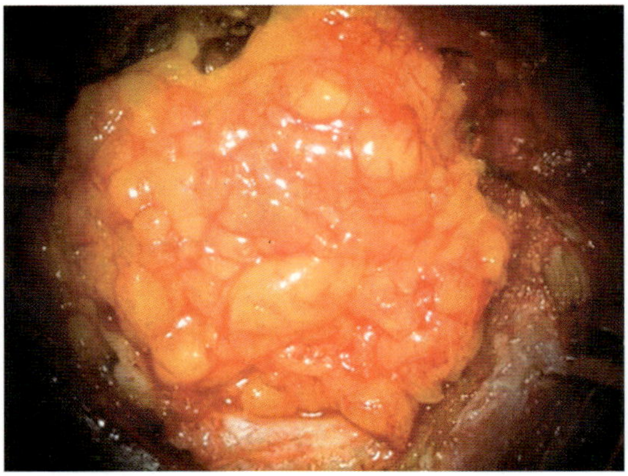

Fig. 19.6: The temporal bone cavity is filled with fat harvested from the abdomen

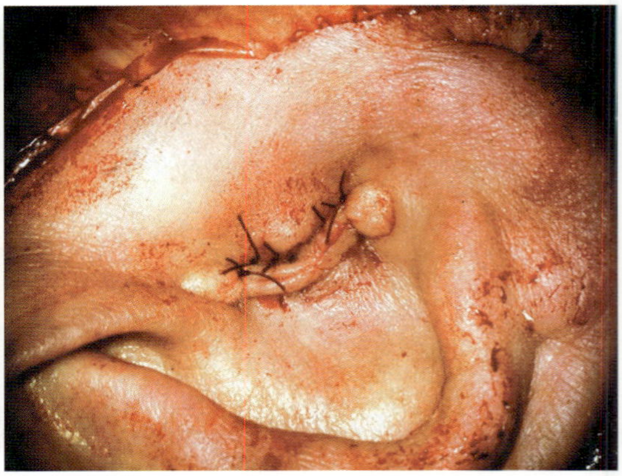

Fig. 19.7: The external auditory canal is closed in a blind sac fashion in two layers

bone. Drilling must be lateral to the eustachian tube to avoid inadvertent damage to the internal carotid artery. The parotid tissue on the tympanic bone is mobilized and an osteotomy is made taking care not to tear through the anterior annulus. The EAC is resected en bloc along with the tympanic membrane, the malleus, with the medial limit defined at the level of the incudostapedial joint[2] (Figs 19.4 and 19.5). The temporal bone cavity is filled with abdominal fat (Fig. 19.6). The external auditory canal is closed in two layers (skin and cartilage) after ensuring a negative margin with frozen section (Fig. 19.7). Some authors advocate that routine superficial parotidectomy (SP) be done with LTBR, especially in T2 tumors[22–24] however we reserve it for cases in which there is invasion of the anterior periosteum and if there are any lymph nodes in the parotid or retroparotid tissues.

Sub-Temporal Bone Resection (STBR)

This is used in T3 and T4 tumors and is an extension of the LTBR. After the steps of LTBR are performed, this procedure extends medially in a piecemeal fashion and includes IAC identification, FN exposure, and removal of the otic capsule with preservation of the petrous apex. Care must be taken to remove adequate bone around the tumor. The capsule of the temporomandibular joint and, if necessary, the condyle of the mandible is resected when found involved. If the tumor extends into the mastoid and dural involvement is suspected, middle and posterior fossa craniotomies might be necessary to achieve adequate exposure. Generally the dura is a good barrier for tumor spread and it must be removed only when necessary. If the dura is found infiltrated, its incision is undertaken and it is excised until free margins are reached. If the FN is invaded by the tumor, it should be included in the specimen. The FN may otherwise be re-routed to give access to the tumor. The sigmoid sinus and jugular bulb are preserved unless infiltrated. If there is any area of uncertain tumor clearance around the jugular bulb or the lower cranial nerves it is advisable to leave a vascular clip in situ for the site to be identified and targeted during postoperative RT (Figs 19.8 to 19.10).

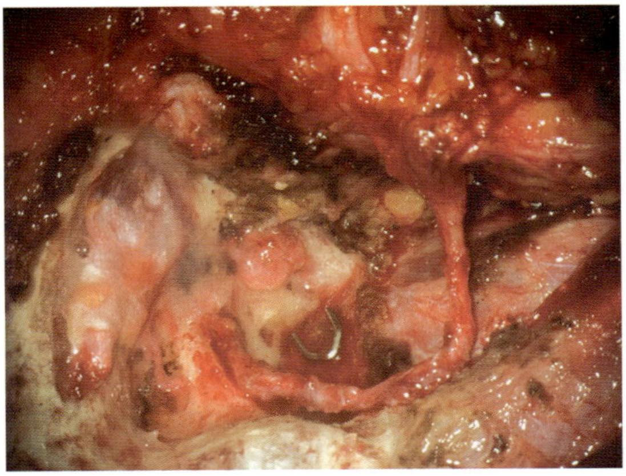

Fig. 19.8: STBR with exposure of the middle fossa dura, mobilization of the facial nerve, superficial parotidectomy. The jugular bulb was not resected due to its dominance on the affected side. A vascular clip was placed at the area of the jugular bulb where there was an element of suspicion of residual tumor to target the area during postoperative RT

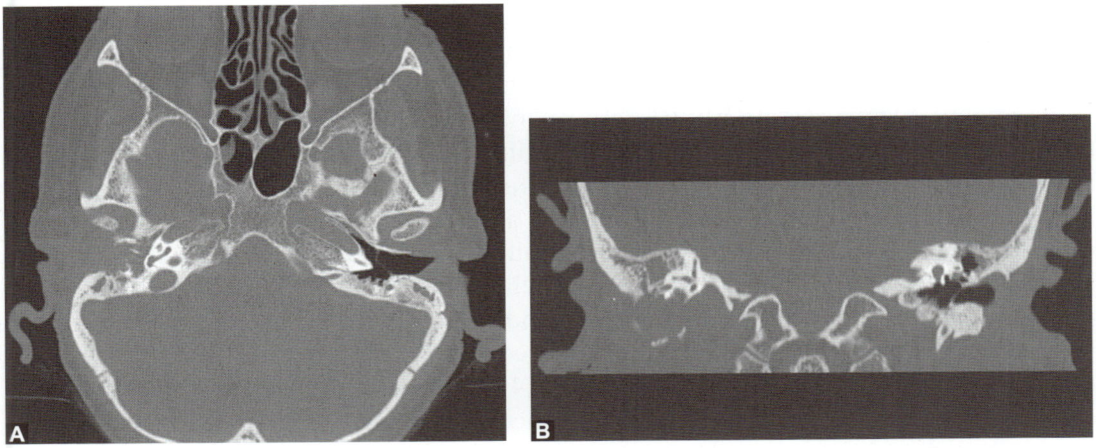

Fig. 19.9: Preoperative axial **(A)** and coronal **(B)** views of the same with T3 tumor of the EAC

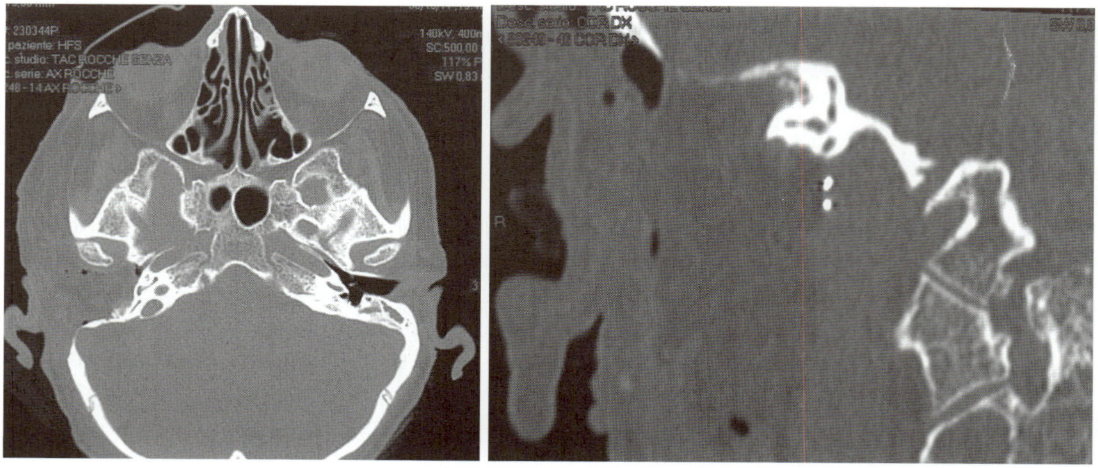

Fig. 19.10: (A) Postoperative axial and **(B)** coronal views of the same patient as in Figs 19.6 and 19.7 after STBR. The vascular clip can be identified near the jugular bulb in the coronal plane

Total Temporal Bone Resection (TTBR)

This procedure is used in advanced T4 tumors. It may be performed with or without resection of the pinna. Bone is resected superiorly for 3 cm above the temporal line to expose the middle fossa dura and behind the sigmoid sinus by a similar amount to leave a residual margin of healthy bone. Medial dissection extends through the labyrinth and exposes the intrapetrous carotid artery. Inferiorly, the sigmoid sinus and jugular bulb are mobilized from surrounding bone. The sternocleidomastoid and digastric muscles are freed from the mastoid tip. At this stage in the procedure, the ascending ramus of the mandible is transected with a Gigli saw or a drill, and this and the head and coronoid process are dissected free and removed. A total parotidectomy is completed, and the specimen is removed en bloc. The residual tip of the petrous bone is then removed with a high-speed drill.[24] Resection of the carotid artery can also be accomplished if the contralateral cerebral blood supply has been proven to be adequate by angiography and preoperative balloon occlusion.[25,26]

Selection of Surgical Procedure

The optimal surgical strategy for SCC of the TB remains controversial. A review of the literature (including papers with a study population of 15 and over) shows that many authors often adopt an individualistic approach to primary tumor and neck nodes management. Sleeve resection (SR) with retention of the pinna is still supported as a treatment of T1 tumors of the EAC[11,27] but it is difficult to believe that excision of the cancer field is not compromised.[24] Zhang et al,[11] have reported recurrence rates of 46.2% with SR for T1 and T2 lesions. We do not perform SRs at our center where LTBR is the accepted mainstay for T1 and T2 tumors. While most authors[2,4,22] agree that LTBR alone or with SP is adequate for T1 and T2 tumors, Moffa al[24] believe that LTBR with excision of the entire pinna, head, and ascending ramus of the mandible and with SP is mandatory for these tumors, but their assumption is based on a limited number of cases. Both LTBRs and STBRs are accepted techniques in T3 tumors.[2,24,28] In T4 tumors, although STBR is the surgery of choice,[2,20,22,29] the application of TTBR in advanced T4 tumors is a matter of debate.

The management of more advanced tumors (T4) is particularly challenging as a result of the complex anatomy and the proximity of intracranial structures. In early studies, the surgical attempt to remove these lesions was associated with high rates of morbidity and mortality[30,31] but this is no longer true in the context of modern skull base surgery. The palliative benefits of TTBR like decreased pain and improved hygiene in comparison with RT have also been emphasized by Moffat et al.[32] Although recent studies reported an improvement in terms of surgical morbidity and survival in patients who have undergone TTBR,[25,32,33] this procedure is still associated with significant postoperative deficits. As previously reported by several authors, the surgical morbidity of STBR is usually limited to FN palsy, and loss of hearing and balance, whereas additional morbidities of TTBR include potential damage to the cavernous sinus and internal carotid artery and postoperative deficits involving the IIIrd, IVth, Vth, and VIth cranial nerves.[28,34,35] In agreement with other authors,[9,36–40] we believe TTBR is unjustified because of the increased risk of morbidity and no proven survival benefit. STBR performed by a combination of en bloc and piecemeal resection techniques followed by postoperative RT could be a reasonable choice in patients with T4 tumors.[28,35,39] Prasad and Janecka,[41] in their review of the English literature, reported that patients with carcinomatous invasion of the petrous apex, IAC, dura, and brain had a poor estimated survival rate, although TTBR or dural excision was used.

En Bloc versus Piecemeal Resection

Performing an en bloc resection according to fundamental oncological principles to obtain clear negative tumor margins but would involve more danger to the surrounding intracranial structures and the cranial nerves while the FN would have to be sacrificed. The alternative is to do a piecemeal resection wherein drilling is continued around the tumor till healthy bone appears after gross tumor removal. This is our preferred treatment policy in T3 and T4 tumors. The advantage of a piecemeal resection is that while the same amount of bone could be removed as in en bloc resection, exposure is better under a microscope with less hazard to the cranial nerves. It is not always possible to obtain clear margins with piecemeal resection but this does not compromise tumor clearance if adequate bone is removed around the lesion. Though many reports[2,9,24,28,42] indicate poorer survival rates in resections with positive margins, this must not be viewed as a factor against piecemeal resection but more as a result of advanced nature of the disease. Further, Zanoletti et al[43] raise the questions of how 'free' negative margins must be in order to be considered oncologically safe in the case of SCC of the TB, to what extent the surgery must be enlarged beyond the presumably free margins to ensure oncological radicality and whether 'free' margins can really be considered negative in bone. These are pertinent issues towards which future studies must focus upon.

The Role of Parotidectomy

Tumors of the EAC can involve the parotid gland either by direct extension or through nodal dissemination of the disease because one of the first echelon[24] lymph nodes involved in SCC of the TB are the intraparotid or periparotid nodes. Preformed pathways around the EAC like the cartilaginous fissures of Santorini, the petrosquamous suture line and the bony foramen of Huschke are suspected to facilitate easy spread of tumor anteriorly. This is the main reason why some surgeons[29,44,45] prefer to associate SP with LTBRs, especially if tumor is found to be eroding the anterior wall of the EAC. The incidence of parotid involvement in SCC of the EAC has been reported to be between 10–62% of patients.[11,13,46–48] But there is no recorded benefit of performing a routine SP in terms of better survival rates. It is well known that nodal dissemination in TBMs is uncommon and hence many authors avoid performing a routine SP for the sake of nodal clearance.[49] We do not include

SP as a routine procedure in all T2 cases and prefer to perform it in T2 tumors only if there is evidence of involvement of the anterior wall of the EAC. However, in T3 tumors we routinely perform a SP. In T4 tumors and when there is evidence of involvement of the parotid gland per se, we perform a total parotidectomy.

The Role of Neck Dissection

Lymph nodes draining the EAC and the middle ear are the parotid and periparotid, pre- and postauricular, submandibular, upper deep cervical and the retropharyngeal lymph nodes. Though lymph nodes involvement is relatively rare (10–36%)[9,22,24,50,51] in TBMs, the presence of nodal metastasis, seen in advanced stages, has an adverse outcome on survival. While some studies have reported a poor survival rate in the presence of nodal metastasis,[43,45,49,51] others have not found this to be statistically significant.[2,5,22,52] With this background it is difficult to justify a routine neck dissection in a N0 neck, especially in T1 and T2 tumors. A positive neck at presentation is a sign of aggressiveness of the primary tumor. Therefore, when there is clinical or radiological evidence of neck nodes involvement one must pursue an aggressive neck dissection. Zanoletti et al.[53] concluded that the prognosis of the clinically positive neck is bad even though failures never occurred in the neck but at the site of the primary. Hence they recommend a more extended and adequate approach to the primary tumor. In N0 neck we perform a frozen section of the level II lymph nodes and proceed with neck dissection only when this is positive for metastasis. In N+ necks we perform routine neck dissection to involve the parotid and the level II lymph nodes.

The Role of Adjuvant Therapy

While RT has proven to be effective an adjuvant therapy, its role as a primary treatment modality for TBMs is not established. Postoperative RT is used to improve local and regional control of the disease. It is indicated in T3 and T4 tumors and also in T1 and T2 tumors where there is evidence of bone invasion, a positive margins, perineural invasion or nodal metastasis. In T3 and T4 tumors, many studies have reported better outcomes with adjuvant RT when compared to surgery alone.[9,11,24,51,54–56] Moreover, patients whose advanced tumors could not be fully resected showed little benefit from adjuvant RT in terms of survival.[42] Cristalli et al[54] applied intraoperative RT and reported a high global local control rate of 73.3%. In important studies by Shiga et al[57] and Sugimoto et al[58] where concomitant chemoradiotherapy (CRT) was used to treat advanced tumors, 5-year survival of 78% and a 2-year survival of 80% were reported respectively. Despite the disadvantage of toxicity associated with this protocol, the high survival rates in advanced cancers indicate that this could be an effective treatment modality and further studies could be pursued in this direction.

Our therapeutic guidelines according to T-staging is compared with those proposed by the Belgium Consensus Conference of March 2002 and by Kunst et al[27] in Table 19.1.

Conclusion

Despite the fact that significant attention has being focused on TBMs in the last few decades, there is still need to comprehensively study the entire gamut of histological varieties, refine existing tumor staging system or develop novel ones and standardize treatment protocols. Radical surgery is the mainstay of treatment of TBMs in all tumor stages. Advances in neuroradiology, skull base surgical techniques and neuroanesthesia have made surgical resection of even advanced tumors in this area feasible with minimal

Table 19.1: Treatment strategies for SCC of the EAC

Tumor staging	*Belgium consensus conference*	*Kunst et al[27]*	*Our guidelines*
T1	LTBR and ND	○ LTBR and RT if margins are positive	○ LTBR and RT if margins are positive
T2	LTBR and ND followed by RT	○ LTBR and RT	○ LTBR and SP if tumor breaches periosteum of AW-EAC, followed by RT
T3	STBR and ND followed by RT	○ LTBR/STBR and RT. If N+ then ND; if parotid+ then TP	○ STBR+SP and RT. If N+ then ND; if parotid+ then TP
T4	Palliative treatment	○ Palliative treatment (T4b and c) or in T4a and some b ○ Tumors: STBR/TTBR and SP, followed by RT. If N+ then ND; if parotid+ then TP	○ T4a and b–STBR with TP and ND, if necessary MCR or skin excision and reconstruction, followed by RT ○ T4c-Palliative treatment. *No TTBR for petroclival extension*

LTBR: Lateral temporal bone resection, STBR: Subtemporal bone resection, TTBR: Total temporal bone resection, ND: Neck dissection, RT: Radiotherapy, SP: Superficial parotidectomy, TP: Total parotidectomy, MCR: Mandibular condylar resection, AW-EAC: Anterior wall of external auditory canal

T4a indicates involvement of extracranial infratemporal fossa, skin, parotid; T4b involvement of intrapetrous bone and extradural extension; T4c, meningeal or intradural involvement

morbidity. Adjuvant RT is indicated in T2, T3 and T4 tumors and is considered in T1 only in case of incomplete resection.

REFERENCES

1. Prasad SC, D'Orazio F, Medina M, Bacciu A, Sanna M. State of the art in temporal bone malignancies. Curr Opin Otolaryngol Head Neck Surg 2014; 22:154–65.
2. Bacciu A, Clemente IA, Piccirillo E, Ferrari S, Sanna M. Guidelines for treating temporal bone carcinoma based on long-term outcomes. Otol Neurotol 2013; 34:898–907.
3. Yin M, Ishikawa K, Honda K, et al. Analysis of 95 cases of squamous cell carcinoma of the external and middle ear. Auris, nasus, larynx 2006; 33:251–57.
4. Nakagawa T, Kumamoto Y, Natori Y, et al. Squamous cell carcinoma of the external auditory canal and middle ear: an operation combined with preoperative chemoradiotherapy and a free surgical margin. Otology and neurotology : official publication of the American Otological Society, American Neurotology Society [and] European Academy of Otology and Neurotology 2006; 27:242–48; discussion 249.
5. Gidley PW. Managing malignancies of the external auditory canal. Expert review of anticancer therapy 2009; 9:1277–82.
6. Arriaga M, Hirsch BE, Kamerer DB, Myers EN. Squamous cell carcinoma of the external auditory meatus (canal). Otolaryngology--head and neck surgery: official journal of American Academy of Otolaryngology-Head and Neck Surgery 1989; 101:330–37.
7. Arriaga M, Curtin H, Takahashi H, Hirsch BE, Kamerer DB. Staging proposal for external auditory meatus carcinoma based on preoperative clinical examination and computed tomography findings. The Annals of otology, rhinology, and laryngology 1990; 99:714–21.
8. Arriaga M, Curtin HD, Takahashi H, Kamerer DB. The role of preoperative CT scans in staging external auditory meatus carcinoma: radiologic-pathologic correlation study. Otolaryngology--head and neck surgery : official journal of American Academy of Otolaryngology-Head and Neck Surgery 1991; 105:6–11.

9. Moody SA, Hirsch BE, Myers EN. Squamous cell carcinoma of the external auditory canal: an evaluation of a staging system. The American journal of otology 2000; 21:582–88.
10. Hirsch BE. Staging system revision. Archives of otolaryngology--head and neck surgery 2002; 128:93–94.
11. Zhang T, Li W, Dai C, Chi F, Wang S, Wang Z. Evidence-based surgical management of T1 or T2 temporal bone malignancies. The Laryngoscope 2013; 123:244–48.
12. Goodwin WJ, Jesse RH. Malignant neoplasms of the external auditory canal and temporal bone. Arch Otolaryngol 1980; 106:675–79.
13. Leonetti JP, Smith PG, Kletzker GR, Izquierdo R. Invasion patterns of advanced temporal bone malignancies. The American journal of otology 1996; 17:438–442.
14. Stell PM, McCormick MS. Carcinoma of the external auditory meatus and middle ear. Prognostic factors and a suggested staging system. The Journal of laryngology and otology 1985; 99:847–50.
15. Clark LJ, Narula AA, Morgan DA, Bradley PJ. Squamous carcinoma of the temporal bone: a revised staging. The Journal of laryngology and otology 1991; 105:346–48.
16. Zhang F, Sha Y. Computed tomography and magnetic resonance imaging findings for primary middle-ear carcinoma. The Journal of laryngology and otology 2013; 127:578–83.
17. Schmalfuss IM, Tart RP, Mukherji S, Mancuso AA. Perineural tumor spread along the auriculotemporal nerve. AJNR American journal of neuroradiology 2002; 23:303–11.
18. Chang PC, Fischbein NJ, McCalmont TH, *et al*. Perineural spread of malignant melanoma of the head and neck: clinical and imaging features. AJNR American journal of neuroradiology 2004; 25:5–11.
19. Wippold FJ, 2nd. Head and neck imaging: the role of CT and MRI. Journal of magnetic resonance imaging : JMRI 2007; 25:453–65.
20. Hosokawa S, Mizuta K, Takahashi G, *et al*. Surgical approach for treatment of carcinoma of the anterior wall of the external auditory canal. Otology and neurotology : official publication of the American Otological Society, American Neurotology Society [and] European Academy of Otology and Neurotology 2012; 33:450–54.
21. Sanna MS, E; Khrais, T; Mancini, F; Piazza, P; Russo, A; Taibah, A. Atlas of Microsurgery of the Lateral Skull Base. Stuttgart: Thieme Publishers, 2007.
22. Leong SC, Youssef A, Lesser TH. Squamous cell carcinoma of the temporal bone: Outcomes of radical surgery and postoperative radiotherapy. The Laryngoscope 2013; 123:2442–48.
23. Lassig AA, Spector ME, Soliman S, El-Kashlan HK. Squamous cell carcinoma involving the temporal bone: lateral temporal bone resection as primary intervention. Otology and neurotology : official publication of the American Otological Society, American Neurotology Society [and] European Academy of Otology and Neurotology 2013; 34:141–50.
24. Moffat DA, Wagstaff SA, Hardy DG. The outcome of radical surgery and postoperative radiotherapy for squamous carcinoma of the temporal bone. The laryngoscope 2005; 115:341–47.
25. Graham MD, Sataloff RT, Kemink JL, Wolf GT, McGillicuddy JE. Total en bloc resection of the temporal bone and carotid artery for malignant tumors of the ear and temporal bone. The Laryngoscope 1984; 94:528–33.
26. Piazza P, Di Lella F, Bacciu A, Di Trapani G, Ait Mimoune H, Sanna M. Preoperative Protective Stenting of the Internal Carotid Artery in the Management of Complex Head and Neck Paragangliomas: Long-Term Results. Audiology and neuro-otology 2013; 18:345–52.
27. Kunst H, Lavieille JP, Marres H. Squamous cell carcinoma of the temporal bone: results and management. Otology and neurotology : official publication of the American Otological Society, American Neurotology Society [and] European Academy of Otology and Neurotology 2008; 29:549–52.
28. Chi FL, Gu FM, Dai CF, Chen B, Li HW. Survival outcomes in surgical treatment of 72 cases of squamous cell carcinoma of the temporal bone. Otology and neurotology : official publication of the American Otological Society, American Neurotology Society [and] European Academy of Otology and Neurotology 2011; 32:665–69.

29. Lavieille JD, C; Kunst, H; Deveze, A; Magnan, J; Schmerber, S. Management of carcinoma of the temporal bone. The Mediterranean Journal of Otology 2005; 1:1–9.
30. Conley JJ, Novack AJ. The surgical treatment of malignant tumors of the ear and temporal bone. Part I. AMA archives of otolaryngology 1960; 71:635–52.
31. Lewis JS. Temporal bone resection. Review of 100 cases. Arch Otolaryngol 1975; 101:23–5.
32. Moffat DA, Grey P, Ballagh RH, Hardy DG. Extended temporal bone resection for squamous cell carcinoma. Otolaryngology--head and neck surgery : official journal of American Academy of Otolaryngology-Head and Neck Surgery 1997; 116:617–23.
33. Asano K, Somekawa Y, Yoshioka I, Ikeda H. En bloc resection of the temporal bone by the lateral approach in carcinoma of the middle ear associated with skull base infiltration with reference to the resection of the petrous apex. Skull base surgery 1998; 8:195–204.
34. Yeung P, Bridger A, Smee R, Baldwin M, Bridger GP. Malignancies of the external auditory canal and temporal bone: a review. ANZ journal of surgery 2002; 72:114–120.
35. Chang CH, Shu MT, Lee JC, Leu YS, Chen YC, Lee KS. Treatments and outcomes of malignant tumors of external auditory canal. American journal of otolaryngology 2009; 30:44–8.
36. Kuhel WI, Hume CR, Selesnick SH. Cancer of the external auditory canal and temporal bone. Otolaryngologic clinics of North America 1996; 29:827–52.
37. Austin JR, Stewart KL, Fawzi N. Squamous cell carcinoma of the external auditory canal. Therapeutic prognosis based on a proposed staging system. Archives of otolaryngology--head and neck surgery 1994; 120:1228–32.
38. Zhang B, Tu G, Xu G, Tang P, Hu Y. Squamous cell carcinoma of temporal bone: reported on 33 patients. Head and neck 1999; 21:461–66.
39. Moore MG, Deschler DG, McKenna MJ, Varvares MA, Lin DT. Management outcomes following lateral temporal bone resection for ear and temporal bone malignancies. Otolaryngology--head and neck surgery: official journal of American Academy of Otolaryngology-Head and Neck Surgery 2007; 137:893–98.
40. Pensak ML, Gleich LL, Gluckman JL, Shumrick KA. Temporal bone carcinoma: contemporary perspectives in the skull base surgical era. The Laryngoscope 1996; 106:1234–37.
41. Prasad S, Janecka IP. Efficacy of surgical treatments for squamous cell carcinoma of the temporal bone: a literature review. Otolaryngology--head and neck surgery : official journal of American Academy of Otolaryngology-Head and Neck Surgery 1994; 110:270–80.
42. Nyrop M, Grontved A. Cancer of the external auditory canal. Archives of otolaryngology--head and neck surgery 2002; 128:834–37.
43. Zanoletti E, Marioni G, Stritoni P, *et al*. Temporal bone squamous cell carcinoma: Analyzing prognosis with univariate and multivariate models. The Laryngoscope 2013.
44. Kinney SE. Squamous cell carcinoma of the external auditory canal. The American Journal of Otology 1989; 10:111–16.
45. Morris LG, Mehra S, Shah JP, Bilsky MH, Selesnick SH, Kraus DH. Predictors of survival and recurrence after temporal bone resection for cancer. Head and neck 2012; 34:1231–39.
46. Gillespie MB, Francis HW, Chee N, Eisele DW. Squamous cell carcinoma of the temporal bone: a radiographic-pathologic correlation. Archives of otolaryngology–head and neck surgery 2001; 127:803–07.
47. Yoon M, Chougule P, Dufresne R, Wanebo HJ. Localized carcinoma of the external ear is an unrecognized aggressive disease with a high propensity for local regional recurrence. American journal of surgery 1992; 164:574–77.
48. Freedlander E, Chung FF. Squamous cell carcinoma of the pinna. British journal of plastic surgery 1983; 36:171–75.
49. Madsen AR, Gundgaard MG, Hoff CM, *et al*. Cancer of the external auditory canal and middle ear in Denmark from 1992 to 2001. Head and neck 2008; 30:1332–38.
50. Stell PM. Carcinoma of the external auditory meatus and middle ear. Clinical otolaryngology and allied sciences 1984; 9:281–99.
51. Dean NR, White HN, Carter DS, *et al*. Outcomes following temporal bone resection. The Laryngoscope 2010; 120:1516–22.

52. Marioni G, Nucci R, Marino F, *et al*. Neoangiogenesis in temporal bone carcinoma: the prognostic role of CD105. Otology and neurotology : official publication of the American Otological Society, American Neurotology Society [and] European Academy of Otology and Neurotology 2012; 33:843–48.
53. Zanoletti E, Danesi G. The problem of nodal disease in squamous cell carcinoma of the temporal bone. Acta otolaryngologica 2010; 130:913–16.
54. Cristalli G, Manciocco V, Pichi B, *et al*. Treatment and outcome of advanced external auditory canal and middle ear squamous cell carcinoma. The Journal of craniofacial surgery 2009; 20:816–21.
55. Bibas AG, Ward V, Gleeson MJ. Squamous cell carcinoma of the temporal bone. The Journal of laryngology and otology 2008; 122:1156–61.
56. Pfreundner L, Schwager K, Willner J, *et al*. Carcinoma of the external auditory canal and middle ear. International journal of radiation oncology, biology, physics 1999; 44:777–88.
57. Shiga K, Ogawa T, Maki A, Amano M, Kobayashi T. Concomitant chemoradiotherapy as a standard treatment for squamous cell carcinoma of the temporal bone. Skull base : official journal of North American Skull Base Society [et al] 2011; 21:153–58.
58. Sugimoto H, Ito M, Yoshida S, Hatano M, Yoshizaki T. Concurrent superselective intra-arterial chemotherapy and radiotherapy for late-stage squamous cell carcinoma of the temporal bone. The Annals of otology, rhinology, and laryngology 2011; 120:372–76.

Chapter

20

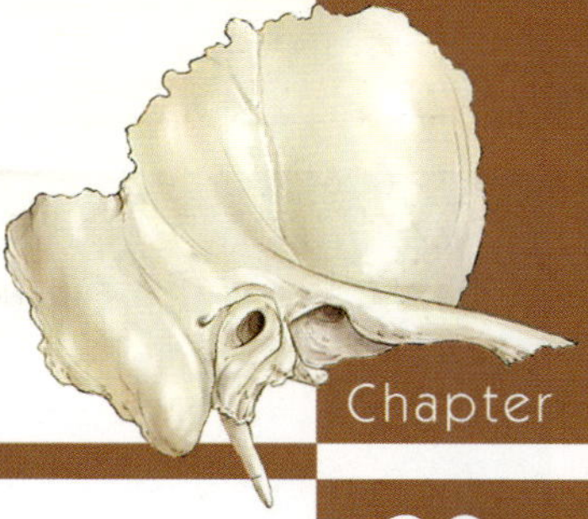

Complications of Mastoidectomy: A Short Review

Dipak Ranjan Nayak • Khageswar Rout • Swetapadma Nayak

Introduction

Mastoidectomy is a routine procedure done in otology, for exenteration of mastoid air cells. Knowledge of the anatomy of temporal bone is critical for performing mastoid surgeries safely. Most complications occur due to inadequate exposure of structures, failure to identify anatomical landmarks, granulations or bleeding obscuring the surgical field. Anticipating complications at all times and taking appropriate measures help prevent disasters. Despite taking all the measures, complications can occur even with the most experienced surgeons. So knowing the complications and its management technique is just as important as the steps of the surgery. Each complication must be evaluated thoroughly for immediate medical/surgical intervention and one has to learn how to avoid them in the future (Khan et al, 2014).

Complications

Hemorrhage

Hemorrhage usually does not cause problem during surgery unless significant vessels are injured. But even small amount of bleeding causes obscured field of view for surgery which in turn increases the risk of injuring underlying structures. Bleeding should be controlled as much as possible using adrenaline soaked gel foam for packing and wait for sometime for bleeding to reduce. Slow oozing can be easily controlled using this method.

The superficial temporal artery is commonly injured while harvesting the graft or while placing the opening incision of the periosteum over temporal line near EAC. This can be prevented by carefully cauterizing the anterior extent of the periosteal incision.

Vessels in the mastoid bone can be controlled by using diamond drill if they are small. Larger vessels can be cauterized using bipolar cautery or bone wax can be used to seal the vessel (Shambaugh, 2010).

Sigmoid sinus injury (Fig. 20.1)**:** If the injured vessel is the sigmoid sinus, often small injuries can be controlled with bipolar cautery. But in case of sizeable injuries care must

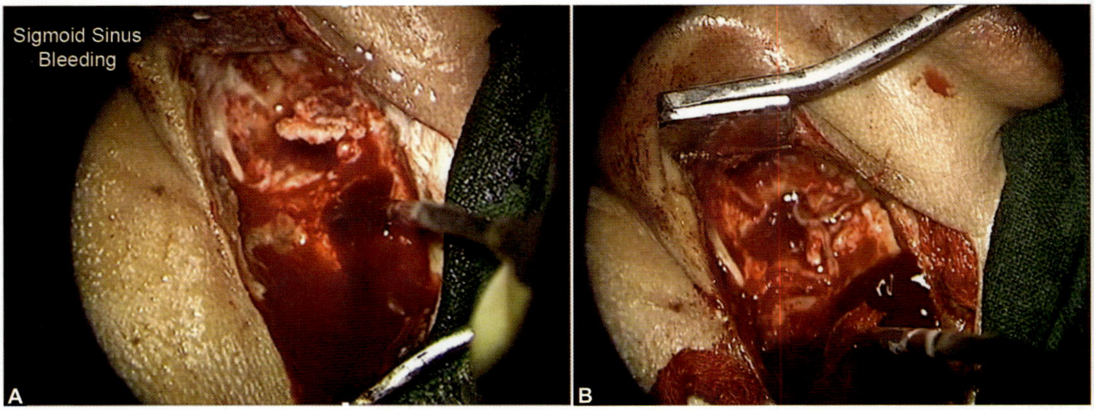

Fig. 20.1: (A) Showing bleeding from the sigmoid sinus, **(B)** showing Gelfoam® being applied to control the bleeding

be taken to prevent air embolism. Placing a finger over the tear in the sinus to prevent further bleeding. While the finger applies pressure to prevent bleeding, the head of the patient should be rotated towards you and the head should be lowered, after which the torn sinus can be repaired. Gelfoam or oxidized cellulose can be placed over the injury site and left in place. Although this technique can give rise to intracranial venous hypertension in case the dominant sinus is involved (Moore, 1994). Studies have shown that the tomographic distance between sigmoid sinus and EAC measuring less than 9 mm complicated the procedure causing torrential bleeding (Periera, 2012). In case of dominant venous sinus injury, there is a risk of development of lateral sinus thrombosis, which can result in fulminant intracranial hypertension which warrants for repair of the tear and the posterior fossa dura and direct thrombocytes techniques in order to prevent major neurological complications (Shekhar, 1997).

Injury to ICA: The damage to ICA can occur in case the bony shell is dehiscent (Hasebe et al, 2003), congenital anomaly (Shambaugh, 1967), persistence of embryonic vessels (Barrett, 1960), bone absorption, or inflammatory changes (Walshe et al, 2002, Sauvaget, 2006). One should keep in mind in case of a retrotympanic mass with aberrant ICA characteristics like anterior pulsatile red colored mass is observed during surgery, one should do a CT scan of the temporal bone should be done before puncturing it or taking a biopsy, in order to avoid injury due to misdiagnosis, or to look for any aberrant carotid artery. It is best advised to do a preoperative CT scan of the temporal bone before attempting any middle ear surgery. In case profuse bleeding occurs during surgery without any identifiable source of bleeding, then the procedure should be abandoned and a tight ear pack should be given and the patient should be subjected to MR angiography to identify the hemorrhage and localize the injury site or any other vascular abnormality. The resulting pseudoaneurysm should be treated at the earliest. The options include proximal and distal carotid artery ligation or embolization can be done, stenting of the artery using self expanding wall graft or occlusion of the pseudoaneurysm using micro coils.

Postaural hematomas can be prevented by the use of tight mastoid bandage which prevents bleeding during postoperative period when the patient strains or coughs.

Facial Nerve Injury

It is one of the most significant complications during mastoid surgery and the most common site 2nd genu where it is closely related to the lateral semicircular canal. Often both the strctures are injured together. Although the risk of facial nerve injury during surgery has drastically reduced with advent of micro drill and microscope but the facial nerve remains at risk during surgery even today with the incidence of 1%. It is of utmost importance to know the facial nerve course and its anatomical variants, specially in the vertical segment from 2nd genu to stylomastoid foramen (Yadav et al, 2006). Initial assessment of facial nerve during postoperative should always be done in the operating room itself, by looking for flaring of nasal ala during the reversal of anesthesia.

Management of iatrogenic facial nerve injury can be divided into three categories (Shambaugh, 2010)

A. Intraoperative recognition of facial nerve injury.
B. Early postoperative recognition of facial weakness.
C. Delayed postoperative recognition of facial weakness.

A. Intraoperative Recognition of Facial Nerve Injury

In case of minimal injury recognized during the surgery, distal and proximal to the injury bony covering should be removed to prevent postinjury edema. The steps of facial nerve decompression (Fig. 20.2) can be read from Chapter 9.

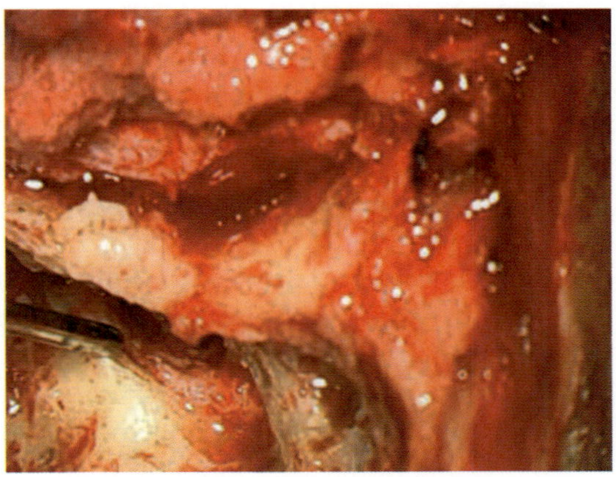

Fig. 20.2: Facial nerve decompression progress

When there is partial transection, it is recommended to preserve the remaining intact fascicles. Anastomosis of separated fascicles can be done. And the site distal and proximal to the injury should undergo decompression. In cases of subtotal transection of nerve, the injured areas of the nerve are brought together without tension using 9–0 nylon suture and the facial nerve function is serially assessed for the next 1 year.

If a complete transection, which is very rare, recognised during the surgery then primary anastomosis should be attempted. In case of loss of tissue, a cable (interpositional) nerve graft can be done using sural nerve or greater auricular nerve depending on the length of tissue loss (Fig. 20.3). Injured lateral canal (Fig. 20.3A) and lateral canal covered with bone dust (Fig 20.3B), the color difference has to be followed as in original figure provided.

B. Early Postoperative Recognition of Facial Nerve Weakness

If during intraoperative period no facial nerve injury is noted but paralysis is noted during immediate postoperative, it could be caused due to local anesthetic effect. This generally subsides within 4 hours. But if the paralysis does not subside within 4 hours, surgical exploration is needed during which the geniculate ganglion to the stylomastoid foramen should be explored. Suspicious areas should be decompressed. Postoperative steroid should be supplemented.

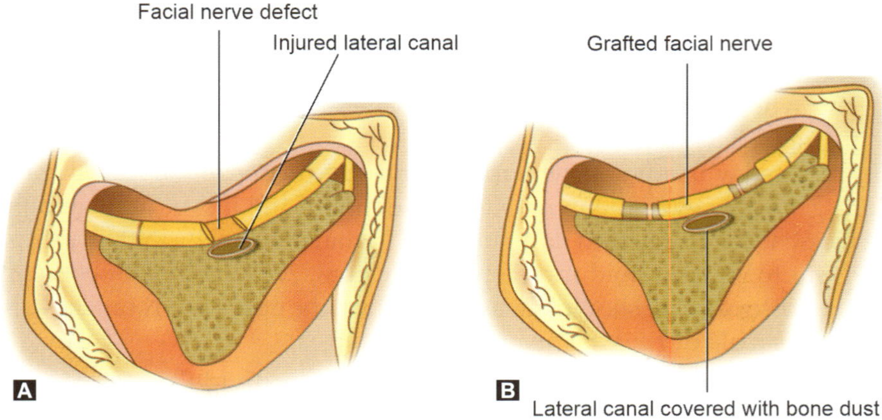

Fig. 20.3: (A) Injured facial nerve along with lateral semicircular canal. **(B)** Grafting of the nerve with great auricular nerve graft and sealing of lateral canal with bone dust

C. Delayed Postoperative Recognition of Facial Nerve Weakness

It is considered to be delayed if the paralysis occurs after 8 hours. Generally managed with steroids, antibiotics and antivirals. Antivirals with better blood–brain barrier penetration is preferred if the delay of onset is after 72 hours. Surgical intervention is very rarely required.

Labyrinthine Injury and Sensory Neural Hearing Loss

Although iatrogenic labyrinthine injury and sensorineural hearing loss are infrequent, the 3 sites which are at maximal risk during surgery are LSCC, promontory and oval window, with injury to oval window being more common (0.5–1.4%, Palva et al)

As in case of cholesteatoma fistula, iatrogenic injury to membranous labyrinth need not be associated with hearing loss. With injury to LSCC being a total incidence of 0.08– 0.1% as noted by Palma et al and Canalis et al. Postinjury an acute, moderately severe sensorineural hearing loss was noticed which reverted to preoperavie levels within 3–6 weeks, but most cases mild, permanent high frequency hearing loss can be noted with their speech discrimination scores returning to normal. Other occasional symptoms include unsteadiness, positional vertigo, spontaneous nystagmus which can have delayed onset going onto start as late as 1–2 years after surgery.

Based on the location of damage, Canalis et al believed injuring the posterior limb would be associated with hemorrhage and serous labyrinthitis where as injuring closer to vestibule would result in permanent damage following contamination of perilymph by endolymph.

It is to be noted that cochlear preservation occurs most of the time due to the collapse of the membranous labyrinth following sudden loss of endolymph causing the fistula to be sealed. It is recommended to seal the iatrogenic fistula with a fascia plug, although bone wax, bone dust and muscle plugs can also be used.

Injury to oval window can occur due to avulsion of the footplate, dislocation of the footplate and fracture without dislocation. Chances of sensorineural hearing loss is rare in these cases.

In any case the dictum of repair should be to cover any opening with fascia and to avoid suctioning. Palva et al also recommend that until the area heals, ossicular reconstruction should be deferred.

Labyrinthine injury can cause sensorineural hearing loss but major damage of hearing is done as a result of excessive manipulation of the ossicular chain, drilling on the ossicles, noise of the drill and other unidentified factors. The incidence of sensorineural hearing loss postsurgery goes up to 2.5% with a 10% reduction in speech discrimination score as reviewed by Smyth.

Injury to Chorda Tympani

The overall reported prevalence of iatrogenic chorda tympani injury is 15–22%. The consequences of injury is variable. The mechanism of injuries includes transection, ischemia, stretching, thermal injury, excessive handling and desiccation. Injury to nerve although does not always cause symptoms. The main symptoms include loss or alteration of taste +/- dryness of mouth. Other associated symptoms include tingling and numbness and postoperative touch evoked dysgeusia (Michael and Raut, 2007). Majority of the studies show that transection of the nerve leads to postoperative gustatory symptoms which most likely will persist than those which preserve the nerve. It is to be noted that the nerve regeneration was more likely to be seen in children and higher recovery rates. Subjective taste disturbances resolve more rapidly as compared to the electrogustometry taste threshold (Kveton and Bartoshuk, 1994).

Injury to Dura

Limited dural exposure usually does not require any repair but dural injury requires adequate management. As compared to earlier decades the rates of dural injuries have come down with the advent of microscope and refinements in technique. It is usually caused by drill or misguided curette, indiscriminate usage of diathermy over dural vessels. The latter can be prevented by usage of bipolar cautery on the dura (Palva, 1971 and 1976). CSF fluid can be noted leaking from the site of injury, but in case the injury is in the middle fossa dura, small injuries are concealed by the dense arachnoid tissue (Sana, 2009). The dictum is to repair any dural injury as soon as it is noticed. Paparella et al recommend that during a middle fossa dura injury, one should remove 5 mm of bone and inspect the dura and brain. Mascerated muscle when placed in the defect in a plugging fashion stops majority of the leaks. A fascia graft may be placed between the dura and the bone. Other approaches include repair using fascia, bone and skin through middle fossa craniotomy, and pressure can be provided no tight intramastoid packing. Other options include cartilage perichondrial grafts, rotational flaps, free flaps or fat obliteration. If it is a linear injury, the tear can be sutured. But if a brain injury is suspected, then neurosurgical consultation should be sought.

Posterior fossa dural injuries do not close spontaneously, hence torrential leaks are likely. Repair involves exposure of normal dura and then placement of graft. The patient is advised not to strain, and is on bedrest for a couple of days with the head end elevated so as to reduce pressure over the repair. In case of persistent leak then serial lumbar puncture can be opted (Paparella et al., 1991).

Once the CSF leak is controlled bone cement (hydroxyapatite) can be used to seal the defect with fascia so that the mucosa grows over it (Catalano, 2000). Fibrin glue can also be used for repair.

Meningoencephalocele

The dural defects when caused as a result of mastoid surgery, the complications include CSF otorrhea or otorhinorrhea, seizures, meningitis, brain abscess, epidural abscess and sometimes meningoencephalocele (Patel, 2008). This is a rare complication where in the brain with its meninges, covering herniates into the mastoid cavity or middle ear cavity (Fig. 20.4). The herniation occurs in cases of CSOM, following surgery, chronic inflammation, trauma, neoplasia, congenital defects, irradiation and degenerative conditions.

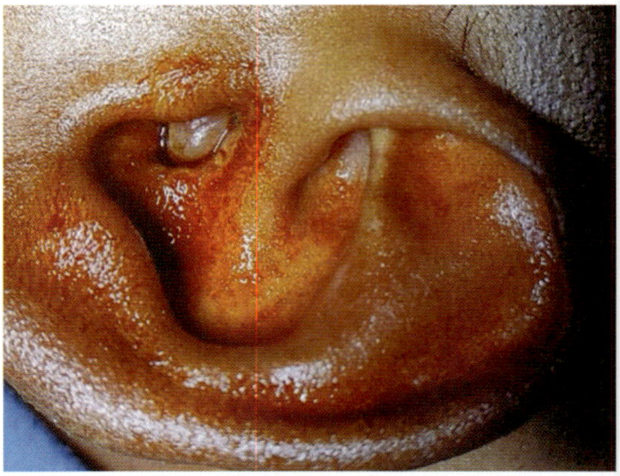

Fig. 20.4: Iatrogenic meningocele following mastoid surgery

Meningoencephalocele +/- CSF leak can be clinically silent, or may present with hearing loss, chronic otorrhea, tinnitus and vertigo, meningitis, temporal lobe epilepsy, aphasia or facial paresis (Fig. 20.5).

High degree suspicion should be kept in order to arrive to diagnosis by using HRCT and MRI to assess the extent of the lesion. CT and MRI with radionuclide cisternography is useful but is not done routinely on every patient (Neely, 1985). Surgery is the treatment of choice. The various approaches include transmastoid approach, minicraniotomy, combined transmastoid and middle fossa approach (Fig. 20.5). The latter provides maximal exposure of the tegmen plate defect. The herniated brain tissue is generally nonfunctional, hence is removed with half of diathermy (Fig. 20.5). The defect is sealed by using temporalis fascia, cartilage, titanium mesh, cadaveric dura, muscle, bone, proplast and fibrin glue. Main aim is to secure a firm and complete closure of the defect in layers (Fig. 20. 6). Some times partial or compete obliteration of mastoid cavity may be required (Figs 20.6 and 20.7).

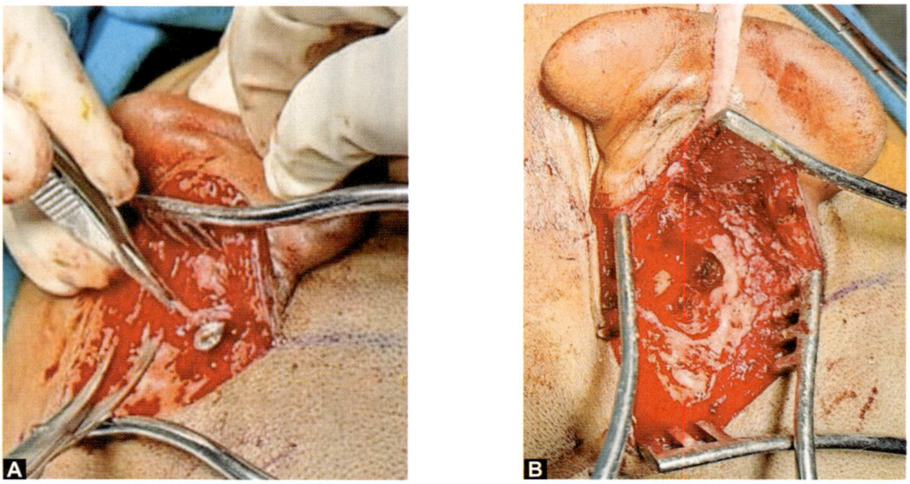

Fig. 20.5: **(A)** Exposure of meningoencephalocele, **(B)** Defect in the tegmen plate and dura after resection

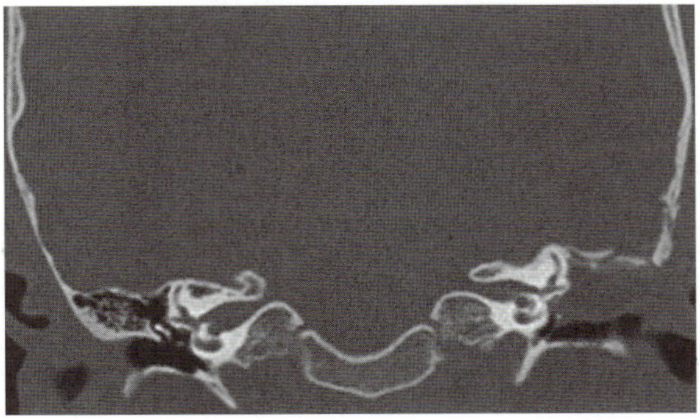

Fig. 20.6: Postoperative ct after reconstruction of tegmen and dural defect with temporalis fascia and bone graft and partial mastoid obliteration

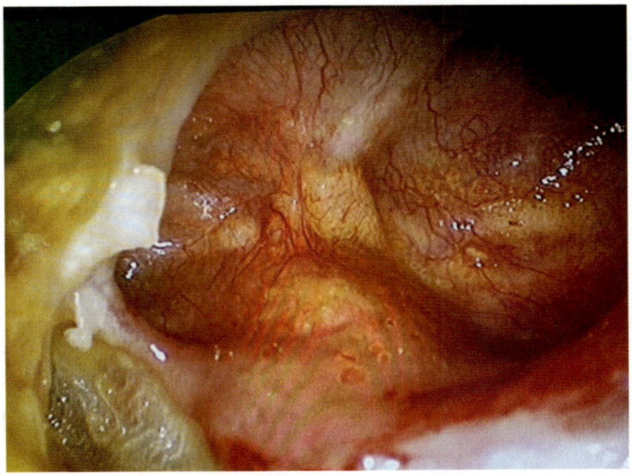

Fig. 20.7: Healed mastoid cavity after reconstruction of dura and partial obliteration and tympanoplasty in the same patient

REFERENCES

1. Khan SU, Tewary RK, O'Sullivan TJ. Modified radical mastoidectomy and its complications--12 years' experience. Ear Nose Throat J. 2014 Apr-May;93(4–5):E30–6.
2. Wormald PJ & Nillsen EN. Do the complications of mastoid surgery differ from those of the disease? Clin Otolaryngol Allied Sci. 1997 Aug;22(4):355–7
3. Shambaugh GE Jr. Surgery of the ear 6th ed.. Philadelphia WB Saunders. 511–13, 2010
4. Moore PJ. The high jugular bulb in ear surgery: three case reports and a review of the literature. J Laryngol Otol. 1994;108(09):772–775. doi: 10.1017/S0022215100128087. [PubMed] [CrossRef] [Google Scholar]
5. Sekhar LN, Tzortzidis FN, Bejjani GK, Schessel DA. Saphenous vein graft bypass of the sigmoid sinus and jugular bulb during the removal of glomus jugulare tumors: report of two cases. J Neurosurg. 1997;86(6):1036–41. doi: 10.3171/jns.1997.86.6.1036. [PubMed] [CrossRef] [Google Scholar]
6. Hasebe S, Sando I, Orita Y. Proximity of carotid canal wall to the tympanic membrane: a human temporal bone study. Laryngoscope 113 802–07, 2003.
7. Shambaugh GE Jr. Surgery of the ear 5nd ed. Philadelphia WB Saunders. 55–56, 1967.

8. Barrett JH, Lawrence V. Aneurysm of the internal carotid artery as a complication of mastoidectomy. Arch Otolaryngol 72 366–368, 1960.
9. Walshe P, McConn R, Brennan P. The role of computerized tomography in the preoperative assessment of chronic suppurative otitis media . Clin Otolaryngol 27 95–97, 2002.
10. Sauvaget E. Aberrant internal carotid artery in the temporal bone--imaging findings and management . Arch Otolaryngol Head Neck Surg 132 86–91, 2006.
11. Rodgers G, Applegate L, de la Cruze A. Magnetic resonance angiography: analysis of vascular lesions of the temporal bone and skull base . Am J Otol 14 56–62, 1993.
12. Laitinen L, Servo A. Embolization of cerebral vessels with inflatable and detachable balloons. J Neurosurg 48 307–308, 1978.
13. Diethrich EB, Ndiaye M, Reid D. Stenting in the carotid artery: initial experience in 110 patients. J Endovasc Surg 3 42–62, 1996.
14. Yadav SP, Ranga A, Sirohiwal BL, Chanda R. Surgical aatomy of tympano-mastoid segment of facial nerve. Indian J Otolaryngol Head Neck Surg. 2006; 58: 27–30.
15. VrabecJT. Delayed facial palsy after tympanomastoid surgery. Am JOtol 1999;201(1):26–30.
16. Weber, P. Iatrogenic complications from chronic ear surgery. Otolaryngol Clin North Arn 2005;38(4):711–22.
17. Palva T, Kårjå J, Palva A. Immediate and short-term complications of chronic ear surgery. Arch Otolaryngol. 1976;102:137–39.
18. Palva T, Kårjå J, Palva A. Opening of the labyrinth during chronic ear surgery. Arch Otolaryngol. 1971;93:75–8.
19. Canalis RF, Gussen R, Abemayor E, Andrews J. Surgical trauma to the lateral semicircular canal with preservation of hearing. Laryngoscope. 1987;97:575–81.
20. Smyth GL. Sensorineural hearing loss in chronic ear surgery. Ann Otal Rhinol Laryngol 1977;86(1 Pt 1):3–8. DOI: 10.1177/000348947708600102.
21. Palva A, Sorri M. Can an operation on a deaf ear be dangerous for hearing? Acta Otolaryngol 1978;360:155–157. DOI: 10.3109/00016487809123503.
22. Palva T, Kårjå J, Palva A. High-tone sensorineural losses following chronic ear surgery. Arch Otolaryngol. 1973;98:176–78.
23. Michael P, Raut V.Chordatympani injury:operativefindingsand postoperative symptoms. Otolaryngol Head Neck Surg 2007;136: 978–81
24. Kveton JF, Bartoshuk LM. The effect of unilateral chorda tympani damage on taste. Laryngoscope 1994;104:25–9
25. Paparella MM, Meyerhoff WL, Morris MS, DaCosta SS. Mastoidectomy and tympanoplasty. In: Paparella MM, Shumrick DA, Gluckman JL, Meyerhoff WL, eds. Otolaryngology, vol. 2. Philadelphia, PA: Saunders; 1991:1405–39.
26. Glasscock ME, Dickins JR, Jackson CG, *et al.* Surgical management of brain tissue herniation into the middle ear and mastoid. Laryn-goscope. 1979;89:1743–54.
27. Bellucci R. Iatrogenic surgical trauma in otology. J Laryngol Otol. 1983;8(Suppl):13–17.
28. Catalano PJ, Post K, Sen C, *et al.* Prevention of cerebrospinal fluid rhinorrhea in neurotologic surgery. Am J Otol. 2000;21:265–69.
29. JG Neely and JR Kuhn, "Diagnosis and treatment of iatrogenic cerebrospinal fluid leak and brain herniation during or following mastoidectomy," Laryngoscope, vol. 95, no. 11, pp. 1299–1300, 1985.
30. M Sanna, F. Paolo, A. Russo, and M. Falcioni, "Management of meningoencephalic herniation of the temporal bone: personal experience and literature review," Laryngoscope, vol. 119, no. 8, pp. 1579–1585, 2009.
31. CR Souliere Jr. and AW Langman, "Combined mastoid/middle cranial fossa repair of temporal bone encephalocele," Skull Base Surgery, vol. 8, no. 4, pp. 185–89, 1998.
32. Rakesh B. Patel, Jed A. Kwartler, Richard M. Hodosh, Soly Baredes. Spontaneous cerebrospinal fluid leakage and middle ear encephalocele in seven patients. Ear, Nose Throat J May, 2008
33. Lundy LB, Graham MD, Kartush JM, LaRouere MJ. Temporal bone encephalocele and cerebrospinal fluid leaks. Am J.

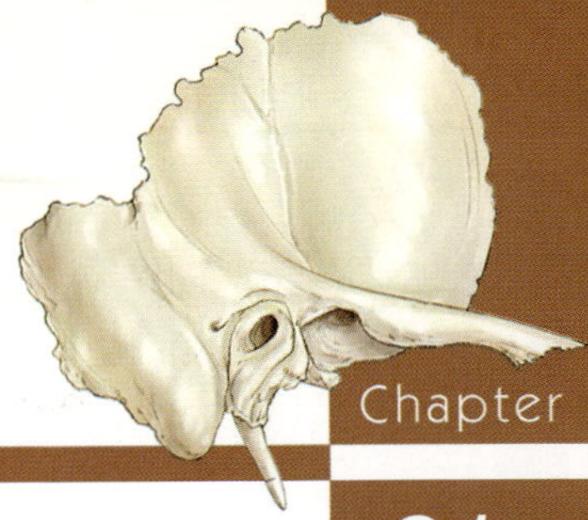

Chapter 21

MIRA: Cerebellopontine Angle and Vascular Conflicts

HN Udayabhanu • Dipak Ranjan Nayak

Introduction

Minimally invasive retrosigmoid approach (MIRA) is a microsurgical endoscope assisted technique for cerebellopontine angle tumor removal. It is done with combined use of microscope and endoscopes. It is aimed at effective microvascular decompression, enhanced grade of CP angle tumor resection with preservation of function, minimal manipulation of neurovascular structures and cerebellar retraction. Cerebellopontine angle (CPA) comprises cerebellopontine and cerebellomedullary cisterns. Cisterns form natural cavities for the introduction of endoscope whereas crossing neurovascular structures delimit anatomical working spaces. Pulsatile compression of vascular structures produces mechanical aggression on both peripheral and central nervous tissues. Persistence leads to demyelination of nerve. Thus topographical knowledge with meticulous evaluation with preoperative magnetic resonance imaging play a vital role.

History

Dandy proposed that neurovascular conflicts exist in cerebellopontine angle as a possible disabling disorder.[1] In the 1970s, it was a surgical challenge to approach the CP angle area.

Peter Jannetta as a neurosurgery resident noticed a microvascular compression of the facial nerve through a subtemporal transtentorial approach using microscope in 1966. The same year he performed the first planned microvascular decompression for hemifacial spasm through a retromastoid approach. Reflecting on potential similarities between facial and trigeminal nerve compressions. Jannetta developed the surgical technique and advocated the retrosigmoid approach because it is associated with better visibility and fewer complications, compared with the subtemporal transtentorial approach.[1]

Anatomical Perspective: Rhotons Rule of 3

Three pairs of cerebellar arteries arise from the vertebrobasilar system and establish specific neural relationships during the course (Table 21.1). Each artery is associated with a cerebellar surface, a fissure and a cranial nerve. This rule simplified the study and

TABLE 21.1: Cerebellopontine angle with neurovascular relationships

Neuro-vascular complex	*Artery*	*Nerve*	*Brain stem*	*Cere-bellar peduncle*	*Fissure*	*Cerebellar surface*	*Neurovascular syndrome*	*Approaches*
Upper	SCA	CNs IV, V	Midbrain	Superior	Cerebello-mesencephalic	Tentorial	○ Trigeminal neuralgia	○ Supracerebellar/ retrosigmoid ○ MIRA
Middle	AICA	CNs VII, VIII	Pons	Middle	Cerebello-pontine	Petrosal	○ Hemifacial spasm ○ Geniculate neuralgia ○ Intractable vertigo, tinnitus	○ Retrosigmoid/presigmoid ○ MIRA
Lower	PICA	CNs IX–XI	Medulla	Inferior	Cerebello-medullary	Subo-ccipital	○ Glosso-pharyngeal neuralgia	○ Retrosigmoid ○ Suboccipital ○ Far-lateral ○ MIRA

surgical approach to the cerebellopontine angle and to tailor the craniotomy and cerebellar retraction to the specific target.

The retrosigmoid approach is the workhorse for posterior fossa surgery. It is a versatile approach to tackle different type of lesions in the cerebellopontine angle. Rhotons rule of 3 is the key to unlock difficult neurovascular relationships. There is wide variability in description of its general setup, involved steps, and potential extensions.

MIRA which is minimally invasive retrosigmoid approach in lateral skull base surgery for otoneurological procedures is one such modification of retrosigmoid approach. It is an extralabyrinthine approach behind the otic capsule.

The retrosigmoid approach is a technical modification of the suboccipital approach to the cerebellopontine angle. This approach carries the craniotomy more anterolaterally, to lie just posterior to the sigmoid sinus. This approach provides access to the cerebellopontine angle without sacrificing the labyrinth.[1]

With increasing life expectancy, a growing number of elderly patients suffer from vascular conflicts and acoustic tumors. Careful clinical assessment, with onset, intensity, duration and frequency of symptoms should be documented with assessment of psychological profile.

MIRA is a key hole approach which is a safe and efficient procedure for even elderly patients. The use of endoscopes has also paved the way for minimally invasive surgery. Smaller craniotomies reduced retraction of the cerebellum.[3] So that patients can resume their daily lives sooner.

Investigations

3D MRI (Fig. 21.1), i.e. 3D–Fourier transform special T2-CISS, T1 weighted turboflash, electrophysiological studies, videoendoscopy of the CP angle.

Progress in otoneurosurgical techniques with the introduction of endoscopic procedures, improvements in anesthesia techniques, and the increasingly widespread use of intraoperative nerve monitoring devices have expanded the range of elderly patients for surgery, for whom the retrosigmoid approach offers less invasiveness and a significant decrease in operating time and morbidity.[2]

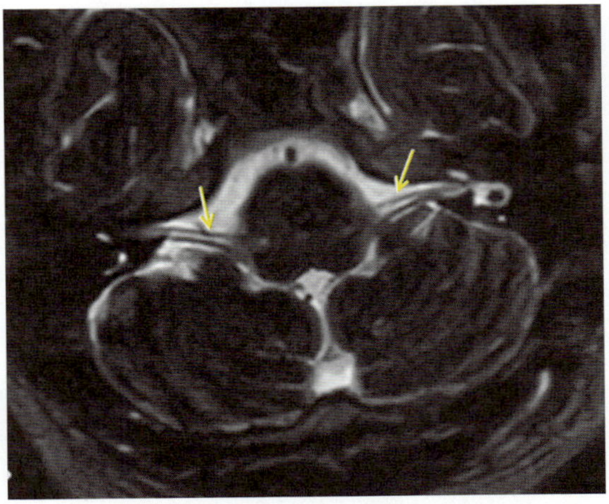

Fig. 21.1: MRI imaging of the CP angle showing vascular loop

Neurovascular Conflicts

Ectatic arteries or prominent veins compressing the nerves in either Redlich-Obersteiner's zone known as root entry zone or within a few millimetres from the origin root exit zone of the nerve causes demyelination of the nerve in long term.[4] It has been explained by following theories:

Ephaptic theory: Development of true short circuit electric activity in and around the area of nerve compression.

Nuclear theory: Hyper reactivity at the core of cranial nerves in brainstem.

Kindling effect: Central hyperexcitability of cranial nerves, could have an associated peripheral origin (site of compression).

Procedure: This includes a retrosigmoid approach with 2 cm craniotomy (Fig. 21.2). Direct view of cerebellopontine angle and exposure of cranial nerves. Endoscope gives panoramic view. There are three types of major incision that can be used the C-shaped, the lazy S and the straight line incision.

Landmarks are the Frankfort line and line following the posterior margin of mastoid process. C shaped skin incision from tip of mastoid process to 2 fingers behind the pinna (Fig. 21. 3 and 21.4). To raise the skin flap anteriorly and muscle flap posteriorly following periosteal incision (Fig. 21.5). Then identify the retromastoid bone, we have to identify the digastric ridge and emissary vein which is a main landmark. We drill around the emissary

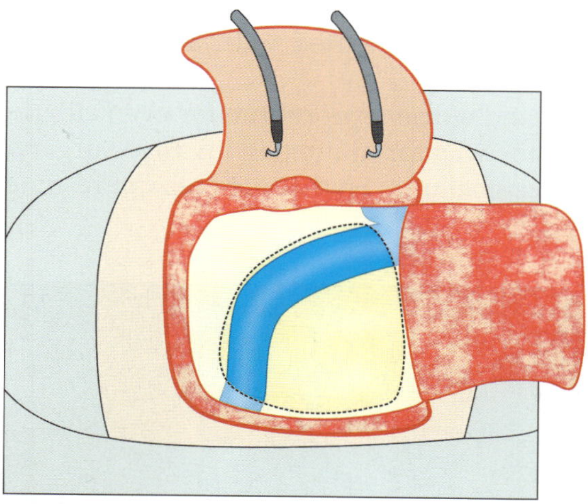

Fig. 21.2: Schematic diagram for retrosigmoid approach

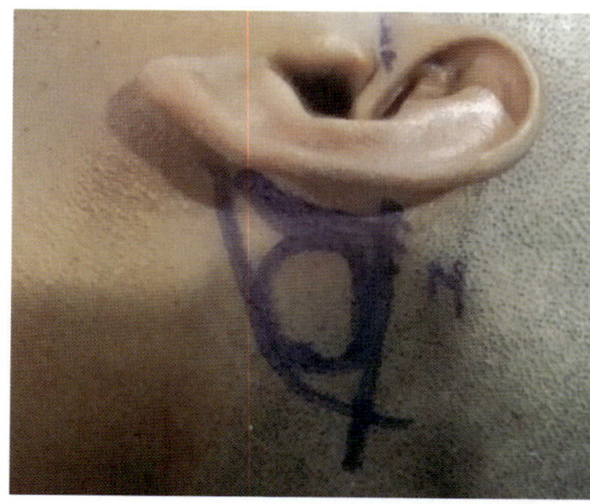

Fig. 21.3: C shaped incision mark, the circle indicates the craniotomy site

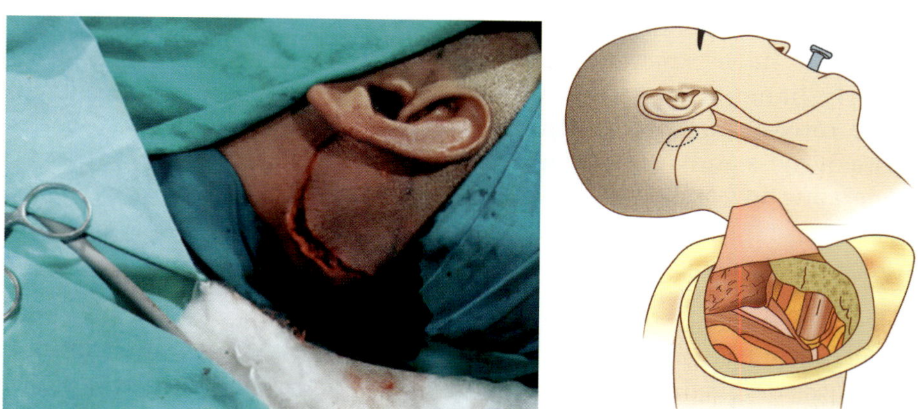

Fig. 21.4: Picture C shaped incision and elevation of skin flap and illustration showing structures exposed in retrosigmoid approach

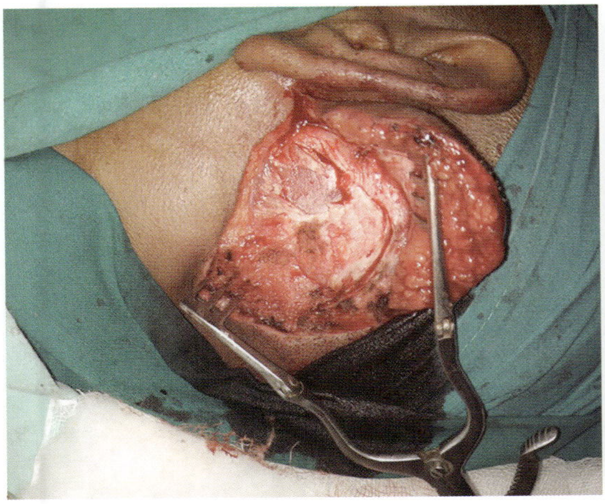

Fig. 21.5: Periosteal incision after skin flap elevation

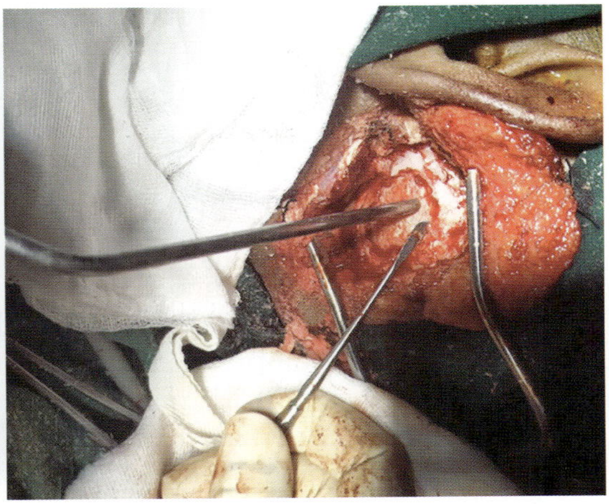

Fig. 21.6: Exposure of the posterior fossa dura after craniotomy

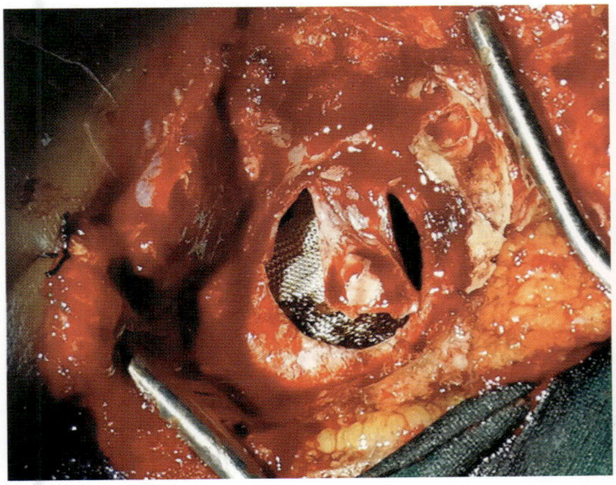

Fig 21.7: Incision of the dura to expose the CP angle

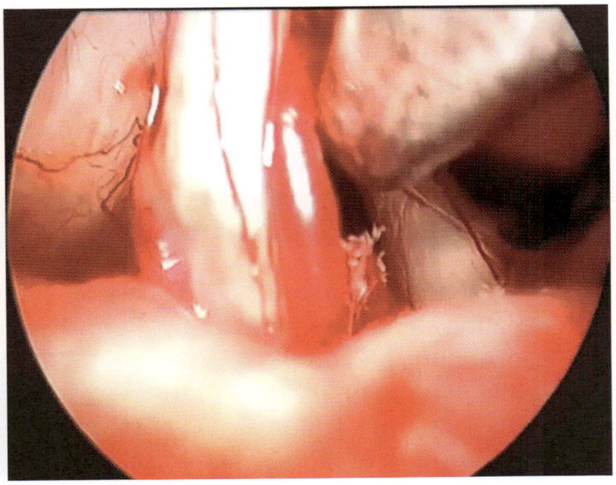

Fig 21.8: Image of the acoustico-facial bundle through MIRA on endoscopy

vein to remove the bone till we reach the posterior border of sigmod sinus. To prevent an inadvertent opening of the transverse and sigmoid sinuses, different landmarks to be identified to map the course of these structures. So we make a 1–2 cm craniotomy (Fig. 21.6). Before opening dura mater, a deeper anesthesia with hyperventilation is required with pCO_2 <25. The axis of microscope should be inferior in CP angle (Figs 21.7 and 21.8). The cisterna has to be opened at the level of the lower cranial nerve to let out the CSF. To emphasize and improve this approach endoscope is used 4 mm, 30 degree endoscope is preferred. Closure is important in layers with dura patch, bone pate and muscle flap to avoid CSF leak.

ET CO_2 (end tidal CO_2) is kept less than 25 mm Hg to hyperventilate patient creating hypocapnia so that CSF pressure is reduced. The endoscope used is a 14 cm in length nasal endoscope and a side port suction or Brackmann suction is used once the dura is open.

Complications

- CSF collection/leakage, wound infection, deep venous thromobosis.
- Indications of otoneurological procedures by retrosigmoid approach
- Trigeminal neuralgia
- Hemifacial spasm
- Mènière's disease
- Intractable tinnitus
- Cerebellopontine angle tumors
- Vestibular neurotomy in incapacitating mènière's disease
- Neurovascular decompression
- Glossopharyngeal neuralgia
  Tumor removal <2 cm acoustic neuroma, meningioma
- Facial palsy/paresis

Advantages

- Retrosigmoid approach is keyhole approach one of the easiest approach to acoustic facial bundle in the cerebellopontine angle when compared to the retrolabyrinthine and middle fossa approach.[2] Less invasive with safety. Efficacy similar or better than other approaches. Shorter recovery time. Its most cost effective and technically feasible.
- Extended retrosigmoid approach is implemented in transmeatal extension, and suprameatal extension in CP angle tumor surgery.

REFERENCES

1. Basma J, Anagnostopoulos C, Tudose A, Harty M, Michael LM 2nd, Teo M, Porter DG. History, Variations, and Extensions of the Retrosigmoid Approach: Anatomical and Literature Review. J Neurol Surg B Skull Base. 2021 Jul 5;83(Suppl 2):e324-e335. doi: 10.1055/s-0041–1729177. PMID: 35832939; PMCID: PMC9272236.
2. Betka J, Zv ina E, Balogová Z, Profant O, Sk ivan J, Kraus J, Lis J, Syka J, Chovanec M. Complications of microsurgery of vestibular schwannoma. Biomed Res Int. 2014;2014:315952. doi: 10.1155/2014/315952. Epub 2014 May 28. PMID: 24987677; PMCID: PMC4058457.
3. Lazard DS, Tosello M, Bozorg-Grayeli A, Vitte E, Bouccara D, Kalamarides M, Sterkers O. Early complications and symptoms of cerebellopontine angle tumor surgery: a prospective analysis. Eur Arch Otorhinolaryngol. 2011 Nov;268(11):1575–82. doi: 10.1007/s00405–011-1539–5. Epub 2011 Mar 4. PMID: 21373897.
4. Tatagiba MS,Roser F,Hirt B,Ebner FH.The retrosigmoid endoscopic approach for cerebellopontine-angle tumors and microvascular decompression.World Neurosurg.2014 Dec; 82(6 Suppl): S171–6. doi:10.1016/j.wneu.2014.08.001.PMID:25496630.

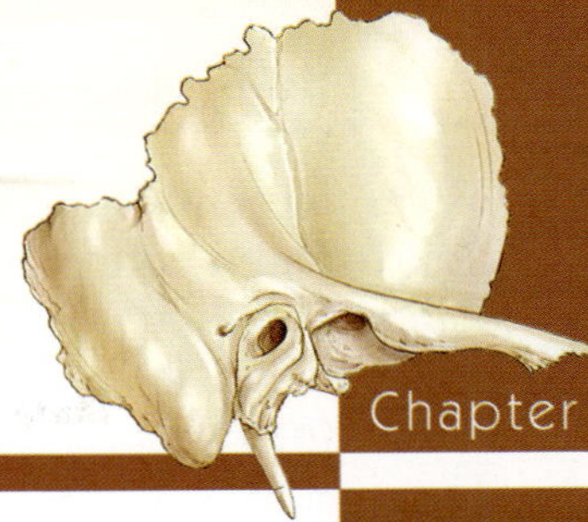

Chapter 22

Mastoid Obliteration

Balakrishnan Ramaswamy • Kailesh Pujary • Dipak Ranjan Nayak

Surgery like radical/modified radical mastoidectomy are known to create large mastoidectomy cavity following cholesteatoma surgery, which is then exteriorized and communicated with external auditory canal by means of a suitable meatoplasty for better healing and periodic inspection. The management of middle ear disease with cholesteatoma by open cavity mastoidectomy is plagued by a number of cavity problems. A chronically discharging cavity besides being a frustrating dilemma to the surgeon is also a social handicap to the patient. Obliteration of such discharging cavities seems to be an effective therapeutic modality.[1] Various methods have been described to obliterate the mastoid cavity partially or completely to reduce postmastoidectomy cavity and its problems. Necessity of regular follow up following mastoid surgery and discharge from the mastoid cavity is the main problem associated with canal wall down procedure. The presence of a potential space in the tip region of the mastoid bowl has been implicated as a cause for collection of debris and subsequent discharge (Balakrishna et al., 2005).

Historical Perspective

Mosher in 1911 was the first person to describe cavity obliteration following radical mastoidectomy with a superiorly based musculoperiosteal flap. Popper in 1935 described the use of a periosteal flap used to line, rather than obliterate, the mastoid cavity. Rambo in 1958 used posteriorly based on posterior branch of temporal artery, pedicle temporalis muscle flap for mastoid obliteration. Palva et al in 1968 described anteriorly base musculo-periosteal flap for mastoid obliteration. East et al (1991) describe temporoparietal flap for mastoid obliteration. Weiss et al., 1992 described mastoid tip amputation and turning the mastoid periosteum into the cavity. Hong Kong flap (Pedicled vascularized superficial temporoparietal flap) based on the posterior branch of superficial temporal artery was described by Van Hassaelt in 1994, which provides the optimal substrate for epithelial resurfacing while separating the mucosa and bone of the middle ear and mastoid from the surface epithelium facilitating excellent healing even under unfavorable circumstances. Yung in 1996, used hydroxyapatite granules for mastoid obliteration. Ramsay et al (2004) described postauricular pericranial and periosteal flap and Yung and Smith (2007) described mid temporal pericranial and inferiporly based periosteal flap. Recently BioAlive bioactive glass have been used for mastoid obliteration.

Classification

Chan and Chan (2012) classified the obliteration technique into free flaps including biological materials like bone paste, cartilage, etc. and local flaps that were already discussed under historical perspective. Yung and Benette (2013) classified mastoid obliteration into soft tissue flaps and fillers. The classification can be further modified as follows:

Mastoid Obliteration Technique

Materials

- **Biologic**
  - Bone paste (Fig. 22.5)
  - Cartilage
  - Fascia
- **Non-Biologic biocompatible**
  - Hydroxyapatite
  - BioAlive bioactive glass (Fig. 22.6)

Soft Tissue Flaps

1. Meatally-based musculoperiosteal flap (Palva flap)
2. Middle temporal artery flap (Hong Kong flap)
3. Temporoparietal fascial flap (TPFF)
4. Pedicled superficial temporalis fascial flap
5. Periosteal-pericranial flap
6. Temporalis muscle flap
7. Inferiorly based fascioperiosteal flap
8. Inferiorly based musculoperiosteal flap

Technique of some commonly used methods for mastoid obliteration:

Palva flap: It is a meatally based periosteal flap can be used for the mastoid obliteration and reconstruction of external auditory canal. After postauricular incision and exposure of soft tissue, a musculoperiosteal flap is raised between linea temporalis and mastoid tip from the lateral aspect, towards pinna to exposed the mastoid bone. After completing the canal down procedure, this flap is rotated into the mastoid cavity for obliteration. It can also be used along with filler materials like bone dusts or bone chips, etc (Fig. 22.1).

Inferiorly-based musculoperiosteal flap: Technique of postauricular incision is given as in case palva flap and the skin with subcutaneous tissue elevated. A rectangular shape incision mark of size 30 × 15 mm is given over the postaural periosteum, soft tissue overlying the conchal cartilage and postaural muscle. The flap with its pedicle base inferiorly is elevated (Fig. 22.2A). Following the canal wall mastoidectomy, this flap is place over the inferior recess (Fig. 22.2B).

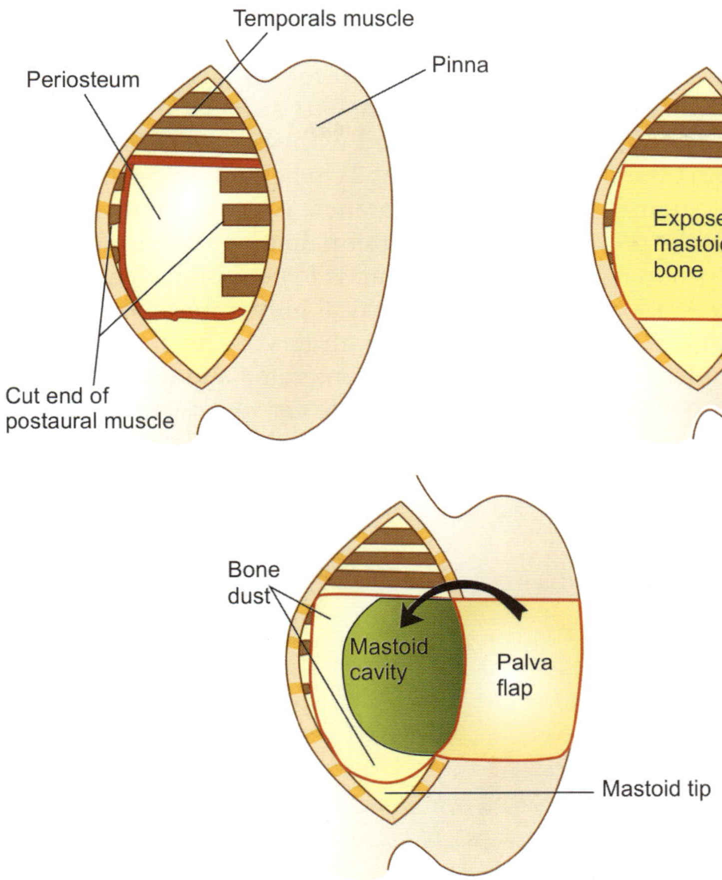

Fig. 22.1: Steps of Palva flap

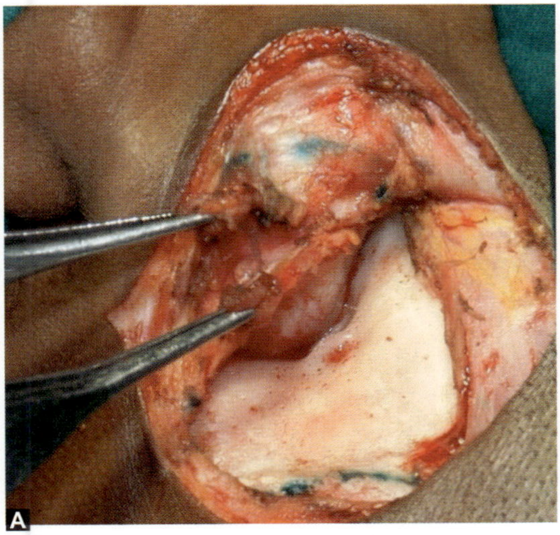

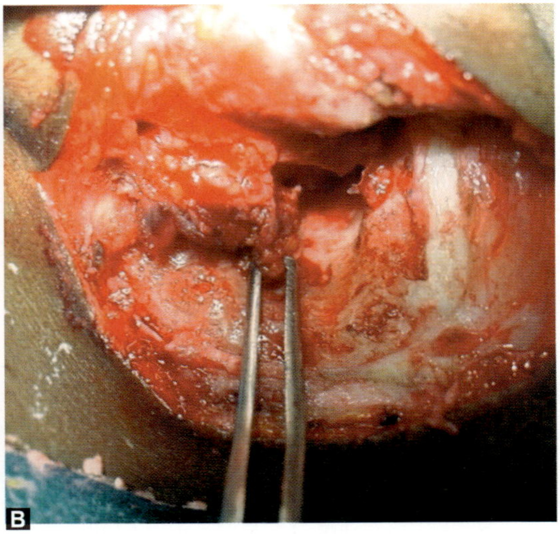

Fig. 22.2: (A) Musculoperiosteal flap being raised, **(B)** Flap being used for inferior recess after MRM

Superficial Temporoparietal Fascial Flap

Brown in 1898 used the temporoparietal fascia flap for reconstruction of the external ear following a defect due to horse bite. Brent in 1983 successfully used this flap for secondary ear reconstruction. The skin is prepared with shaving of the hair 4 cm above the auricle and extending the shaving area at least 2 cm behind the postauricular region. This flap is based on temporal artery posterior branch. A 'Y' incision is given with the inferior limb starting at the preauricular region after palpating the location of superficial temporal artery as shown in Fig. 22.3. The skin flap is to be raised superiorly, anteriorly and posteriorly after the mastoid surgery. The vertical limb can be joined to a good and wide postauricular Wilde's incision for mastoid surgery. After the canal wall down mastoidectomy is completed and all the aircells excenterated and granulations removed with complete clearance of cholesteatoma, the middle ear reconstruction is done. Then the temporoparietal flap can be raised. The middle fossa dural plate is skeletonized and the root of zygoma is drilled and removed. This step prevents compression of the pedicle when the flap is rotated posteriorly. The entire mastoid bowl is saucerised well.

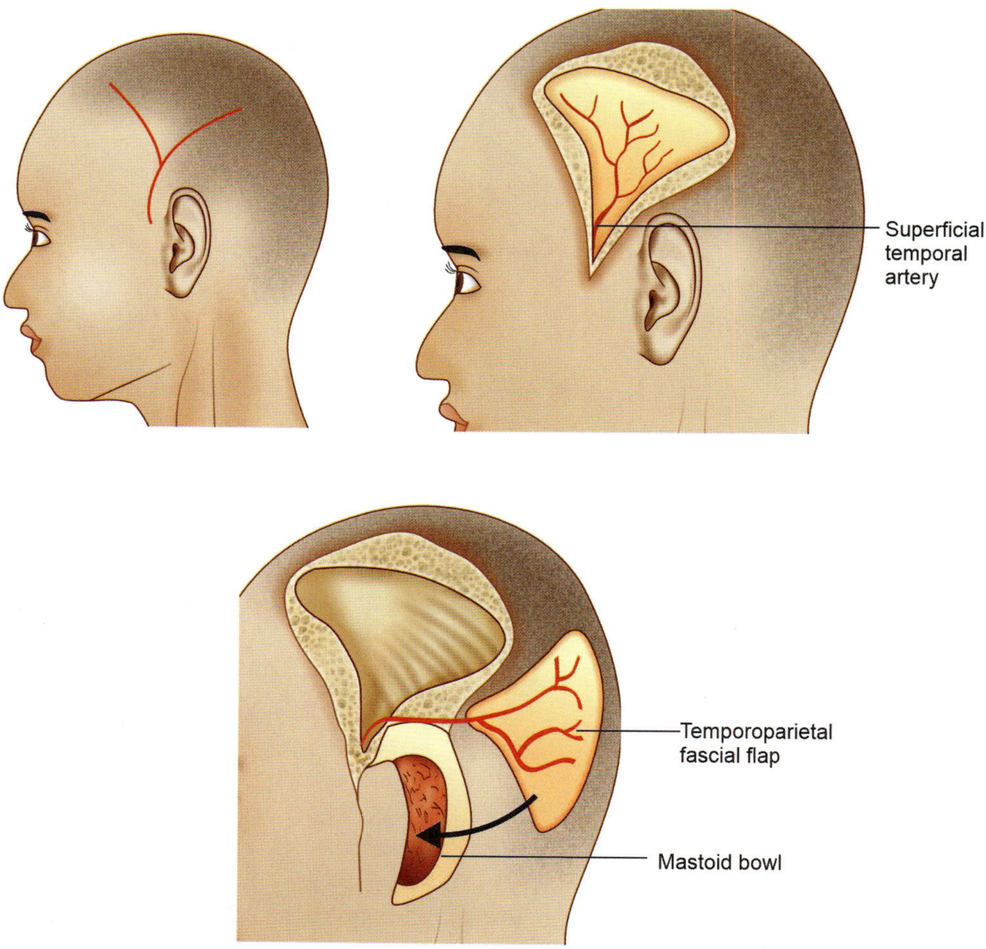

Fig. 22.3: Mastoid obliteration with temporoparietal fascial flap

The skin flap is raised with sharp dissection with 15 blade Bard Parker knife. Diathermy should be avoided for this step as it can compromise blood supply to the flap. While elevating the skin flap, the hair follicle of the skin is identified and the temporoparietal flap area remains just beneath the hair follicle along with superficial temporal vessels. The skin flap is secured anteriorly–superiorly and posteriorly while taking care not to damage the hair follicle. Bipolar cautery is used for hemostasis. The triangular flap with its narrow pedicle including the posterior branch of superficial temporal vessels raise till the temporalis muscle and temporalis fascia and this triangular flap is now ready for reconstruction and obliteration (Fig. 22.4).

Posterior Canal Wall Reconstruction

This may be done to deepen the middle ear space which gives favorable results if ossiculoplasty is being considered. It can be staged or can be done in the same sitting. Reconstruction can be done using autologous material like bone dusts (Fig. 22.5) and chips, cortical bone graft, tragal or scaphoid cartilage. Synthetic material like hydroxyapatite may be used however extrusion can be a problem. The best way is to cover bioactive material with suitable flap as described above (Fig. 22.7). Bioactive glass S53P4 is being used recently to obliterate the mastoid cavity after and to seal CSF leak (Fig. 22.6) (Sarin et al 2012)

Middle Ear Mastoid Cavity Augmentation Following Blind Sac Closure

It is necessary to provide complete seal of mastoid or mastoid and middle ear and external auditory canal to provide complete seal to prevent CSF leak following major surgery like translabyrinthine approach or lateral skull base approaches. Fat is a good source for augmentation and obliteration in such cases. Alternatively temporalis muscle can be rotated to augment the mastoid cavity. But is very effective in provide seal to prevent CSF leak.

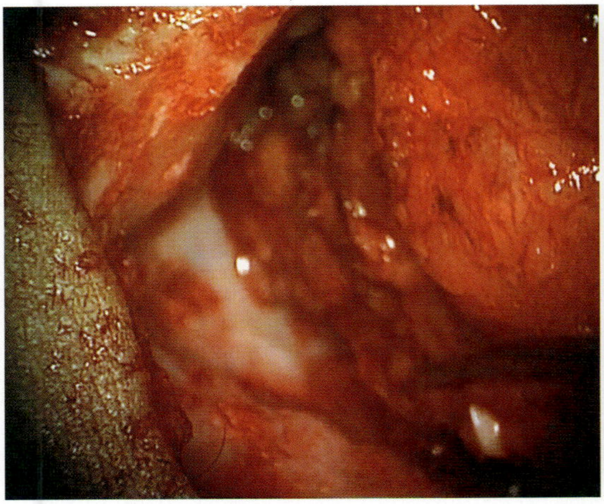

Fig. 22.4: Obliteration with musculoperiosteal flap

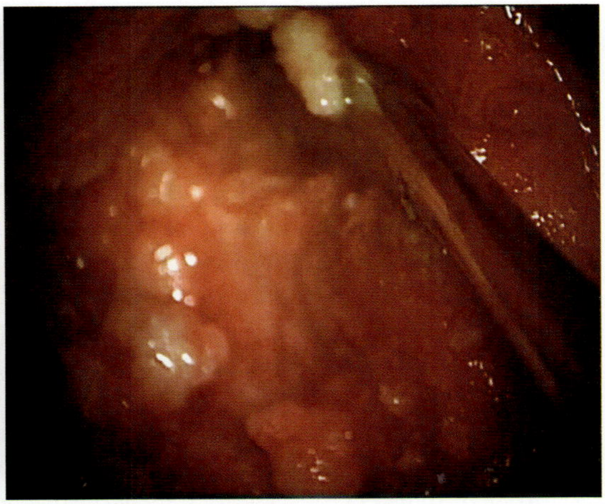

Fig. 22.5: Bone dust being used to obliterate mastoid cavity

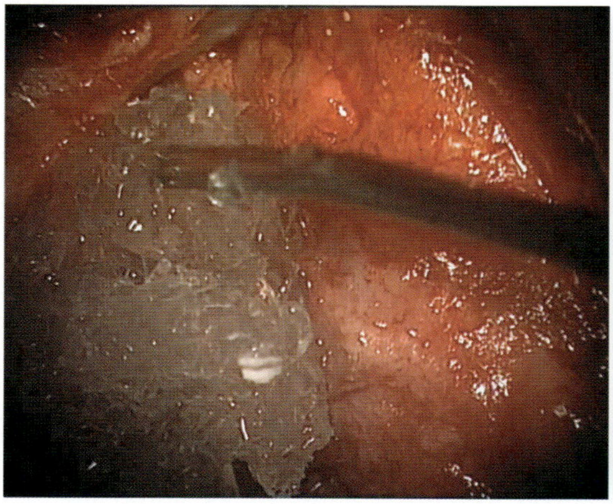

Fig. 22.6: Obliteration with bioactive glass

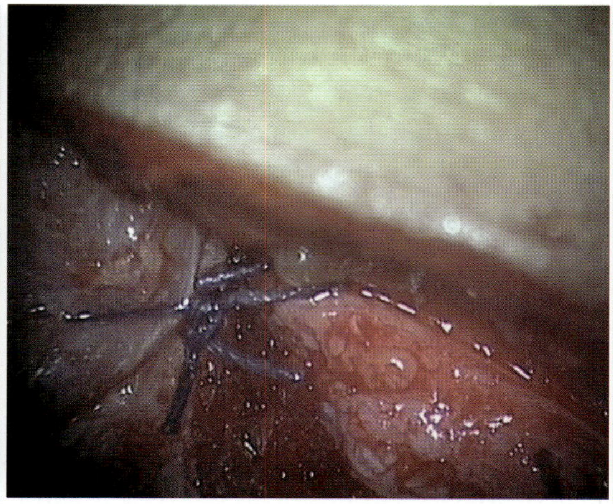

Fig. 22.7: Closure of flap after obliteration of mastoid cavity

REFERENCES

1. Parmekar S, Hazarika P, Vishwanathan A, Balakrishnan R(1997). Mastoid obliteration using temporpareital flap-Our experience; IJOHNS, , 49(2),pp117–121
2. Ramaswamy, B, Kailesh, P, Parul, P and Dipak, R N (2005). Inferior recess obliteration in open cavity mastoidectomy: Indian Journal of Otology. 11, SEP., p. 5–9 5
3. Mosher HP (1911). A method of filling the excavated mastoid with a flap from the back of the auricle. Laryngoscope 21(12): 1158–1163.
4. Popper O. Periosteal flap grafts in mastoid operations. S Afr Med J 1935;9:77.
5. Kisch J (1928). Temporal muscle grafts in the radical mastoid operation. J Laryngol 43: 735–36.
6. East CA, Brough MD, Grant HR (1991) Mastoid obliteration with the temporoparietal fascial flap. J Laryngol Otol 105(6): 417–20.
7. Weiss MH, *et al.* 1992: Surgery of recurrent and residual cholesteatoma. Laryngosope (102) pp 145–51
8. Van Hasselt CA, Liu KC, Tong MC. The Hong Kong vascularized temporalis fascia flaps for optimal, mastoid cavity reconstruction. Rev Laryngol Otol Rhinol (Bord). 1995;116(1):57–60.
9. Yung M W. The use of hydroxyapatite granules in mastoid obliteration. Clin Otolaryngol Allied Sci 1996;21(6):480–4
10. Ramsey MJ, Merchant SN, McKenna MJ. Postauricular Periosteal-Pericranial Flap for Mastoid Obliteration and canal wall down tympanomastoidectomy. Otol Neurotol 2004; 25(6):873–8.
11. Yung M, Smith P. Mid-temporal pericranial and inferiorly based periosteal flaps in mastoid obliteration. Otolaryngol Head Neck Surg 2007; 137:906– 12.
12. Mark Adams, Ekembar Reddy, Ted McNaboe. Mastoid obliteration with BioAlive Bioactive glass, JLO, Volume 130, Supplement S3 (Abstracts for the 10th International Conference on Cholesteatoma) May 2016 , pp. S15–S16
13. Brown WJ. Extraordinary case of horse bite: the external ear completely bitten off and successfully replaced. *Lancet*. 1898. 1:1533.
14. Brent B, Byrd HS. Secondary ear reconstruction with cartilage grafts covered by axial, random, and free flaps of temporoparietal fascia. *Plast Reconstr Surg*. 1983 Aug. 72(2):141–52.

Index

F

G

H

I

J

K

L

M

R

S

T

U

V

W

X

Y

Z